RECOVERING THE BODY

To Jannah Brown,
Rachel's aunt,
I hope you like the
ideas expressed
in my book.

Carol Caroline

RECOVERING THE BODY
A Philosophical Story

CAROL COLLIER

The University of Ottawa Press
2013

The University of Ottawa Press acknowledges with gratitude the support extended to its publishing list by Heritage Canada through the Canada Book Fund, by the Canada Council for the Arts, by the Federation for the Humanities and Social Sciences through the Awards to Scholarly Publications Program, by the Social Sciences and Humanities Research Council, and by the University of Ottawa.

We also gratefully acknowledge the University of Sudbury's Research and Publication Fund, whose financial support has contributed to the publication of this book.

www.press.uottawa.ca

Library and Archives Canada Cataloguing in Publication

Collier, Carol, 1943-
Recovering the body : a philosophical story / Carol Collier.

Includes bibliographical references and index.
Issued also in electronic formats.
ISBN 978-0-7766-0799-3

1. Human body (Philosophy)--History. I. Title.

B105.B64C64 2013   128'.6   C2013-900538-2

To Mackenzie, Alli, Graeme and Eric

TABLE OF CONTENTS

FOREWORD

Never has it been more urgent to be enlightened by a philosophical reflection on the body. Confronted with such crucial issues as organ traffic, organ donation, assisted suicide and biomedical research, citizens, politicians and policy makers certainly need solid scientific evidence to justify their decisions. But, first and foremost, actors in the public forum need to identify what the real issues are. This cannot be accomplished without getting at a problem's philosophical underpinnings. Too often, solutions address only pseudo-problems. Take this line of reasoning, for example: there is a shortage of organs; therefore we should implement policies and programs for the purpose of increasing the availability of organs. While this assertion makes sense in and of itself, most politicians, policy makers and citizens fail to see that this kind of assertion results from a philosophical discourse on the body, which itself rarely becomes the subject of an enlightened public discussion. Why? Because philosophy itself is part of the problem.

First of all, philosophy has obliterated the question of the body. This obliteration, far from being a simple oversight, is the result of philosophy as a system of inquiry. A systemic approach to the philosophical treatment of the body over time, such as Dr. Collier so brilliantly outlines for her readers, clearly shows the impact of modernity as a turning point (or point of no return) beyond which the body is merely understood as a discrete object of knowledge like any other material object. No doubt the modern turning point, and the vision of the body that ensued, would allow for the formidable development of science and technology. But has it not become too evident that modernity came at a hefty price? This price can be intuited from the many profound ethical conundrums in which we now find ourselves.

To write a philosophical book about the body, and to try, in so doing, to recuperate some philosophical views that may contribute to the reconstitution of the body, as we would a precious work of art, is not only courageous: it is indeed truly visionary. The body is not a scientific or social construct; it is a meaningful fact. The body is always someone's body. It is experienced or "lived," as phenomenologists say. My body signifies me in a unique way. It announces and proclaims my existence with authenticity. Here I am—body and flesh! My body is also a microcosm within a macrocosm. Bodies discovered in common trenches signify many persons' ultimate fates within violent political systems possibly sustained by a global political community. Someone's tumour is not only a malignant organization of cells; it is the result of a dynamic relationship with her environment, habits and genes. Surrogate motherhood is not only hosting a baby within a womb, and transplanting a lung does not simply mean transferring one person's organ into another's body. Life involves an intricate network of interconnected forces (objective) and intentions (subjective). As a society, we must stop making decisions as if we were dealing with discrete pieces of a puzzle. To paraphrase Ricoeur (and no doubt Aristotle), real ethics begins when one has to discriminate not between black and white, but between grey and grey.

Finally, by capturing philosophically relevant meanings that emanate from alternative medicine and traditional yoga practices, Dr. Collier courageously takes up Stephen Toulmin's project to "humanize modernity." As a philosopher and a concerned citizen, I am greatly indebted to philosophers like Dr. Collier, who strive to undertake such a philosophically sustainable endeavour.

Chantal Beauvais, PhD
Rector and Member, Faculty of Philosophy, Saint Paul University

Acknowledgements

This book is the result of many years of reflection on the body in philosophy and medicine, but its structure developed over the last decade through my teaching, first at St. Paul University in Ottawa and then at the University of Sudbury. I am grateful to Chantal Beauvais, who, in 2002 as head of the Philosophy Department at St. Paul's, encouraged me to teach a summer course on the body-machine. The students, who came from different disciplines, responded very well to the philosophical and historical aspects of the course, and participated with great enthusiasm in the second part of the course dealing with contemporary questions of the body, all of which helped me in the development of Part II of this book.

I am also grateful to my colleagues in the Philosophy Department of the University of Sudbury (Paolo Biondi, Réal Fillion, Lucien Pelletier and Rachel Haliburton) for their support, encouragement and flexibility in allowing me to develop my body-machine course further under the rubric of Topics in Early Modern Philosophy. I am grateful to all the students who enthusiastically participated in this course over several years, many of whom provided fresh ideas regarding contemporary attitudes toward the body. I am also grateful to those same philosophy colleagues, and to the University of Sudbury, for supporting my sabbatical project in 2010, during which time I was able to complete the manuscript.

For the places and spaces in which I was able to write during that sabbatical year, I am grateful to the Yasodhara Ashram at Kootenay Lake, BC, for providing both teachings and tranquillity; to Beth Penny for her peaceful Kootenay cabin with its ever-inspiring view of the mountains; to Ilse and Giles Stevenson for the use of their beautiful Victoria house; to Gwynneth Evans and Deb Cowley for the use of their Ottawa houses; and to Larry Heald and Joanne Dale for their hospitality and moral support during my many trips to Toronto over years of research and writing.

Thanks to the many friends and colleagues who read and commented on my project at different stages and who provided comments, support and helpful criticism of various chapters. Special thanks to Danièle Letocha and Syliane Charles for their helpful support at the very beginning of my proposal; to Swami Sivananda, Carlean Fisher and Patricia Hurdle for reading Chapter 8; to Paolo Biondi for helpful comments on Chapters 1 and 2; to Réal Fillion and Erik Stephenson for sharing their knowledge of Spinoza and keeping me on track in Chapter 6; to Alicia Batten for correcting my errors in Chapter 3; and to Rachel Haliburton for commenting on Chapter 7—as well as for many supportive conversations along the way. Thanks to Peter Saunders for his help in developing the proposal and presenting it to publishers, to Jen Groundwater for her very professional editing assistance, and to the reviewers at the University of Ottawa Press for their helpful comments. A special thanks to the University of Sudbury for financial support from its Research and Publication Fund.

INTRODUCTION

The purpose of this book is to tell a story, to uncover the history of the body in our Western philosophical tradition leading up to the modern conception of the body as a machine. It is also a work of recovery, bringing to light many aspects of this history that have been lost or forgotten in the West since the Scientific Revolution. At a time when our biological knowledge of the body has never been greater, a philosophical void exists in our understanding of the body's relation to mind, soul, nature and cosmos.

Surprisingly, this is not a story that has already been told—at least not by philosophers and not in the English language.[1] Philosophers have had much more time for the soul and the mind (the latter being the modern conception of the former), and even now, in philosophy of mind or cognitive science debates continue as to whether consciousness or mind actually exists. The body has not generally been considered a serious philosophical subject, perhaps because there appears to be no philosophical problem in it, perhaps because it has been left to the scientists to dissect, both literally and figuratively. Whatever the reasons, philosophers have generally been quite silent on the subject to the point that Chantal Jaquet refers to the body as the phantom limb of philosophy.[2]

As a result of this neglect of the body by philosophy and philosophers, one must often extrapolate from definitions and descriptions of soul—something that is done sometimes by the philosophers themselves.[3] An excellent example of this is Plato's description of the soul in the *Phaedo* as "that which is divine, immortal, indestructible, of a single form, accessible to thought, ever constant and abiding true to itself," followed by his description of the body as "that which is human, mortal, destructible, of many forms, inaccessible to thought, never constant nor abiding true to itself"—in other words, the exact negative opposite of the soul. Reading such a description one cannot help but think that the body, for Plato, is simply 'not-soul.' In the final analysis, the body can be seen as a leftover, an ungainly offshoot of the philosophical pursuit of the soul (now mind). Thus, part of my goal in this narrative is to give the body a place in the history of philosophy by bringing to the fore what the various schools of philosophy and philosophers did say—explicitly or implicitly—about the body.

Some might argue that much is now being written on the subject, especially in areas such as sociology, psychology and feminist studies. While this is true, it does not fill the gap in the philosophical literature. The social sciences themselves have their presuppositions about mind and body and do not necessarily make them known. Further, many such books take critical aim at the post-Cartesian mechanistic view of the body, which forms the basis of modern biology and medicine, without any extensive explanation either of how the mechanistic concept of the body—and the body-machine—came about, or of what preceded it in the Western tradition.

A story is a narrative; it has a beginning, middle and end. This story has a beginning and middle in the history of Western thought, but it does not have an end. The narrative is still being played out in the world of ideas—and in the popular imagination—and many of its twenty-first-century chapters are, in some ways, winding their way back to its early Greek beginnings. In other words, certain ideas, which had been like dropped threads at the beginning of modernity, are reappearing in current attitudes toward and writings about the body—though little of this can be found in the mainstream philosophical literature.

The words 'story,' 'narrative' and 'threads' suggest a unity of progression that might make academic philosophers nervous. A narrative is written from a point of view, and has a plot, a theme, as well as a direction, and this is the case with this book. The history of ideas is neither smooth nor direct, but if one wants to tell a story, one has to choose what fits the narrative, and this is what I have chosen to do. The story does not claim to be exhaustive or complete; it is a point of view on the development of the modern conception of the body-machine, a conception that forms the basis of modern biology and medicine, and one that is more and more subject to questioning and revision.

I will be following two major threads through the history of the philosophy of the body: a dualistic thread and a monistic (holistic) thread. While not all the philosophers discussed fit neatly into this dichotomy, and the threads become knotted and intertwined in some of them, the separation of themes is consistent enough to paint a cohesive picture of different (and sometimes opposing) visions of the body that helps to explain conflicting elements of our attitudes toward the body today.

I will also be following three epistemological threads throughout my story, three different ways of conceiving the relation between knowledge (the goal, after all, of philosophy) and the body: the body as an obstacle to knowledge (shown most clearly, but not by any means exclusively, in Plato's *Phaedo*); the body as an object of knowledge (shown most clearly in the culture of dissection of the Renaissance and in Descartes' dualism and mechanism); and the body as a source of knowledge (shown in both the Stoics and Spinoza with their notions of living in accordance with nature).

One objective of my story is to demonstrate that it *matters* what metaphysical and epistemological view of the body is at work in our personal and collective lives. Whether we recognize it or not, we have metaphysical presuppositions regarding the body that determine our approach to many practical issues of the day. The latter part of my story will look at some of these: the dream of the downloading of consciousness into robots (a modern-day version of the body as an obstacle to knowledge); contemporary practices of extreme body modification; and examples of high-tech medicine, such as reproductive technologies and organ transplantation (which assume a dualistic vision of mind and body and a belief in the body as an object of scientific knowledge—and manipulation). This will be followed by an examination of alternative approaches to the body—specifically yoga and alternative medicine—approaches which are, in some ways, a revival of ancient holistic visions of body and soul, and which have as their underlying epistemological principle the body as a source of knowledge.

In his book *Cosmopolis*, Stephen Toulmin states that philosophy has reached a dead end with respect to modernity and that it has three choices:

> It can cling to the discredited research program of a purely theoretical (i.e. 'modern') philosophy, which will end by driving it out of business;
> it can look for new and less exclusively theoretical ways of working, and develop the methods needed for a more practical ('post-modern') agenda;

or *it can return to its pre-17th century traditions, and try to recover the lost ('pre-modern') topics that were sidetracked by Descartes, but can be usefully taken up for the future.*[4]

Toulmin is not making reference to the body in his statement; however, since the mechanistic vision of the body forms part of the philosophical enterprise of modernity, it can be argued that the same comments apply. The so-called New Age or non-scientific notions of the body that I will discuss (as demonstrated in alternative medicine or yoga, for example) will be treated as presenting the possibility of recovering notions of the human body that, like other lost pre-modern topics, were "sidetracked by Descartes." Advances in science and technology have made possible the discovery and application of techniques for investigating certain ancient notions that until recently were seen as absurd in the West (acupuncture meridians, to give just one example). Reconsidering pre-modern notions of the body and its relation to the cosmos in light of new knowledge is not only philosophically interesting; it should be seen as a scientific imperative. The late philosopher of science Paul Feyerabend said, "There is no idea, however ancient and absurd that is not capable of improving our knowledge. The whole history of thought is absorbed into science and is used for improving every single theory."[5] Further, he points out that the idea that the Earth moves was not so much discovered by Copernicus as rediscovered. It was Pythagoras' theory until it was confined to the dustbin of history by Ptolemy and finally revived centuries later by Copernicus. Science is not necessarily a history of the progression of ideas. Some ideas are discarded without being properly understood and, in the process, become anathema to the scientific establishment. Feyerabend points to Traditional Chinese Medicine (to be discussed in Chapter 9) as an example of a science that was discarded in China and then revived as a result of the anti-Western political bent of the 1950s. This was a politically enforced scientific dualism, according to Feyerabend, but it "led to most interesting and puzzling discoveries both in China and in the West and to the realization that there are effects and means of diagnosis which modern medicine cannot repeat and for which it has no explanation. It revealed sizeable lacunae in Western medicine."[6]

In reading about the human body from the perspective of the pre-modern philosophers, the reader should bear in mind that the question is not *Were they right or wrong?* or even *Does this make sense to us?* The real questions to ask are: *What were they trying to explain? What was their purpose in describing the body this way?* Invariably, those philosophers' elaborate descriptions of the body were designed to accommodate a perceived *connection* between body and nature, or body and cosmos, that to them was a necessary component of any explanation of the body.[7] The body was not perceived as being limited or bounded by the skin (which to us serves as a kind of envelope separating us from the world around us). To them, the body was porous, allowing spirits (sometimes known as *pneuma*, sometimes by other names) to enter and leave, but, more importantly, allowing a connection between the body and the cosmos. For want of a better term, I refer to these notions as 'cosmic connectors.' In looking at the cosmic connectors that thread their way through this narrative, both as ancient concepts in Western philosophy and as enduring concepts in Eastern philosophy, it is useful to bear in mind Feyerabend's main principle, which he calls "anything goes," a principle that he sees not as inhibiting knowledge but as "both reasonable and *absolutely necessary* for the growth of knowledge."[8]

Thus, the purpose of my philosophical story is to track these cosmic connectors and to understand just what explanatory framework was in play in different philosophical periods. Perhaps the explanations of the Stoics or the Renaissance philosophers were fanciful to our understanding of nature and the body. At the same time, as pointed out above, we now have methods that allow us to begin to understand that bodily energies and forces are not bounded by the skin. Further, given the popularity of practices like yoga and alternative therapies within the general population today, there may also be a collective *need* to explore and understand the connection of body, mind and nature that was severed with the Scientific Revolution. The time may be opportune to consider recuperating certain old ideas using a new vision and new methods. In the spirit of Feyerabend, quoted above, it may not only be opportune, but absolutely necessary.

The focal point of my narrative is the body-machine of Descartes, which is the subject of Chapter 5. I maintain throughout that this conception of the body, which assumes a dualistic and mechanistic vision of nature and of the human body, is still with us and forms the basis of modern medicine. This vision is both metaphysical (the human body, like the natural world, is strictly material, devoid of mind or soul) and epistemological (knowledge of the body comes through purely physical explanations, ultimately reducible to the laws of physics and chemistry). While Descartes was not the first dualist, he was the first to combine dualism and mechanism in such a way as to provide the metaphysical and epistemological underpinnings of the modern vision of the body-machine. Chapter 5 offers an explanation and a critique of the Cartesian project.

The first four chapters provide a narrative outlining several roads that culminated in Descartes' conception of the body machine. Chapter 1 traces the dualism of Plato and how this ancient philosopher attempted to explain body, soul and cosmos in ways that were not always consistent, but that nonetheless served as influences for later, especially Christian, thought about soul and body. The immortality of the soul and the predominance of reason in Plato leave the body in a secondary and sometimes denigrated position. In much of Plato's discussion of mind and body, the body is seen as an obstacle to knowledge. In opposition to Plato's dualism, Chapter 2 looks briefly at Aristotle's transformation of Plato's ideas of form and matter, and then examines the monism of the Stoics, in particular their view of living in accordance with nature. Through the Stoic concept of *oikeiosis*, we learn how the body is the foundation of all our knowledge of nature and ourselves, as well as the foundation for rational development, morality and wisdom.

An examination of the Christian view of the body in Chapter 3 provides a glimpse of, and an explanation for, the ambiguity and ambivalence toward the body that persists in many ways to this day. Here, because of the importance of the body to the central mysteries of the Christian faith, in particular the founding mystery of the Incarnation (whereby God took on a human body in the form of Jesus), the status of the body is raised from being an obstacle to knowledge as seen in Plato, for example. On the other hand, because of the Christian religion's emphasis (not unlike Plato's) on the temptations of the flesh, the body can also be perceived as an impediment to knowledge of God. It is thus a source of sin *and* salvation, underlining a fundamental ambivalence that left its mark on Western thought about and attitudes toward the body.

The Renaissance marks a pivotal point along the road to the body-machine, and Chapter 4 traces a history of the body from an exalted position as part of a living cosmos to an object among others in a disenchanted universe—an object of knowledge for the rising scientific mind. This chapter discusses the double influence of Copernicus and Vesalius, the former leading to a mechanized picture of the cosmos, the latter to a mechanized picture of the human body. By delineating the move from naturalism to mechanism, Chapter 4 demonstrates how the path was opened for Descartes and his body-machine.

Closing Part I of the narrative is a discussion of Spinoza's philosophy of the body, which I present as the 'road not followed.' Spinoza's ideas of the body can be linked to those of the Stoics. In his monistic metaphysics, the body is not separate from the mind, and both are part of nature. Like the Stoics, Spinoza professes a philosophy of living in accordance with nature, and of the body as a source of knowledge and self-knowledge. While I present Spinoza as the road not followed, I also point to the renewed interest in his philosophy as a corrective to the dualistic and mechanistic enterprise, and thus worthy of serious reconsideration.

Concluding Part I with Spinoza as the road not followed is based on my assumption that it was Descartes' mechanistic road that *was* followed—by the sciences of physiology and biology, psychology and medicine, to name the most important from the point of view of the body. Part II thus begins, in Chapter 7, with a discussion of the legacy of mechanism, which I present through an analysis of a number of contemporary practices (organ transplantation, reproductive technologies, biotechnology, robotics, extreme body modification). I maintain that, in different ways and to differing degrees, these practices paint a picture of a fragmenting and disappearing body to the point that some contemporary thinkers actually write about the body as obsolete. My presentation of these practices is not unbiased: in my view they represent the end of the road that was followed, a road that can only be perceived, from the point of view of the human body, as a dead end. In my analysis of these various practices, I often pose questions of how this road appears when observed from the perspective of the road not followed. In other words, I ask, what would Spinoza think? I do not have an adequate answer to this question, but I do think the question leads us back to my interpretation of Toulmin's point made earlier: philosophy must return to some of the pre-Cartesian ideas of the body that were sidetracked by Descartes. This would mean giving serious consideration to notions of the body as an integral part of the natural world and the cosmos. There are many scientists who are seriously investigating these notions but constitute a minority, somewhat on the fringes. In the spirit of Feyerabend's principle of 'anything goes,' mainstream science could broaden its field of study and look anew at ancient notions such as macrocosm-microcosm, world-soul, sound and vibration, and other discarded and disregarded ideas that serve to connect the human mind, body and nature, in light of new knowledge, updated concepts and new technologies.

It is in this light that I present the book's final two chapters, each providing a perspective on recovering the body and reflecting the title of the book: the body of yoga in Chapter 8, and the body of alternative medicine in Chapter 9. In these two chapters, I point out similarities with earlier themes, such as macrocosm-microcosm and living in accordance with nature, and suggest avenues that could be recuperated for a fresh and more realistic vision of the body. Certain themes hark back to the Stoics and to Spinoza, themes that can be seen as lost threads of the historical tapestry of the body—threads that were dropped in the seventeenth century.

My preoccupation in this narrative is metaphysical and epistemological. In other words, I am telling a story of how, in the history of philosophy, questions about what the body is and how we know the body have been addressed. There are other ways of looking at the body—anthropological, sociological or economic, for example—that would tell quite a different story. I do not reject any of these particular ways of telling the story of the body. Feminists, in particular, regard the body (as do many so-called postmodern thinkers) as a social construction, determined more by political and social forces (fundamentally based on male fantasy and power) than by material and biological ones. Because many feminist thinkers resist the determinism implicit in starting from the body as a biological or material fact, they are strong critics of the Cartesian body-machine. I tend to agree with them here, but I do not join them in the theory that the body is simply a social construction. In this I agree with Lynda Birke, a feminist biologist, when she states that, "in emphasising social constructionism, in opposing it to biological determinism, we have perpetuated the dualism; and have played down the importance of the biological body itself."[9] Playing down the importance of the biological body reinforces some of the practices I analyze in Chapter 7, practices that see the body as increasingly unrelated to the person or the self. Birke points out that even biology is de-emphasizing the body—not in favour of social constructivist theories, but in favour of genetic constructivist ones, emphasizing the genotype (genes) over the phenotype (organism), often with an accompanying narrative "in which the body is irrelevant except as temporary home for the genes."[10] What I am hoping my philosophical story will show is the need for a revised metaphysics and epistemology of the body, and, as I show in Chapter 6, some feminist philosophers agree that this might be possible through a recuperation of certain aspects of Spinoza's monism (to which I would add the monism of the Stoics and some of the Renaissance naturalists).

Since I am telling a story about the body in the history of philosophy, I have selected philosophers and periods that have shaped that story. As a result, many thinkers are left out, and many periods are treated solely from the perspective of the plot that I am trying to unravel. I do not deny that there are other interesting and important perspectives on mind, body and nature presented since Descartes (Nietzsche, Heidegger, Foucault and Merleau-Ponty, for example). Nor do I deny that these philosophers, along with others, recognized many of the problems of dualism and mechanism, and proposed alternative metaphysical and epistemological approaches to the body and its relation to the world. Their views, however, did not have a significant impact on the fundamental premises of the body sciences, which accepted the metaphysical vision of the body as a machine and built their perceptions of the body upon them. In spite of the work of modern philosophers in this area, the model of the body-machine has persisted to this day.

Thus, the historical part of my story stops at the seventeenth century, which I see as the starting point for the body-machine as it is perceived in science and medicine today. The metaphysical underpinnings of the body sciences were set at the time of the Scientific Revolution, and questioning them within those sciences does not appear to have been part of the research agenda up to the present day. The materialistic and mechanistic view of the body has been accepted as a given. I hope to show that it is, in fact, a metaphysical presupposition that has a history—and that this presupposition needs to be rethought.

As with all philosophical questions, there are debates about any historical interpretation of particular philosophies and philosophers, and to take all of these debates into consideration would make for a very long book. In addition, the attitude of many philosophers to the body was one of ambivalence, and their discussions of the body can sometimes be ambiguous or even contradictory. For example, not only do philosophers differ in their interpretation of Plato, but it is clear that Plato himself had different visions of the body in different writings—such that one can ask: how many different platonic bodies are there? Similarly, there are debates about whether or not Aristotle thought the soul was immortal, whether for Augustine the body was a prison or a temple, whether Descartes really believed that animals do not feel pain, and even whether Descartes was really a dualist. Where these interpretive debates are relevant and/or enlightening, they are addressed in the text. Otherwise, they are referred to in footnotes and the reader may pursue them if he or she wishes to do so. As for the ambiguities of the philosophers themselves, these are addressed as part of the analysis of the body as a philosophical problem.

I have attempted to write a book that will be accessible to interested readers who do not have a philosophy background, and who do not wish to wade through pages of philosophical argument or doctrinal dispute. At the same time, I have attempted to write a book that is philosophically accurate and relevant. Because my theme is metaphysical, it delves into areas of thought that some philosophers might find suspect, and tends to use language (especially in the historical part) that non-philosophers might find challenging. As a result, there are copious footnotes designed either to explain some philosophical points for non-philosophers, or to substantiate a philosophical claim for readers more familiar with the concepts and authors dealt with in the text. One of my goals in writing the book has been to provide philosophical support for such alternative practices as yoga and alternative medicine, which are often perceived as too far out of the mainstream to be taken seriously by academics. I have also endeavoured to demonstrate that there is a conceptual base for these practices in our own Western philosophical history, and that serious efforts to recuperate some ancient ideas and concepts could help to bridge the philosophical gap between East and West, a gap that is reflected in the debate between modern scientific medicine and alternative medicine. In order to understand the history of ideas about the body, it is necessary to become familiar with the philosophers and their ideas. It is in this light that I attempt to present the ideas of Plato, Descartes, Spinoza and others in an accessible way, without oversimplifying their philosophies. This has been a tough row to hoe and I hope the reader will judge my efforts worthwhile.

Notes

1.   Note that a number of books have been written in French in the last decade, including, among others, Chantal Jacquet's *Le Corps* and Bruno Huisman and François Ribes' *Les Philosophes et le Corps*. An important exception on the English side is the work of Richard Shusterman, in particular his recent book *Body Consciousness: A Philosophy of Mindfulness and Somaesthetics*, to which I refer in Chapter 8.

2.   Chantal Jaquet, *Le Corps* (Paris: Presses Universitaires de France, 2001), 3: "Le corps devient ainsi le membre fantôme de la philosophie, le spectre qui la hante tant qu'un dieu vérace n'y met pas bon ordre et ne lui donne sa place au sein de l'institution de la nature." [Note: The *Encyclopedia of Philosophy* does not have an entry for 'body' (it refers one to 'mind-body problem'); nor does the *Routledge Encyclopedia*. On the other hand, the *Encyclopédie philosophique universelle* has an extensive entry on 'corps']. Jaquet has recently published a book, *La philosophie de l'odorat* (Paris: Presses Universitaires de France, 2010), in part

to challenge the primacy of the sense of sight in the history of philosophy—the one sense that favours the objectification and distancing of the self from the world. (The primacy of sight is called into question in my Chapters 8 and 9 with the discussion of sound—both in the yogic practice of mantra and in the development of alternative therapies using sound for healing.)

3. Descartes is a rare exception, here; his *Treatise on Man* is dedicated to body, specifically to the "body-machine." This work, which will be discussed in Chapter 5, is a part of his larger work, *The World*, referred to by him as his "physics," and was not published in Descartes' lifetime due to his fears of persecution by the religious authorities. One book that does deal with Descartes' mechanistic physiology is Leonora Cohen Rosenfield's *From Beast-Machine to Man-Machine* (New York: Octagon Books, Inc., 1968), but her work deals mostly with animal automatism or the animal-machine. Rosenfield makes the interesting point that the animal-machine in Descartes was a corollary of the human body-machine, rather than the inverse, but that the controversy raised by this idea centred principally on the question of whether animals have souls, not on the question of whether the human body is a machine: "Yet, and this is one of the strange things about the whole quarrel, none of the ardent defenders of the animal soul in this first period took up the cudgels to preserve the human body from the taint of mechanism" (25).

4. Stephen Toulmin, *Cosmopolis: The Hidden Agenda of Modernity* (Chicago: University of Chicago Press, 1990), 11 (emphasis added).

5. Paul Feyerabend, *Against Method* (London: Verso, 1979), 47. Feyerabend also gives the example of Voodoo, which nobody understands but which everybody considers "a paradigm of backwardness and confusion. And yet Voodoo has a firm though still not sufficiently understood material basis, and a study of its manifestations can be used to enrich, and perhaps even to revise, our knowledge of physiology" (3).

6. Feyerabend, 4.

7. Descartes' purpose was the opposite, of course: to show that no such connections were needed to describe the workings of the human body.

8. Feyerabend, 23. This principle does not mean that nothing should be subjected to scientific analysis or proof. It simply means that science should not exclude anything in advance and should compare its explanations not only against experience and experiment, but also against other theories, including ancient and foreign ones, which should be examined for their explanatory value.

9. Lynda Birke, *Feminism and the Biological Body* (New Brunswick, NJ: Rutgers University Press, 1999), 25.

10. Birke, 139. Birke is here referring particularly to the 'selfish gene' narrative of Richard Dawkins.

PART I

The Road to Mechanism: Ancient Greece to the Scientific Revolution

My story of the body in philosophy begins with Plato; however, there are concepts of the body pre-Plato that are of interest to my narrative. My story focuses on philosophy in the Western world, but later chapters bring in Eastern concepts of body for comparison and contrast. An interesting aspect of the history of the body before Plato is the number of comparisons that can be made between ancient Eastern (particularly Chinese) and Western conceptions of body and cosmos. The most important of these in relation to my narrative is the concept of breath in the two cultures.

In his book *The Expressiveness of the Body: The Divergence of Greek and Chinese Medicine*, Shigehisa Kuriyama writes, "Once upon a time, all reflection on what we call the body was inseparable from inquiry into places and directions, seasons and winds. Once upon a time, human being was being embedded in a world."[1] Part of the way in which the body was embedded in the world was through breath, known in the Greek world as *pneuma* and in the Chinese world as *qi*.[2] But in the case of both the Greeks and the Chinese, Kuriyama notes a "blurriness of the divide separating outer flux and inner vitality, winds from breath," such that there was a unity of outer and inner breath, and disruptions of its flow were the cause of disease.[3] In both cases, the terms referred to wind and only later to breath, a similarity that is remarkable since there was no known contact between the two cultures.[4]

In neither culture had a division between inner and outer been made, and winds, linked to weather, could blow gently or rage violently, controlling the fortunes of individuals and communities. But wind was also linked to the immanent powers of the gods to an extent that blurred the distinction between the individual and the cosmos. In Homeric times, for example, the body of the hero was permeable to forces animating it from the outside, and the powers of the hero were attributed not to the hero himself, but to these external, vital powers: "When a man feels joy, irritation or pity, when he suffers, is bold or feels any emotion, he is inhabited by drives that he senses within himself, in his 'organic consciousness,' but which, breathed into him by a god, run through and across him like a visitor coming from the outside."[5] But the same wind or breath could also be dangerous, being able to inspire madness, cause myriad diseases and even kill. Kuriyama tells us that Chinese physicians "discerned wind's influence everywhere," and that in both Europe and China "winds haunted the imagination."[6]

In both Greek and Chinese cultures, wind became internalized into breath, but there the similarity ends and contrasts begin. The Eastern concept of *qi* continued to function as a link between microcosm and macrocosm, and the notion of vital energy, with its importance to health and healing, survived in what is referred to as Traditional Chinese Medicine (which will be discussed in Chapter 9). The Western internalization of *pneuma* began to be elaborated as "inner *content*," and eventually became linked to the inner core or essence of a person. In so doing, it "redefined the nature of the body."[7] The emphasis shifted from forces to forms, the latter being identified with the organs. The result was that the theory of the body became synonymous with action and human agency: "*Organa* were tools—the original meaning of the term—instruments with specific uses. And they presupposed a *user*."[8] The long-term result of this shift in the two notions of wind/breath was a medicine in the East based on vital forces and one in the West built on musculature and anatomy. The result was also two different conceptions of autonomy, one that in the East "portrayed selves preserving their integrity by resisting the depleting outflow of life, the loss of vital energies...." In the West, on the other hand, "the autonomy of the muscleman lay in the capacity for genuine action, for change due neither to nature nor chance, but dependent on the will."[9] As my story of the body unfolds, we will see the rise of the individual self out of the Western conception of soul (eventually reduced to mind), and its gradual retreat from the forces of the cosmos. We will see a body impervious to external forces, be they wind or breath, operating solely under the principles of matter and mechanism. With multiple shifts in the notions of body, soul and cosmos, the impermeable and objective body, along with the autonomous willing 'self,' will be born.

Notes

1. Shigehisa Kuriyama, *The Expressiveness of the Body: The Divergence of Greek and Chinese Medicine* (New York: Zone Books, 2002), 262.

2. Pronounced *chi* (and sometimes written that way).

3. Kuriyama, 246.

4. The ancient Indian notion of *prana* was similar, as well being both wind and breath: "This cosmic wind was mankind's vital breath (*prana*), the unique manifestation of a person's immortal soul." Kenneth G. Zysk, "Vital Breath (*Prana*) in Ancient Indian Medicine and Religion," in Yosio Kawakita, Shizu Sakai, and Yasuo Otsuka (eds.), *The Comparison Between Concepts of Life-Breath in East and West* (Tokyo and St. Louis: Ishiyaku EuroAmerica, Inc., 1995), 33.

5. Jean-Pierre Vernant, "Dim Body, Dazzling Body," in Michel Feher, Ramona Naddaff, and Nadia Taxi (eds.), *Zone 3: Fragments for a History of the Human Body* (New York: Zone Books, 1989), 29.

6. Shigehisa Kuriyama, "*Pneuma, Qi*, and the Problematic of Breath," in Kawakita et al., 9.

7. Kuriyama, *Expressiveness*, 262.

8. Kuriyama, *Expressiveness*, 264.

9. Kuriyama, *Expressiveness*, 268.

BODY AND SOUL AT WAR: PLATO

The comment has often been made that all of Western philosophy is a footnote to Plato,[1] and this claim is certainly true as it pertains to the Western view of the body. In this narrative, Plato provides the opening chapter of the dualistic story of soul and body that has influenced philosophical and religious thought for over two millennia. His dualism is more complex than our modern version, however, having dimensions that are missing from contemporary mind-body debates. While he appears to have a clear separation of soul and body (and elevates the former at the expense of the latter), there are ambiguities in his approach. Whatever heights the soul can reach in mortal life, it cannot get there without the body (even though the body, by its very nature, renders the elevation of soul difficult, if not impossible).

Plato was born in 427 and died in 347 BCE at the age of eighty. Not much is known about his life except that he was born into an aristocratic family, probably did some military service (during the Peloponnesian Wars), had some involvement in politics and founded a school of philosophy known as the Academy.[2] Although Plato was the first Western thinker to have written a body of philosophical work (including metaphysics, epistemology, politics, ethics, mathematics and religion), he was influenced by thinkers who came before him, such as Pythagoras and Heraclitus, and he also came under the strong influence of Socrates, an itinerant teacher in Athens who was sentenced to death by the authorities because of the perceived danger of his teachings. Socrates did not write any philosophy himself, but he is a character in most of Plato's dialogues, raising the question about whether Socrates the character is speaking for Plato or for the historical Socrates himself—a question that has been debated by scholars for centuries. There is no consensus on this point, but there are earlier dialogues, generally referred to as Socratic dialogues, where the historical Socrates is believed to be speaking through the character Socrates; and there are later dialogues where the character Socrates is taken to be speaking for Plato.[3]

In order to appreciate the different dimensions of the Platonic soul-body dichotomy and the ambiguities attached to the Platonic body, it is important to understand that Plato's dualism is rooted in a fundamental preoccupation regarding the difference between that which is sensible and ever-changing and that which is absolute and immutable; the tension he perceives between these two spheres underlies his theory of Forms. It is also necessary to understand something about his cosmology, including three elements that were influential in subsequent debates about body, mind and cosmos: teleology, world-soul and the very pervasive, influential concept of macrocosm-microcosm.[4]

The Theory of Forms

Plato was not the first to explore the tension between the fleeting and the permanent, between the absolute and the changing. It was Heraclitus who observed before Plato that everything is in flux; a person cannot step into the same river twice, since neither the river nor the person is the same from moment to moment. Plato's way of dealing with this problem of the ever-changing and the immutable is to divide the universe into two realms. First, there is the world of sense—the visible world—characterized by its multiplicity; and, second, the world of Forms—the intelligible world or the absolute—characterized by its unity. This division underlines the difference between *what is in process of becoming* and *what is*, or between what is always changing and what always remains the same. As Plato explains in the *Republic*:

> Let me remind you of the distinction ... between the multiplicity of things that we call good or beautiful or whatever it may be and, on the other hand, Goodness itself or Beauty itself and so on. Corresponding to each of these sets of many things, we postulate a single Form or real essence, as we call it.... Further, the many things, we say, can be seen, but are not objects of rational thought; whereas the Forms are objects of thought, but invisible.[5]

Some philosophers refer to Plato's invisible objects of thought as Ideas, but this word should not be taken in our modern sense of ideas as concepts. It is also often assumed that the Forms are simply Plato's way of conceiving what we call universals (the general idea of 'dog' as opposed to a particular Fido). They have also been explained as a kind of standard for comparison; a drawn circle is compared to the standard of absolute circularity, or a beautiful person to the standard of absolute beauty. However we conceive them, it must be borne in mind that the Forms or Ideas are very real for Plato. They are not just neutral concepts that we apprehend rationally, but "transcendent essences that, when directly experienced by the pure philosopher, evoke intense emotional response and even mystical rapture."[6] The words "pure philosopher" are not accidental, here; the Forms can be apprehended by the soul alone, but only if the soul is unfettered by the body, its senses, needs and desires. As Socrates puts it in the *Phaedo*: "It really has been shown to us that, if we are ever to have pure knowledge, we must escape from the body and observe matters in themselves with the soul by itself."[7] In Socrates' view, it was the philosopher who, by definition, came closest to achieving this goal during mortal life. Because it is impossible to attain this kind of knowledge with the body, true knowledge, even for the pure philosopher, can only come after death. In fact, Socrates tells us in the *Phaedo*, "the aim of those who practise philosophy in the proper manner is to practise for dying and death."[8] In life, the only way one can come even close to this knowledge is to "refrain as much as possible from association with the body."[9] This is as clear a statement as Plato makes (and he makes many) indicating that the body is an obstacle to true knowledge; and true knowledge, for Plato, is knowledge of the Forms. In a conversation with Simmias in the *Phaedo*, Socrates asks:

— Do we say that there is such a thing as the Just itself, or not?
— We do say so, by Zeus.
— And the Beautiful, and the Good?
— Of course.
— And have you ever seen any of these things with your eyes?
— In no way, he said.
— Or have you ever grasped them with any of your bodily senses? I am speaking of all things such as Size, Health, Strength, and, in a word, the reality of all other things, that which each of them essentially is. Is what is most true in them contemplated through the body, or is this

the position: whoever of us prepares himself best and most accurately to grasp that thing itself which he is investigating will come closest to the knowledge of it?

— Obviously.

— Then he will do this most perfectly who approaches the object with thought alone, without associating any sight with his thought, or dragging in any sense perception with his reasoning, but who, using pure thought alone, tries to track down each reality pure and by itself, freeing himself as far as possible from eyes and ears, and in a word, from the whole body, because the body confuses the soul and does not allow it to acquire truth and wisdom whenever it is associated with it. Will not that man reach reality, Simmias, if anyone does?

— What you say, said Simmias, is indeed true.[10]

With our senses we can apprehend individual things: good persons, beautiful things, just decisions, healthy or strong individuals. But these will only provide fleeting and ever-changing knowledge of what is beautiful or good or just, etc. In order to have true knowledge of these things, we must apprehend them in their absolute and unchanging form: the Beautiful in itself, the Just in itself, and the Strong in itself. These are the Forms, the eternal essences to which only the soul has access.

Plato's theory of Forms presupposes his theory of reincarnation and the transmigration of souls. Each soul has lived before in a mortal body, and will live again. In between our mortal incarnations we do have access to the knowledge of essences, the Forms. We had this knowledge before we were born. It is through birth and incarnation that this pure knowledge is hidden from us. But it is not completely hidden; when we learn in life, we are, in fact, *recollecting* what we already knew before we were born. If we did not have this knowledge of Forms, our senses could tell us nothing. For example, in perceiving objects as equal to each other, or greater or smaller than each other, we cannot use these terms properly unless we already know, in some way, what is meant by "equal," or "greater," or "smaller." As Socrates puts it to Simmias: "Then before we began to see or hear or otherwise perceive, we must have possessed knowledge of the Equal itself if we were about to refer our sense perceptions of equal objects to it…." The same applies to "the Beautiful itself, the Good itself, the Just, the Pious and, as I say, about all those things to which we can attach the word 'itself' when we are putting questions and answering them. So we must have acquired knowledge of them all before we were born."[11]

Thus, Plato's theory of Forms is intimately linked to his belief in reincarnation and his theory of Recollection. Only the soul has access to the pure knowledge that is the Forms; it has access to that knowledge between mortal lives, but loses it when it becomes tied to a body. The incarnated soul can attain only partial knowledge of the Forms, and this only with great difficulty, by turning away from the body. In other words, the body is an obstacle in the soul's search for knowledge. We will return to the theme of the body as an obstacle to knowledge later in the chapter. In the meantime, it is necessary to consider the role of Plato's cosmology in his overall philosophy of the body.

Plato's Cosmology

Plato's vision of the universe is set out in his dialogue *Timaeus*. Timaeus, a character in the dialogue, recounts to Socrates the myth of creation, including the creation of human beings. While many or even most of the characters in Plato's dialogues are historical persons, there is, according to F. M. Cornford, no historical evidence that there was a real person named Timaeus. He was likely invented by Plato, who wanted a credible protagonist—a philosopher with knowledge of science—in order to tell his tale of creation convincingly. At the same time, because Timaeus speaks dogmatically but without appeal to any authority, Cornford tells us that "we may regard his doctrine as simply Plato's own."[12]

One very significant fact about the *Timaeus* is that, as one of the few works of Plato available to Christian thinkers, it was very influential among philosophers, physicists, doctors and astronomers until the time of Galileo. Thus, in spite of its mythical character and strangeness to the modern intellect, it provides a very important basis for our exploration of the philosophy of the body from the development of Christianity to the Renaissance.

As a myth, the dialogue does not pretend to be an analytic description of the truth; it is presented as a possible, but hypothetical, scenario. It is also the first Greek account of divine creation, although it must be borne in mind that this is not the creation *ex nihilo* of Christianity; Plato's Demiurge, or craftsman, does not create the world but "brought it from disorder into order."[13] The material of which the cosmos is made is initially *chaos*. The Demiurge creates the order (based on the idea or form of the Good) from the already-created material, which sets certain limits to his work. Being neither omnipotent nor creator, he is not responsible for any disorder in the universe, "but only for those features of order and intelligible design which he proceeds to introduce, 'so far as he can.'"[14] At the same time, Plato's cosmos is both beautiful and good, following the Forms of the Beautiful and the Good. It is a living organism that possesses a soul and intelligence.

Teleology

Following the form of the Good, Plato's universe is *teleological*; the natural order is moving toward the Good, and each thing within the universe has an end in relation to the totality. Everything is moving toward the perfection of the whole. Because of this, Plato favours teleological over mechanical explanations. He is less concerned with causal explanation about how things work; he is interested in why they work the way they do. For Plato, the ultimate explanation of a cause of something is its purpose, its end, its relation to the perfect whole. Thus, an event is not caused by antecedent events, but by a goal toward which the so-called effect is directed. In other words, the cause is that toward which the effect is moving, not that which physically initiated the change or movement (usually referred to as the efficient cause). As Socrates says in the *Phaedo*:

> I no longer understand or recognize those other sophisticated causes, and if someone tells me that a thing is beautiful because it has a bright colour or shape or any such thing, I ignore these other reasons—for all these confuse me—but I simply, naively and perhaps foolishly cling to this, that nothing else makes it beautiful other than the presence of, or the sharing in, or however you may describe its relationship to that Beautiful we mentioned ... all beautiful things are beautiful by the Beautiful.[15]

World-soul

Plato's teleological principle makes sense only because his cosmos is conceived as an intelligent whole (there is a purpose to the whole and to its parts). But it is also linked with (and dependent upon) another essential element of his cosmology: the world-soul. Being both intelligent and alive, Plato's cosmos is *ensouled*. The universe and all beings in it partake in, or are a part of, a world-soul. As explained in the *Timaeus*,

> And in the centre [of the world's body] he set a soul and caused it to extend throughout the whole and further wrapped its body round with soul on the outside; and so he established one world alone, round and revolving in a circle, solitary but able by reason of its excellence to bear itself company, needing no other acquaintance or friend but sufficient to itself. On all these accounts the world which he brought into being was a blessed god.[16]

Although not everyone would agree, one could say that, not only does the material world *have* a soul, but that the material world is *in* the world-soul. Plato offers an elaborate description of the composition of the world-soul based on the Forms of Existence, Sameness and Difference, an analysis of which is not necessary for our purposes.[17] But what is interesting is that his description of the three ingredients is such that the world-soul is spoken of "as if it were a piece of malleable stuff—say, an amalgam of three soft metals—forming a long strip, which will presently be slit along its whole length and bent round into circles."[18] The whole is then divided proportionally into parts in such a way that the harmony created corresponds to the intervals of a musical scale, leading to the notion, expressed by some, of the music of the heavens.[19] Another important aspect of the world-soul is that it represents the principle of life of the universe and, ultimately, of every being in it. The Greek word *psyche* refers not primarily to mind but to the principle of life, which pertains to all living beings. Because the entire cosmos is a living, intelligent being, everything in it possesses soul to varying degrees. Human beings are endowed with intellect, the highest and most noble (and also immortal) part of the soul, but soul cannot be reduced to mind in the Platonic universe.

The human soul is similar to the world-soul; both are fashioned out of the same substance by the Demiurge who "turned once more to the same mixing bowl wherein he had mixed and blended the soul of the universe, and poured into it what was left of the former ingredients, blending them this time in somewhat the same way, *only no longer so pure as before*."[20]

Macrocosm-Microcosm

This brings up another fundamental element of Plato's cosmology: the notion of macrocosm-microcosm. The human soul is a reflection in miniature of the world-soul; it is the microcosm and the world-soul is the macrocosm, just as the human is the microcosm and the cosmos is the macrocosm. Both the world-soul and the human soul represent reason and life; as the world-soul is the principle of life of the universe, so the human soul is the principle of life of the human being. As pointed out above, rationality permeates the universe and there is soul in everything to varying degrees.

Breath is another example of the microcosm-macrocosm relation; in humans, as well as in the cosmos, breath is composed of air and fire, the most active elements. The inner fire of the human unites with the exterior fire of the cosmos, and the exterior air enters the body to take the place of the air that escapes. The human head copies the round shape of the universe; the human heart is like the sun. Man is intimately linked to the cosmos, body and soul. This concept will be central to a metaphysic of the body until the time of Descartes.

In spite of the fact that the soul is intimately linked to the cosmos, Plato's description of the creation of the human soul in the *Timaeus* sets the stage for a less-than-perfect union of the soul with the body, and for the dominance of the former over the latter. In Plato's view, the human soul has three parts, only one of which is immortal and divine. To underline this difference, Plato's myth has the Demiurge create only the immortal part of the soul from the same bowl as the world-soul; it leaves the creation of the mortal parts of the soul—along with the body itself—to lesser divinities. The Demiurge created as many souls as there were stars, and each soul was distributed to a star:

> There mounting them as it were in chariots, he showed them the nature of the universe and declared to them the laws of Destiny. There would be appointed a first incarnation one and the same for all, that none might suffer disadvantage at his hands; and they were to be sown into the instruments of time, each one into that which was meet for it, and to be born as the most god-fearing of living creatures; and human nature being twofold, the better sort was that which should thereafter be called 'man.'[21]

Meanwhile, the lesser gods set about the task of creating the human body and plunging the immortal soul into "the turbulent tide of bodily sensation and nutrition."[22] For this task,

> they borrowed from the world portions of fire and earth, water and air ... and cemented together what they took ... welding them with a multitude of rivets too small to be seen and so making each body a unity of all the portions. And they confined the circuits of the immortal soul within the flowing and ebbing tide of the body.[23]

The confinement of the immortal soul within the mortal body was accompanied by "a strong and widespread commotion ... violently shaking the circuits of the soul" and disrupting and twisting the harmony of the circles of the Same and Different, causing "infractions and deformations."[24] The gods house the immortal part of the soul in the head of the human they are creating; the lesser parts of the soul are housed in the lower regions of the body. This tripartite structure of the soul and its relation to the body will be discussed a little later. The important point, here, is that the ontological status of the human soul and body and their relation to the cosmos and world-soul have been established in the creation myth, which serves as a basis for the fundamental tension and opposition of body and soul in Plato's philosophy. The soul does not go happily into the body, which comes to be seen as a prison or a tomb from which it will ultimately seek to escape. It longs to return to its happy state where it acquired the knowledge of the whole universe.

The Platonic Body: An Obstacle to Knowledge or a Way to Knowledge?

It is impossible to overestimate the importance of knowledge in Plato's philosophy. The reason for this is its intimate connection with virtue; for Plato, goodness is knowledge and people err only out of ignorance. G. M. Grube tells us that the historical Socrates "wished to reduce all excellence to some kind of knowledge and was profoundly convinced that 'no man does wrong on purpose' because no man is willingly ignorant."[25] Knowledge is both the object of the good life and the means to achieving it. True knowledge, as we have seen, is knowledge of the Forms, and it is achieved through the soul alone. But humans are composed of a soul and a body, which poses a problem that Plato attempts to resolve in different ways, leading to ambiguities or even contradictions in his philosophy of the body, although these may be more apparent than real. We will look at three different versions of the relation of soul and body in the human quest for knowledge: 1) the radical dualism of the *Phaedo*, where it is not an exaggeration to assume that Plato sees body and soul almost at war, and where the body is presented as an obstacle to knowledge; 2) the tripartite soul of the *Phaedrus* and *Timaeus*, where one can conclude that the three parts of the soul actually can live in harmony and the body is not necessarily an obstacle to knowledge; and 3) the route to knowledge through love set out in the *Symposium*, where the body serves, in effect, as a source of knowledge for the soul.

Body and Soul in Conflict

Unlike the *Timaeus*, there is nothing mythical about the *Phaedo*, which is an account of what took place at a meeting between Socrates and a number of his close friends just before his death. Plato was unable to be there due to illness, but some commentators believe that the story was actually relayed to him by Socrates' friend, Phaedo, who was present. While the theory of Forms coupled with a rather strong denigration of the body are ideas presented by Socrates in the dialogue, R. Hackforth points out that this is a dialogue in which Socrates is Platonized, with Plato attributing to Socrates a more metaphysical stand regarding the soul and a more hostile attitude toward the body than is usually seen in the historical Socrates.[26] The theory of Forms does not come from Socrates; however, while the tendency to denigrate the body is extreme in this dialogue, it is based on Socratic teachings about the importance of tending to the soul and of seeking knowledge in the pursuit of virtue. Even the setting of this dialogue reflects the Platonic view of the soul as a prisoner of the body: Socrates is in prison; he is condemned to die, but he appears quite unconcerned about his imminent death, which will simply be the release of his soul from his body. When asked by his friends how they should bury him, he simply says, "In any way you like," making the further point that he, Socrates, is not the thing that they will soon be looking at as a corpse.[27] He tells them that, where he is going, he "shall acquire what has been our chief preoccupation in our past life," that is, pure knowledge, which he is certain can only be attained after death. Thus, the journey that he is now forced to undertake "is full of good hope."[28]

Plato's concern with the Forms and with the immortality of the soul motivates his many derogatory comments about the body in this dialogue. The body can only give knowledge of visible, or material, things, while the Forms are invisible and immaterial.[29] Bodily knowledge is sensory knowledge, fleeting and changing. It is not true knowledge; it actually leads us away from true knowledge. As Socrates says to Cebes:

> Haven't we also said some time ago that when the soul makes use of the body to investigate something, be it through hearing or seeing or some other sense—for to investigate something through the senses is to do it through the body—it is dragged by the body to the things that are never the same, and the soul itself strays and is confused and dizzy, as if it were drunk, in so far as it is in contact with that kind of thing?[30]

If we want true knowledge, we have to turn away from the senses, which actually lead us astray, making us believe what is false; in other words, the senses—and the body—are an impediment to knowledge. For Socrates, the way out of the ignorance caused by the senses is through philosophy, or the love of learning. Philosophy can get hold of the soul, even though it is imprisoned in the body. It "gently encourages it and tries to free it by showing [the lovers of learning] that investigation through the eyes is full of deceit, as is that through the ears and the other senses. Philosophy then persuades the soul to withdraw from the senses...."[31]

But the notion of the body as an obstacle to knowledge extends further. It is not just that the senses can misinform us about reality; they are also at the root of physical pleasure and the desire that such pleasure instils in the soul. "Every pleasure and every pain provides, as it were, another nail to rivet the soul to the body and to weld them together."[32] The body leads the soul astray and drags it down, not only in this world but also in the next, because there the soul's next incarnation will pay the price for its previous attachment to the material world and its pleasures. So the true philosopher "keeps away from pleasures and desires and pains as far as he can."[33]

Thus, the body and the soul are in a constant battle, with the soul needing to be vigilant in order not to succumb to the body's lusts, desires and pains. But the soul must even do battle with the body in ordinary everyday ways, since it "keeps us busy in a thousand ways because of its need for nurture," and if it becomes ill, it impedes our search for truth.[34] The body represents a never-ending battlefield for the wise soul, according to Socrates, arguing against Simmias and Cebes, who think that the soul and body actually work in harmony—that they are naturally attuned to each other. In his view, whatever harmony exists is only the result of the domination of the soul,

> ruling over all the elements of which one says it is composed, opposing nearly all of them throughout life, directing all their ways, inflicting harsh and painful punishment on them, at times in physical culture and medicine, at other times more gently by threats and exhortations, holding converse with desires and passions and fears as if it were one talking to a different one....[35]

This all seems to be at odds with the cosmic harmony that we have seen in Plato's cosmology. If the cosmos is an intelligent, living whole, one would think its parts, while not perfect, must be directing themselves toward perfection. The *Phaedo* makes it appear that there is a constant battle going on and that universal harmony is impossible. This may be the reason that many commentators find the dualism of the *Phaedo* extreme; Richard Shusterman refers to it as "Plato's most body-despising dialogue."[36] Further, while Plato's soul is supposed to have three parts, it seems to be treated in this dialogue as having only one, or only one that really counts (the intellect). This is not the case in other dialogues, and while Plato appears to be arguing against the possible harmony of soul and body in the *Phaedo*, he approaches the matter a little differently in other dialogues, such as the *Phaedrus* and the *Timaeus*.

Body and Soul in Harmony

In our discussion of the *Timaeus*, above, it was pointed out that, while the Demiurge fabricated the highest, or immortal, part of the soul, "the task of the generation of mortals, he laid upon his own offspring,"[37] who were the lesser gods. They first fashioned a round head to house the immortal part of the soul, as we have seen. Then, as Timaeus explains,

> For a vehicle they gave it the body as a whole, and therein they built on another form of soul, the mortal, having in itself dread and necessary affections: first pleasure, the strongest lure of evil; next pains that take flight from good; temerity moreover and fear, a pair of unwise counselors;

passion hard to entreat, and hope too easily led astray. These they combined with irrational sense and desire that shrinks from no venture, and so of necessity compounded the mortal element.[38]

In order to keep the immortal and mortal parts of the soul separate, and the latter from polluting the former, the gods placed the neck "as an isthmus and boundary" keeping the two apart.[39] The mortal parts of the soul are also of two types, the first, the spirited part, being nobler and housed closer to the head (in the heart); and the second, the appetitive part, being baser and housed "between the midriff and the boundary towards the navel," where "they tethered it like a beast untamed."[40] The diaphragm acts as a separation between the spirited and the appetitive parts of the soul; housed in the middle, between Reason and Appetite, the spirited part of the soul can go either way, aiding Reason against the power of the appetites, or, alternatively, falling under the sway of the appetites and working against the rational part of the soul.

It is extremely important for the health of the individual that the soul and body be in harmony, and this is a question of *proportion*:

> For health or sickness, goodness or badness, the proportion or dispro-
> portion between soul and body themselves is more important than any
> other.... When the soul in [a body] is too strong for the body and of
> ardent temperament, she dislocates the whole frame and fills it with
> ailments from within.... On the other hand, when a large body, too big
> for the soul, is conjoined with a small and feeble mind ... the motions of
> the stronger part prevail and ... [making] the powers of the soul dull and
> slow to learn and forgetful, they produce in her the worst of maladies,
> stupidity.[41]

In order to prevent disproportions of this sort, both the body and the soul must be exercised in the right way; those who are involved in intellectual pursuits must make sure the body receives adequate athletic training, while anyone whose principal activity is physical must "compensate his soul with her proper exercise in the cultivation of the mind and all higher education."[42]

When the proper proportion between soul and body is not maintained, disease is the result. Diseases of the body are of many types, but usually arise because of an imbalance in the primary bodily elements of fire, water, air and earth, which are associated, respectively, with the bodily fluids of yellow bile, blood, phlegm and black bile. Plato is following the principles of the medicine of his time, which held that health is a question of harmony of the constituents of the body, and illness is a breakdown of that harmony. Bodily illness can also cause illness in the soul. A buildup of phlegm or bitter bilious humours, for example, can induce disorder at all levels of the soul and "beget many divers types of ill-temper and despondency, of rashness and cowardice, of dullness and oblivion."[43] Similarly, excess of pleasures or pains causes illness in the soul that is often interpreted, according to Plato, as badness, when in fact the "soul is rendered sick and senseless by the body." For Plato, people do not err intentionally, but "because of some faulty habit of body and unenlightened upbringing, and these are unwelcome afflictions that come to any man against his will."[44] Keeping order and proportion in the three parts of the soul and the corresponding parts of the body is not a small accomplishment. But, as Plato's detailed discussion of soul-body harmony in the *Timaeus* tells us, it is possible with care of both body and soul.

The anatomical description in the *Timaeus* of the three parts of the soul and the need for harmony among them is set out metaphorically in the *Phaedrus* in the myth of the winged charioteer and his team of two horses:

> Let us ... compare the soul to a winged charioteer and his team acting together. Now all the horses and charioteers of the gods are good and come of good stock, but in other beings there is a mixture of good and bad. First of all we must make it plain that the ruling power in us men drives a pair of horses, and next that one of these horses is fine and good and of noble stock, and the other the opposite in every way. So in our case the task of the charioteer is necessarily a difficult and unpleasant business.[45]

While this metaphor emphasizes that the mortal parts of the soul are influenced by bodily needs and desires, these needs and desires are not necessarily all bad or evil. There is a mixture of good and bad in the horses—one of them, representing the spirited part of the soul, is described above as "fine and good and of noble stock" and the other, representing the appetites, "the opposite in every way." The former, of high stature, agile and white in colour, can either control or be controlled by the latter, which is short, heavy and black in colour. And while it is up to the charioteer to keep the horses in check and not be run by them, he also depends on them to move forward. He needs their cooperation, in other words, and they can work in harmony. Even the lower soul, representing the appetites, can show virtue in moderation.

In fact, in the myth, the charioteer—the immortal part of the soul—is actually trying to move upward; thus the wings. Before being embodied, the soul is part of the winged procession of the gods, surveying the heavens or "the abode of the reality with which true knowledge is concerned, a reality without colour or shape, intangible but utterly real, apprehensible only by the intellect which is the pilot of the soul"[46]—in other words, the world of Forms. The soul that is embodied has shed its wings, and during its time in an earthly life must try to get them back by nourishing itself with beauty, wisdom and goodness, the qualities which "are the prime source of nourishment and growth to the wings of the soul, but their opposites, such as ugliness and evil, cause the wings to waste and perish."[47] It is up to the charioteer to guide the horses and not be guided by them; at the same time, regaining his wings and moving them upward is, as Socrates said, necessarily a difficult and unpleasant business. Some charioteers may rise and fall due to the restiveness of the horses; they may from time to time glimpse a part, but not the whole, of reality. The majority, however, fail to reach the upper world "and are carried round beneath the surface, trampling and jostling one another, each eager to outstrip its neighbour ... many souls are lamed and many have their wings all broken through the feebleness of their charioteers...."[48]

The main point to note, here, is that the possibility for harmony between the parts of the soul does exist, and the spirited part of the soul can contribute to that harmony. While it is up to the charioteer to do most of the work, the white horse can be brought in to support him in his battle with the black horse. This still leaves most bodily needs in the realm of what is bad or evil, but it does allow for the cultivation of virtues that aid in the establishment of equilibrium between the parts of the soul and, thus, between soul and body. This allows the charioteer to rise higher toward the realm of the Forms from which he descended, although "the unruly behaviour of its horses impairs its [the soul's] vision of reality."[49] As in the *Phaedo*, it is those who work hardest at recollecting the things that the soul once perceived (and thus, at the pursuit of knowledge) who succeed in rising this high—which is "why it is right that the soul of the philosopher alone should regain its wings."[50] However, while the philosopher of the *Phaedo* is in constant battle with his body, the philosopher of the *Phaedrus* must overcome passions in his own soul. The division of the soul into three parts means that the struggle for the Good represents not the domination of soul over body, but the overcoming of conflict within the soul itself, thus extending the notion of *psyche* to include passions and desires, rather than simply intellect.

The improvement on the extreme dualism of the *Phaedo* that is evident in the *Phaedrus* is not a small one. Nor is the tripartite soul a primitive idea, according to Grube, who sees it, rather, as very advanced: "one of the most startlingly modern things in Platonic philosophy is just this discovery of the importance of conflict in the mind."[51] In other words, it's not all the body's fault. The body is not the source of everything evil, nor is it always dragging the soul down; rather, following the analogy of the charioteer and his horses, the body can even serve to help raise the soul upward, toward the realm of true knowledge: the Forms. Each part of the soul has its virtues and its temptations, and harmony can be achieved only when the three parts work together, each performing according to its proper function. This, of course, really means that the lower parts of the soul must work in harmony with the highest part, and Plato does not waver on the idea, even in the tripartite soul, that the highest level, Reason, is in charge. But it represents a softening the extreme language of the *Phaedo* regarding the body, and a recognition that the mortal parts of the soul, and the parts of the body to which they correspond, have a role to play in the soul's harmony, keeping the "head of its charioteer above the surface"[52] as it rides the journey of its earthly life. Plato has brought a few nuances to his conception of the body, and, rather than simply condemning it as the source of earthly pleasures that lead the soul astray, he chooses to try to understand the pleasures of the body and to set out ways to control them. Perhaps in his later dialogues Plato understands that even the highest pleasures linked to learning and the quest for knowledge must pass by the body. This understanding permeates the *Symposium*, where Plato is quite clear that the only way to ascend to the Form of Beauty is to experience true beauty in its earthly form: human love.

Body as a Way to the Forms

The *Symposium* takes place at a banquet in honour of Dionysus, after which various participants provide discourses on the theme of love.[53] Love is discussed from the point of view of its baser form (which is limited to sexual gratification and the procreation of children) and its nobler form (which, in Plato, applies to men only and "is directed exclusively towards young men"[54]). This latter form of love is an ideal that transcends sexual attraction and involves a shared search for knowledge and the Good. The most important speech of the dialogue is that of Socrates, but his speech is, in fact, a reiteration of the speech of someone else, someone from whom Socrates admits that he himself learned about the meaning of love. It is a discourse about Socrates' education in love at the hands of Diotima, a woman of Mantinea who was, in Socrates' words, "my instructress in the art of love."[55]

Before examining Socrates' discourse on Diotima, it is interesting to take note of another important and well-known discourse of the dialogue, that of Aristophanes, whose speech "constitutes almost the most brilliant of all [Plato's] achievements as a literary artist."[56] It is the rather whimsical story of how, originally, human beings came in three forms: male, female and hermaphrodite. In these forms, they were complete in themselves:

> [E]ach human being was a rounded whole, with double back and flanks forming a complete circle; it had four hands and an equal number of legs, and two identically similar faces upon a circular neck, with one head common to both the faces, which were turned in opposite directions. It had four ears and two organs of generation and everything else to correspond. These people could walk upright like us in either direction, backwards or forwards, but when they wanted to run quickly they used all their eight limbs, and turned rapidly over and over in a circle, like tumblers who perform a cart-wheel and return to an upright position.[57]

They were very strong and vigorous, but also very proud; their exaggerated pride caused them to do battle with the gods, who, as punishment, decided to weaken them by cutting them in two. The dissection necessitated some fine-tuning, including the turning of the face toward the dissected side, and a healing of the wounds, which the gods accomplished, leaving "a few wrinkles on the belly itself round the navel, to remind man of the state from which he had fallen."[58] Since then, men and women have been searching for their other halves, something that explains, according to Aristophanes, "the innate love which human beings feel for one another, the love which restores us to our ancient state by attempting to weld two beings into one and to heal the wounds which humanity suffered."[59] Those who were of the original hermaphrodite sex are looking for their other half in the opposite sex; those who were of the male or female sex are searching for a person of the same sex—although, in a twist that Aristophanes does not adequately explain, males tend to look for men in their boyhood, but become "lovers of boys in manhood, because they always cleave to what is akin to themselves."[60]

While this story should perhaps not be given too much weight in an analysis of the Platonic body, it is interesting from several points of view. It gives the same value to homosexual as to heterosexual love (perhaps downgrading the latter—at least in relation to the married state, to which the male is naturally disinclined, according to Aristophanes). But, more importantly, it explains the very strong, natural attraction of one person to another in purely *physical* and bodily terms. It is the body that was originally a whole (if a rather cumbersome one), which, in separation, is in constant search of its other half. Of course, the attraction to, and the need for, the other is only truly satisfied at the level of soul: "It is clear that the soul of each has some other longing which it cannot express, but can only surmise and obscurely hint at." But the attraction is initially physical; the longing (the basic expression of love) is physical before it is spiritual; and the spiritual longing itself is obscure, not explicit. Further, while the heterosexual love that guarantees procreation cannot attain the heightened status of the perfect intellectual love between two men, this is seen as a limitation, not degradation. It is also in keeping with the belief held at the time that women were not capable of true intellectual or spiritual communication with anyone.

This makes Socrates' speech all the more interesting. Socrates is admitting that he learned all he needed to know about love from a woman—and the love that he will ultimately refer to in his speech is that very superior kind of love that takes place only between kindred souls, not simply bodies. Susan Hawthorne remarks that, "in spite of the marked social and political differences in rights between women and men in Ancient Greek culture, Socrates presents the teachings of Diotima in a way that make it very clear that he held her in high regard."[61] Further, the feminine and bodily imagery used by Diotima serves to underline a certain ambiguity in Plato in relation to both women and the body, something that has already been pointed to in this chapter.

According to Diotima, Love is a spirit, half-god and half-man, who bridges the gap between men and the gods. This placement of love as an intermediate space between the mortal and the immortal is noteworthy in itself, given the extreme dichotomy shown in the *Phaedo* between the heavenly and the earthly realms. It is also interesting because it follows a short exposition by Diotima in which she admonishes Socrates for his tendency to think in opposites. That something is not beautiful does not mean that it is ugly; that a person does not have the whole truth does not mean that he is ignorant. There is a halfway position between knowledge and ignorance, which is called having true convictions. Socrates has maintained that Love cannot be beautiful or good, because, if he were, he would not desire the beautiful and the good; he would possess them already. But, as everyone knows, Love does desire the beautiful and the good. However, Diotima insists that this does not mean that Love is ugly and bad. "Do not suppose," she says, "that because, on your own admission, Love is not good or beautiful, he must on that account be ugly and bad, but rather that he is something between the two."[62] Love is a lover of beauty, and wisdom is one of the most beautiful things, so Love is a lover of wisdom—even though he is in a state between wisdom and ignorance. Love desires to move toward the Good, the Beautiful—in other words, the Forms. The object of love is, ultimately, the Good, or, more precisely, according to Diotima, "love is desire for the perpetual possession of the good."[63] In his intermediate state, Love is always in a state of *becoming*, and Diotima uses both bodily and feminine metaphors to describe Love's activity and Love's goal. Hawthorne points out that Diotima uses "a great number of metaphors which relate to the process of birth: from conception, to pregnancy, to giving birth, then to processes of becoming; to initiation, to death and to rebirth," all metaphors showing a concern "for the ongoing process of life" linked more with women's than men's experience.[64] And, one might add, more with the bodily than the intellectual realm.

A side issue, here, relates not to Plato's own ambiguity regarding the body and women in general, but to that of his translators. Hawthorne points to "misogynist translations," which tend to avoid the starker references to female anatomy and processes. For example, where Rouse translates the phrase at 208e1–3 as "those who are pregnant in body ... turn rather to women," Walter Hamilton (whose translation is used here) translates the same phrase as "those whose creative instinct is physical have recourse to women."[65]

However, even Hamilton cannot avoid the pregnancy metaphor completely. The offending phrase is referring to the fact that there are two different ways of procreating: the usual way of begetting children through sexual intercourse between the sexes, and another way by those "whose creative desire is of the soul, and who long to beget spiritually, not physically, the progeny which is the nature of the soul to create and bring to birth."[66] Both are seeking immortality, the former through begetting children, the latter through creating lasting works of poetry, crafts or inventions. All men, Diotima tells Socrates, have the creative impulse, and this can be satisfied either physically or spiritually. If we ask why procreation is the object of love, Diotima answers:

> Because procreation is the nearest thing to perpetuity and immortality that a mortal being can attain. If, as we agreed, the aim of love is the perpetual possession of the good, it necessarily follows that it must desire immortality together with the good, and the argument leads us to the inevitable conclusion that love is love of immortality as well as of the good.[67]

What is interesting about this metaphor of pregnancy and birth is the association, on an apparently equal level, of creations of the body and those of the soul. This may strike us as an inappropriate equation and as a devaluation of the importance of bearing and raising children, but we must bear in mind that in Plato's male-oriented world—and particularly in light of his preference for intellectual over physical pursuits—this actually raises the level of creations of the body to that of creations of the mind. Not a small step for the Plato of the *Phaedo*. No lesser a step is putting the words of a woman into the mouth of his preferred protagonist, Socrates, even if this does leave these words two steps removed from the author himself. "Diotima speaks from her experience of the body, as a woman, and it is from this experience that her perceptions, and her metaphors, derive."[68] The fact that Plato is calling on her to speak at all is a nod in the direction of the body that one must recognize, if not actually applaud.

An even more important reason for seeing in the *Symposium* a more nuanced view of the body than Plato has shown in his other dialogues is the recognition, through the discussion of love, that knowledge of Beauty comes about through the love of beauty in a loved one. One must begin by falling in love with a beautiful person and, through that love, "beget noble sentiments in partnership with him."[69] Through the recognition of physical beauty in one person, one will gradually come to the realization that "physical beauty in any person is closely akin to physical beauty in any other."[70] This way, the lover becomes a lover of all physical beauty, and will begin to focus on beauty itself, as opposed to one beautiful person.

> The man who has been guided thus far in the mysteries of love, and who has directed his thoughts towards examples of beauty in due and orderly

succession, will suddenly have revealed to him as he approaches the end of his initiation a beauty whose nature is marvellous indeed, the final goal, Socrates, of all his previous efforts. This beauty is first of all eternal ... he will see it as absolute, existing alone with itself, unique, eternal, and all other beautiful things as partaking of it....[71]

This is referred to as the 'ascent passage,' where it is shown that a man, "starting from this sensible world and making his way upward by a right use of his feeling of love for boys,"[72] ascends continually to meet absolute Beauty itself. It is almost astounding, to a reader of the *Phaedo*, to see that knowledge of the form of Beauty is achieved not by turning away from the body, but, in fact, by starting from the body. In other words, the sensible world becomes the means by which the lover ascends to the world of Forms. Here, the body is not an obstacle to knowledge of the Forms, as it is in the *Phaedo*, but can actually be seen as a source of such knowledge, at least in the sense that it is through knowledge of the body that one arrives at true knowledge of the Forms. Diotima rejects the implied constant battle between the bodily and the intellectual realms in favour of an integration of the two. Transformation, here, begins in the body. "Diotima recognizes degrees of change, rather than simply seeing only those qualities at each end of the spectrum."[73] The body, at least momentarily in the Platonic corpus, has been given its due, and, with this, through the feminine metaphors used by Diotima, the intellect is brought to recognize the flesh, bringing both into harmony.[74]

The Lasting Influence of the Platonic Body

Reference was made at the beginning of this chapter to the fact that Plato's dualistic vision of soul and body had great influence over subsequent ideas of the body right up to, and following, the time of Descartes. His influence can still be perceived in our own dualistic vision of mind and body, although his dualism is much more complex than our own mind-body split, as I hope to have shown in this chapter.

Even in its extreme form as set out in the *Phaedo*, Plato's dualism has one very important difference from modern notions of mind and body: the soul is the principle of life—and this is not restricted to human beings. Animal and vegetable life is also endowed with soul, although to varying degrees, something that Plato does not treat in detail in his work, but which is taken up by Aristotle. The fact that the human soul can be reincarnated in an animal body shows that the difference between animal and human souls must be one of degree and not of kind. Whether animals can be reincarnated as humans is an aspect of the question that is not dealt with in detail by Plato, but one can only assume that, if my punishment for this life is to be a donkey in the next, my soul must have the chance of returning to a human body in a subsequent life. What I have to achieve in my life as a donkey in order to get back to humanity is not discussed, and any attempt at explanation will, of course, strike the modern reader as silly at best. The point to remember, however, is always that one must consider what the theory in question is meant to explain. Plato's account of immortality, his theory of Recollection and his theory of Forms are all linked, and they, in turn, are linked to his idea of the Good. He needs to account in some way for reward and punishment at the end of life. What, for example, happens to the soul that is not pure at the time of death? Reincarnation can be seen as providing an explanation. In the Christian world, a person who leads a bad life goes to the eternal suffering of hell; in Plato's world, he comes back to Earth for another chance, but at a reduced level of being. This can only make sense in a universe where soul is, in varying degrees, in everything.

Soul is also connected with the world-soul. This is another aspect that has been lost or dropped from the modern conception of soul, which, aside from in a church or on the psychotherapist's couch—and maybe not even there—has been reduced to mind, if not simply to brain processes.[75] All life is connected in the Platonic world, and life on Earth is a reflection of cosmic life through the all-important principle of macrocosm-microcosm—the cosmos itself being a living, intelligent whole. This flows over into notions of body, since the body is the receptacle of the cosmic fire, the heart is the sun in miniature, and we take in the breath of the universe with each human breath. For Plato, the body is intimately connected with the cosmos, another notion that will fall by the wayside with the Scientific Revolution.

Plato's tripartite soul will be influential until the time of Descartes, who found it expedient to materialize the lower parts of the soul (dropping the notion of soul from them completely) along with the principle of life, which he will explain in purely mechanical terms. But Plato's ideas about both spiritual and physical health being achieved through harmony among the three parts of the soul will also be very influential in medicine, again up to the time of

Descartes, and these ideas are recovered in many forms of alternative medicine being practiced today. It is interesting to consider Plato's three levels of soul within the context of Eastern energetic systems, especially the chakra system, where the lower chakras can be compared to Plato's lowest level of soul related to physical and sexual needs; the middle chakras to emotions like anger and courage and the ability to act on what is good for oneself; and the upper chakras to insight, reasoning and intellectual activity. Of course, many today will look questioningly at both of these systems, but the question again is: what is being explained, here?

Plato's (or Diotima's) idea of the soul ascending to the world of Forms (Beauty and the Good, in this case) through bodily love gives an importance to the body that appears to be an anomaly in Plato's thought. It is an idea that was more influential in monist thought; it is central to the Stoic idea of living in accordance with nature, where the body serves as a source of knowledge of nature and the divine, notions that were taken up centuries later by Spinoza. We get only a glimpse of this idea in Plato—and it comes through the voice of a woman, another anomaly in Plato's dialogues. But it is important that it is there, at least in that one dialogue, and, intentionally or not, it highlights a fact that should be obvious: any ascent to higher forms of learning or understanding can only come about *through* the body and not by rejecting the body. At the very least, we need our brain to think, and most people have some experience, through love of music or nature, or through the love of another person, of achieving higher levels of understanding and knowledge, if only momentarily. These moments are achieved through bodily, as well as spiritual, understanding.

Perhaps a cautionary note to the modern reader would be helpful here. Before judging Plato's ideas of the body as irrelevant or thinking that his sometimes extreme rejection of the body (in order to achieve knowledge) is a very antiquated notion, one would do well to read Ray Kurzweil, one of the current gurus of the idea of downloading consciousness into robots, whose work will be discussed in Chapter 7. In his view, the body's need for nourishment uses up too much brain energy—energy that could better be used processing information. Ultimately, he tells us, "we will need to port our mental processes to a more suitable computational substrate. Then our minds won't have to stay so small."[76] The computational substrate would appear to be a high-tech version of Plato's prison or tomb, limiting in this case not the soul's capacity for knowledge, but the mind's. For Kurzweil and others, the body is obsolete and will soon not be needed at all. Reading Kurzweil, one gets the feeling that

Plato is alive and well in the dualistic world of computer intelligence. However, whether we are reading the ancient Plato or the modern Kurzweil, we need to remind ourselves that, in spite of these thinkers' lofty ideas about the mind or soul, the body counts in the search for knowledge.

Notes

1. The comment actually comes from Whitehead: "The safest general character-ization of the European philosophical tradition is that it consists of a series of footnotes to Plato." Alfred North Whitehead, *Process and Reality* (New York: The Free Press, 1969), 53.

2. According to Crombie, the Academy was "a community of scholars, young and old, in which instruction was given to the young and in which the older pursued their own studies.... It seems in fact to have been a centre of intellectual activity both theoretical and practical." I. M. Crombie, *Plato: The Midwife's Apprentice* (London: Routledge & Kegan Paul, 1964), 1.

3. It should be pointed out that there are also scholarly debates concerning the grouping of Plato's dialogues into early, middle and later periods.

4. Of the thirty-five dialogues that Plato wrote, those of greatest relevance for my narrative are the *Phaedo, Timaeus, Symposium* and *Phaedrus*. These will be discussed throughout this chapter.

5. F. M. Cornford, *The Republic of Plato* (New York and Oxford: Oxford University Press), VI, 507, 217–218.

6. Richard Tarnas, *The Passion of the Western Mind* (New York: Random House, 1991), 41. If the notion of real essences of things is foreign to the modern mind and thus very difficult to grasp, we should nonetheless realize that for some modern mathematicians numbers are real, in the Platonic sense of the Forms. This is known as conceptual, or mathematical, realism (sometimes referred to as mathematical Platonism) and one of its adherents was the twentieth century's mathematical genius, Kurt Gödel. In writing about Gödel's belief in mathematical realism, Rebecca Goldstein writes, "For Gödel mathematics is a means of unveiling the features of objective mathematical reality, just as for Einstein physics is a means of unveiling aspects of objective physical reality." Referring to Einstein's belief in an objective world 'out yonder,' Goldstein remarks that, for Gödel, 'out yonder' "is out beyond physical space-time; it is a reality of pure abstraction, of universal and necessary truths, and our faculty of *a priori* reasoning provides us—mysteriously—with the means of accessing this ultimate 'out yonder,' of gaining at least partial glimpses of what might be called ... '*extreme*

reality.'" Rebecca Goldstein, *Incompleteness: The Proof and Paradox of Kurt Gödel* (New York: W. W. Norton & Company, 2005), 45.

7. Plato, *Phaedo*, 66e, in *Plato: Five Dialogues*, trans. G. M. A. Grube (Indianapolis: Hackett Publishing, 1981). All quotations from the *Phaedo* are from this edition, unless otherwise indicated.

8. *Phaedo*, 64a.

9. *Phaedo*, 67a.

10. *Phaedo*, 65d–66a. Note: the *Phaedo* is seen as one of the dialogues where what the character Socrates says often goes beyond the teachings of the historical Socrates to reflect the views of Plato himself, particularly in relation to the theory of Forms.

11. *Phaedo*, 75d. The theory of Recollection is Plato's answer to what later became the question of innate ideas in the debate between the rationalists and the empiricists. The empiricist holds that the mind is a blank slate and that all knowledge comes from experience. The rationalist holds that the mind already has some form of knowledge that is awakened or made evident by experience and that without this prior, innate knowledge, what we receive from the senses would not make sense. A child could not grasp that two objects are the same size, or a different colour, unless he already had an idea of 'same' and 'different.' The debate on innate ideas is not closed, but has taken a different form in our time with theories of evolutionary intelligence. Some now refer to our brains as being 'hardwired,' for example, in relation to language structure. Plato's clearest description of the theory of Recollection occurs in the *Meno*, when Socrates explains the Pythagorean theorem to a slave boy in order to show that the uneducated boy already had this mathematical knowledge within him and that Socrates only served to bring it out.

12. F. M. Cornford, *Plato's Cosmology: The Timaeus of Plato* (London: Routledge & Kegan Paul, 1956), 3. All quotations from the *Timaeus* are from this edition, unless otherwise indicated.

13. *Timaeus*, 30b.

14. Cornford, 37. This represents an important difference from the Christian view and avoids the difficulty that Christians have always had in explaining how an omnipotent and benevolent God could allow for evil in the world.

15. *Phaedo*, 100d. This is in stark contrast to what we will see in Descartes and the mechanists of the seventeenth century, who worked very hard to rid explanations of the physical world of teleology or final causes.

16. *Timaeus*, 34b.

17. For an explanation of the circles of Being, Same and Difference (Other), see G. M. Grube, *Plato's Thought* (Indianapolis: Hackett Publishing, 1980), 142, and Cornford, 72ff. Cornford also explains their relation to the planetary circles.

18.   Cornford, 66.

19.   Cornford disagrees with this interpretation, stating that there is nothing in the *Timaeus* referring to the music of the heavens. In his view, the harmony referred to resides in the structure of the soul and not in any audible music. For a complete analysis of the division of the world-soul into harmonic intervals, see Cornford, 66–72.

20.   *Timaeus*, 41d. (Emphasis added). The lesser degree of purity of the human soul accounts for the fact that humans do not match the perfection of the cosmos and are thus subject to error.

21.   *Timaeus*, 41e. The notion that every first incarnation is in the male (as opposed to female) form creates problems that suggest, as Cornford emphasizes, that the myth should not be taken literally. After the first incarnation, a soul wanders until it is again imprisoned in a body, one that resembles the kind of character it was in its previous life. "Those, for example, who have carelessly practiced gluttony, violence and drunkenness are likely to join a company of donkeys or of similar animals." So says Socrates in *Phaedo*, 81e.

22.   Cornford, 147.

23.   *Timaeus*, 43a.

24.   *Timaeus*, 43a.

25.   Grube, *Plato's Thought*, 216.

26.   See R. Hackforth, *Plato's Phaedo* (Cambridge University Press, 1972), 4.

27.   *Phaedo*, 115c.

28.   *Phaedo*, 66b, 66c. In fact, Phaedo reports at the beginning of the dialogue: "Although I was witnessing the death of one who was my friend, I had no feeling of pity, for the man appeared happy both in manner and words as he died nobly and without fear" (58e).

29.   Being invisible does not necessarily mean being immaterial, but Plato does not appear to distinguish the two in the *Phaedo*. See Raymond Martin and John Barresi, *The Rise and Fall of Soul and Self* (New York: Columbia University Press, 2006), 16, on this point.

30.   *Phaedo*, 79c. The idea that the senses deceive us is a persistent one in philosophy and one that Descartes will reiterate strongly in his *Meditations*. It represents a perennial problem for philosophers to distinguish between the world *as it appears to us* and the world *as it really is*.

31.   *Phaedo*, 82e.

32.   *Phaedo*, 83d.

33.   *Phaedo*, 83b.

34.   *Phaedo*, 66b.

35.   *Phaedo*, 94d.

36. Richard Shusterman, *Body Consciousness: A Philosophy of Mindfulness and Somaesthetics* (Cambridge and New York: Cambridge University Press, 2008), 16.

37. *Timaeus*, 69c.

38. *Timaeus*, 69c–d.

39. *Timaeus*, 69e.

40. *Timaeus*, 70e. Monique Labrune points out that, in the *Timaeus*, "le corps se modèle sur les âmes, comme un vêtement s'ajuste au corps qu'il épouse." "États d'âme: Le corps dans la philosophie de Platon," in Jean-Christophe Goddard and Monique Labrune, *Le Corps* (Paris: Vrin, 1992), 34.

41. *Timaeus*, 87d-e.

42. *Timaeus*, 88c.

43. *Timaeus*, 87a.

44. *Timaeus*, 86e.

45. *Phaedrus*, 246a, in Walter Hamilton (ed.), *Plato: Phaedrus & Letters VII and VIII* (New York: Penguin, 1973). All translations from the *Phaedrus* are from this edition, unless otherwise indicated.

46. *Phaedrus*, 247c.

47. *Phaedrus*, 246e.

48. *Phaedrus*, 248b.

49. *Phaedrus*, 248a.

50. *Phaedrus*, 249c.

51. Grube, *Plato's Thought*, 133.

52. *Phaedrus*, 248a.

53. This dialogue is also called the *Dinner-party*, and in French is known as *Le banquet*. The symposium in Greco-Roman society was a banquet, "although it tended to emphasize the latter part of the banquet, the drinking party during which the entertainment of the evening would be presented." In the case of the philosophical banquet, the entertainment was "uplifting conversation on an appropriate subject in which everyone could participate." Dennis E. Smith, *From Symposium to Eucharist: The Banquet in the Early Christian World* (Minneapolis: Fortress Press, 2003), 49–50.

54. Walter Hamilton, ed. and trans., *Plato: The Symposium* (New York: Penguin, 1951), 14.

55. *Symposium*, 201d.

56. Hamilton, *Plato: The Symposium*, 16.

57. *Symposium*, 190b.

58. *Symposium*, 191a.

59. *Symposium*, 191c.

60. *Symposium*, 192d.

61. Susan Hawthorne, "Diotima Speaks Through the Body," in *Engendering Origins: Critical Feminist Readings in Plato and Aristotle*, ed. Bat-Ami Bar On (New York: suny Press, 1994), 83.

62. *Symposium*, 202b. Since Love is being described as a god, it is personified as 'he' (not 'it') and the word is capitalized as in a proper name, although the translation by Hamilton is not consistent in this regard.

63. *Symposium*, 206a.

64. Hawthorne, 85.

65. Hawthorne, 93, note 11.

66. *Symposium*, 209a.

67. *Symposium*, 207a.

68. Hawthorne, 86.

69. *Symposium*, 210b.

70. *Symposium*, 210b.

71. *Symposium*, 210e–211a.

72. *Symposium*, 211c.

73. Hawthorne, 90.

74. That being said, it is still through the love of the body of a man (or boy) by a man that the ascent to the Forms happens.

75. The reduction of soul to mind, accomplished so effectively by Descartes' mechanistic framework of mind and body, will be dealt with in detail later in the book. However, it is useful to point out, here, that dropping explanatory frameworks (such as world-soul or teleology) because they are complex or cumbersome may have the advantage of simplifying explanation, but at the same time the disadvantage of leaving much unexplained. One risks throwing the baby out with the bathwater.

76. Ray Kurzweil, "The Evolution of Mind in the Twenty-first Century," in Jay Richards (ed.), *Are We Spiritual Machines? Ray Kurzweil vs. The Critics of Strong A.I.* (Seattle: Discovery Institute, 2002), 29.

CHAPTER II

Body and Nature:
Aristotle and the Stoics

Naturalizing the Forms: Aristotle

Aristotle (who lived from 384 to 322 BCE) is one of the giants of the history of philosophy. At the same time, he is a philosophical figure who does not fit readily into my narrative of the body. Unlike Plato, he does not fit the dualist stream, since he does not accept that the mind and body are separate entities, and he is indifferent to the question of the immortality of the soul, something that was of primordial interest to Plato. On the other hand, he does not fit neatly into the monist stream, as do the Stoics, whom we will meet next, as he does not admit, and is in fact scornful of, the possibility of a material soul. In the end, he is less interested in questions relating to mind and body than in questions relating to living vs. non-living things. The human body as such, along with what we would now call human consciousness, were not among his philosophical concerns. Further, as much as Plato focused on that which is unchanging as the important work of the philosopher (confining the ever-changing to the world of appearances), Aristotle focused precisely on explaining change, something he believed to be the hallmark of all living things, as well as the proper object of a science of nature.

Several factors render the task of writing succinctly about Aristotle very challenging. First, he wrote on a wide variety of topics (logic, ethics, metaphysics, rhetoric, politics and physics, as well as biology, botany, zoology, astronomy and more). As Jonathan Barnes tells us, "Choose a field of research, and Aristotle laboured in it; pick an area of human endeavour, and Aristotle discoursed upon it. His range is astonishing."[1] Yet less than a quarter of his writings have survived, and, of those that have, it cannot be said that they are systematic. In fact, it is generally agreed that the treatises we do have were lecture notes rather than polished texts written for wide circulation.[2] As a result, there are widely diverging interpretations among specialists about Aristotle's position on matters that are of considerable philosophical importance to a discussion of the body (for example, regarding whether his theory of perception is materialist or dualist, or whether or not the soul is immortal). In sum, it is not easy to find a complete and coherent account of the human body in Aristotle's sizeable volume of work.

On the other hand, a philosophical history of the body minus Aristotle would be incomplete. So much of what came after him was a reaction to, or a modification of, his notions of the soul, which played a role in successive notions about the body—in Christianity, the Renaissance and Descartes, in particular—that not to bring him into my narrative would be a serious omission. In what follows, I will be concentrating on those aspects of Aristotle's work that relate most clearly to my themes about the body, in particular those that diverge from or contradict the teachings of Plato, and those that later philosophers felt obliged to reject in their quest for a new philosophical and scientific paradigm.[3]

One of the most relevant facts of Aristotle's life, from the point of view of this narrative, is that he was a student of Plato. He went to study at the Academy in Athens at the age of eighteen, and remained there for close to twenty years, until the death of his master. He returned to Athens a dozen years later (after having, among other things, served as a tutor to Alexander the Great when the latter was a young teenager) and set up his own school, the Lyceum, where he conducted empirical research and taught both his own selected students and members of the general public.[4] Most of his works were written during this period in Athens. When Alexander died, Aristotle left Athens, fearing that the Athenians might commit a second crime against philosophy (an allusion to the their condemnation of Socrates in 399).[5] He died of natural causes in 322.

Aristotle and Plato

Richard Tarnas puts the relationship between the philosophies of these two ancient masters succinctly: "With Aristotle, Plato was, as it were, brought down to earth."[6] We have seen that, for Plato, the empirical world is the world of appearances, while the real world is the transcendent world of Forms. Aristotle, the empiricist, could not accept Plato's description of the everyday world as fundamentally unreal. On the contrary, for him, it was the empirical world that is real. There is no transcendent world of Forms; individual, particular things have ontological priority over universals. Where, for Plato, there is an ideal form of a dog—of which a particular Fido is an imperfect occurrence—for Aristotle, it is the individual, unique Fido that is real, and the idea of 'dog' only comes about through abstraction from many particular instances (knowing a Fido and a Lassie and a Pug allows us to arrive at the idea of 'dog'). For Plato, the form of red exists, even if there are no (nor have ever been any) red objects; for Aristotle, if there are no red objects, then there is no idea of red. "Aristotle turned Plato's ontology upside-down," says Tarnas. "For Plato, the particular was less real, a derivative of the universal; for Aristotle, the universal was less real, a derivative of the particular."[7] Aristotle does not deny the utility of universals for comprehending the world; he simply denies them real existence. This is a major and fundamental difference between the master and his pupil.

Form and Matter

Aristotle does not do away with the notion of form, but he brings it down to earth; in effect, he naturalizes form by making it an intrinsic part of nature. Like Plato, Aristotle conceives the cosmos as ordered—but there is a difference. For Plato, as shown in the *Timaeus*, the order of the world is *extrinsic*—it comes from outside the world; it is imposed on nature (out of chaos) by the demiurge. For Aristotle, on the other hand, the order of the world is *intrinsic*—it comes from nature itself. It is a first principle of Aristotle's philosophy that "nature is everywhere a cause of order."[8] Nature itself provides the order and intelligibility of the world, and everything in nature is always moving toward the order and perfection of the whole. This order, perfection and intelligibility can also be referred to as form. For Plato, form is imposed on the material world; for Aristotle, it is part of the material world. As explained by Helen Lang, for Plato, "the foundation of the physical world, the receptacle, has no formal character of its own but is something underlying that is able to receive temporarily whatever form is imposed on it."[9] Aristotle rejects this portrayal of form and matter, although, like Plato, he insists on the primacy of form.

For Aristotle, form is "that toward which a thing tends or grows."[10] In other words, every living thing in nature is moving toward the actualization of the form that it is meant to have or to be; it is moving or growing toward becoming what it is (an acorn toward an oak tree, a puppy toward a dog, a baby toward an adult human). In fact, this movement is a kind of impulse: "matter runs after form, it desires and yearns for form … in natural things, matter is never neutral to form, and form never needs to impress itself or be impressed (by another) upon matter."[11] Form moves matter to become what it is, toward its own being. In Aristotelian language, it moves matter from potentiality to actuality: "Matter is potential and is moved by form because it is actively oriented toward its proper form."[12]

This impulse to move from potentiality to actuality pertains only to living things, or, to use Aristotle's language, things that are *by nature*. It does not pertain to man-made things, which have their form imposed from without. There is no innate impulse in bronze to become a statue, and it needs an artist to move it from its potential as a statue to its actualization as a statue. But there is an innate impulse in a seed to become a rose, and it will become a rose unless something interferes with the natural actualization of its potential. Aristotle identifies this actualization of potential with movement; in fact, "an account of motion is nothing other than an account of the relation between what is potential and what is actual."[13] Aristotle's account of potentiality and actuality serves to counteract the Platonic view that the empirical world, because it is always in a state of becoming, is an unreal world of appearances. In effect, Aristotle "gave to the process of becoming its own reality…. Change and movement are not signs of a shadowing unreality but are expressive of a teleological striving for fulfillment."[14]

Form as Soul
This description of form and matter, whereby form is intrinsic to living things and provides the impetus for their striving to become what they are, explains the relationship between body and soul. For Aristotle, soul is form and body is matter. Soul is what moves the body from potentiality to actuality, and, as such, it is the primary principle of life. It is important to underline, however, that form (soul) is not separate from the matter (body) that 'desires' it. For Aristotle, a living individual (plant, animal, human) is a substance, and, as such, is composed of both form and matter.[15] In relation to the human body, this means a substance composed of body and soul. As explained by Paolo Biondi,

"it must be kept in mind from the outset that soul and body form one entity and signify a unity of being bearing, nonetheless, a duality of principles."[16] We would not think of the form of a rose, inherent in the seed, as being a substance separate from the material of the seed that desires it. The form gives the seed the impulse and the capacity to grow into the plant that it is meant to be. Aristotle provides an interesting analogy when he tells us that, "if the eye was an animal, then sight would be its soul … when sight leaves it it is no longer an eye except homonymously, in the way of a stone or painted eye."[17] Similarly, the soul provides the impulse and the capacity for the human being to grow to its potential; the ensouled body "possesses the capacity to live and perform vital functions, and the performance of any one of these vital functions would be its actuality as exercising the vital capacity."[18] Since, as we will see below, humans (and only humans) possess a rational soul, the movement from potentiality to actuality includes the functions and capacities of a rational mind.

But it is not only humans that have souls. At the beginning of *De Anima*, Aristotle tells us that knowledge of the soul is "held to make a great contribution to the complete understanding of the truth and especially towards that of nature. For the soul is, so to speak the first principle of living things."[19] Given that the soul is the first principle of living things, it follows that there must be an account of soul for *all* living things, not just humans—and this is what Aristotle gives us. Aristotle's cosmos is hierarchical, with a ladder of being from primitive matter to rational thought.[20] There are gradations of soul in living things, moving from plants, to animals, to humans. Plants have a nutritive or vegetative soul, which governs nutrition and reproduction; along with the nutritive soul, animals have a sensitive soul, which governs sensation, pleasure, pain, attraction and repulsion, as well as locomotion; humans possess the first two levels of soul, along with a rational soul, which governs the intellect. While the higher species possess the soul levels of the lower ones, these levels of soul are expressed differently, and also hierarchically, as we move up the ladder. For example, the nutritive capacity in plants is of a simpler nature than that of animals or humans, and while both animals and humans possess the capacity of perception, this faculty is generally superior in humans (although some animals will have a range of perception in one sense—e.g., colour perception in bees—that is superior to that particular sense in humans). Similarly, there is a hierarchy of complexity for the nutritive soul in relation, for example, to what kinds of food will nourish what bodies.

The potential for nourishment exists in all living things, but the actualization of that nourishment is a faculty of the nutritive capacity of different souls. The soul, at its different levels and in relation to different beings, is what allows the being to function, to grow and to actualize itself. As explained by Barnes:

> Aristotle's first general account of the soul amounts to this: for a thing to have a soul is for it to be a natural organic body actually capable of functioning. The second general account simply explains what those functions are. Thus Aristotle's souls are not *pieces* of living things; they are not bits of spiritual stuff placed inside the living body; rather, they are sets of powers, capacities or faculties. Possessing a soul is like possessing a skill. A skilled man's skill is not some part of him, responsible for his skilled acts; similarly a living creature's animator or life-force is not some part of it, responsible for its living activities.[21]

Thus, the soul of a human being is the set of powers, capacities or faculties that allow the human being to become the perfect, rational creature that he or she is capable of being. It is the form of the body toward which the latter is actively oriented; it represents the actuality toward which the potentiality of the body is moving. As already pointed out, body and soul are one entity; thus, there is no question of body and soul in conflict. If we think back to Plato we remember that, in the *Timaeus*, the soul resists being dragged down into the body, and the body of the *Phaedo* acts as a prison of the soul. But for Aristotle, the potency of the body desires and is impelled toward the form of the soul immediately and intrinsically, just as the seed desires and is impelled toward the form of the rose. The soul is not something placed inside the body; it is the set of capacities and skills that impel it into actuality.[22]

An important point about body and soul in Aristotle is that the body is not an impediment to knowledge as it is in Plato. For Plato, the soul, having been dragged down into the body, needs to escape the body in order to have true knowledge of the Forms. The senses, being bodily, get in the way of knowledge and lead the soul astray. Not so for Aristotle. Body and soul are both integral to our perception of the world. Knowledge of the world, for all beings with a sensitive soul, begins with the senses. Through the senses, the body actually takes on the form of the sensed objects. The eye, for example, is not a mechanical device through which the soul perceives the world. Like the rest of the body, the eye is both form and matter, its form being its capacity for seeing. Thus sensation is a matter of body and soul by definition. As expressed by R. D. Hicks,

> Sensitivity in the abstract is a form which knows or apprehends sensible forms. Similarly intellect is a form which knows or apprehends intelligible forms. Moreover, in both sensation and intellection alike at the moment of apprehension, there is identity between the form which apprehends and the form which is apprehended.... Sensation cannot dispense with a bodily organ, a part of the body appropriated to its special function.[23]

Strange as this might seem to modern sensibilities, it means that for cognition to take place, the mind in some way actually takes on the form of the object of perception, "even though in the world that form never exists apart from its particular material embodiment."[24] This is less strange if we think in terms of movement, and of the eye, for example, having its potential for seeing stimulated by movement from the form of the sensed object.[25] In the process of sensation, the eye moves from a state of potentiality to one of actuality in relation to the form of the sensed object. Further, sensation cannot be reduced to a purely mechanical physical process (as Descartes will maintain many centuries later). And, although Aristotle calls on the rational soul to explain true cognition and scientific knowledge, he does not denigrate the body or the knowledge that comes first from the senses. Rather, he contends, "that knowledge of the natural world derives first from perception of concrete particulars in which regular patterns can be recognized and general principles formulated."[26]

Aristotle's theory of perception is too briefly summarized here, but a detailed exposition goes beyond the scope of this chapter. What is important is that, unlike Plato before him and Descartes after him, Aristotle does not denigrate the body or the senses. Because concrete particulars are ontologically prior to pure intellectual knowledge of the forms (as in Plato), Aristotle can maintain that our knowledge of the world comes first and foremost from perception. As with his conception of form and matter in general, in relation to cognition, "Aristotle realigned Plato's archetypal perspective from a transcendent force to an immanent one."[27]

Teleology

We have seen that, as potential, matter is actively oriented toward its actual-ization by form. Everything in nature strives toward completion. This is Aristotle's teleology of nature: "form acts as an object of desire—indeed form is a final cause when it acts as a principle of motion—and matter immediately desires form as its nature and definition."[28] But the final cause, here, is immanent in nature and not transcendent, as in Plato. As Aristotle naturalized the Forms, he also naturalized teleology. The end, or completion, toward which every living thing is moving, is not external to nature. It is not a transcendent God or a demiurge that has caused the movement and direction of the world. But in rejecting the design of the demiurge, Aristotle does not fall back on mechanical necessity to explain the order of the world. The directedness toward a goal in nature is non-intentional and unconscious. Natural processes are directed toward a goal, but that goal has not been determined by an external god or creator. The direction comes from within nature itself. This serves to explain the regular occurrence of physical events, since "no description of the physical world that concentrates solely on material and efficient principles can account for the order and repeatability of natural physical processes."[29] It also serves to explain the relation of part to whole in the structure of animals (and humans), since "animals have the parts they have in order to be able to perform the functions for which they are designed."[30] The important point, here, is that the whole is prior to the part in the sense, as Aristotle points out, that a house does not come to be for the sake of the bricks and stones, but the bricks and stones for the sake of the house. Parts are adapted to the whole and not the other way around, and nature is everywhere a cause of order.

It will be important to remember the non-intentional nature of Aristotle's teleology later on in my story of the body, when we see the notion of final causes rejected in seventeenth-century science, at least partly in order to keep religious notions (e.g., God's plan for the world) out of scientific explanations. Aristotle's teleology does not depend on God's plan. Structure (and thus the goal) is built into nature and into every living creature. It should be noted, however, that medieval Christian thinkers altered Aristotle's non-intentional teleology so that it would conform to the Christian belief in creation by a transcendent God. As a result, Aristotle's natural teleology was transformed, becoming imbued with notions of divine purpose and design—a view that would later be rejected by Descartes and ultimately ridiculed by modern science.

The Four Causes

A final aspect of Aristotle's philosophy that will reverberate into the seventeenth century is his doctrine of the four causes. We have seen that, for Aristotle, movement is fundamental to his concept of matter and form; it is the inner dynamism of form that moves any being from potentiality to actuality. Movement is change, for Aristotle, and change comes about through four different types of causality: material, formal, efficient and final. Since any substance is made up of matter and form, the material cause is invoked to explain matter: the material cause of a bronze statue is the bronze; the material cause of an animal is the material of the body—organs, bones, etc. The formal cause is what gives the entity its form (the shape of the statue, the soul of the human being). The efficient cause is what initiates motion or change from outside (the artisan of the statue, the parents of the child). The final cause is the goal or direction of a living being (the seed's change into a rose, the child's flourishing into an adult), or the purpose of a man-made entity (the statue as a beautiful art object, the house as a place to live). In living beings, because of the teleological nature of the forms, the formal and final causes are intricately related, and all causes work together. In effect, the four causes "are four ways of answering different but equally crucial questions about why things are how they are. If we cannot answer these questions, Aristotle holds, we cannot really know the objects of which we speak."[31]

The move to mechanism in the seventeenth century will reduce Aristotle's notion of the fourfold cause to one, the efficient cause. This will be examined in Chapter 5. For the moment, what is important is the idea of dynamism that is integral to Aristotle's notion of cause, which serves to explain the activity of form as an internal organizing principle, and which is a broader notion of cause (with more complex explanatory value) than our own.

The Aristotelian Body

It can be seen that the body of Aristotle is not the body of Plato. It is not a container housing an immortal soul. Soul is an integral part of body and cannot be separated from it.[32] Explanations about mind or soul cannot ignore the body, and explanations of body cannot ignore the soul. In addition to this, and perhaps flowing from it, there is no undervaluing of the body in Aristotle.

The body is not a prison, holding a reluctant soul as prisoner, and bodily senses are not denigrated as leading the soul astray. The body is not an impediment to knowledge, as all knowledge begins with the body and the senses.

While Aristotle does emphasize that humans are rational animals and that the actualization of human potential means the correct use of reason, he does not suggest that the soul must forget the body in order to reason properly, or that it is the philosopher who has privileged access to true knowledge. He extols contemplation as one of the intellectual virtues, but he also emphasizes both practical wisdom and skill, the latter referring to how we make or bring things into being (e.g. making a coat). Practical wisdom entails knowing what is good or bad for us and how to apply such knowledge in the real world. Thus, the intellectual virtues entail knowledge of the body and skill in using both body and mind.

Like Plato, Aristotle has a notion of a hierarchical continuum between plants, animals and humans, and holds that all living things are ensouled. He goes further than Plato, however, in describing the different kinds of soul, and how the higher levels of soul maintain and enhance the capacities and powers attributed to the lower levels, an idea that will be pursued by the Stoics. Unlike Plato, he does not posit a world-soul to connect the heavenly and the earthly realms of being. However, given that there is no transcendent artificer or demiurge, this connection would be rendered redundant. His teleology allows for a relation of parts and wholes, and of an interconnectedness of nature without the need for a world-soul. And, since the body is not a temporary container for an immortal soul, there is no doctrine of reincarnation in Aristotle. This body and this soul are one and live one life together.

Living in Accordance with Nature: The Stoics

To speak of Stoicism is to speak of six centuries of philosophy. Zeno, the founder of Stoicism, was born when Aristotle was still alive, while Marcus Aurelius, whose death in 180 CE marked the end of the Stoic period, was born after the last of the Christian Gospels, the Gospel of John, was written. Thus, the Stoic philosophers do not fit seamlessly into the chronology of my narrative on the body; they span the period from the Greek philosophers we have already discussed through the development of Christian theology and philosophy, which will be discussed in the following chapter. Further, while the early Stoics like Zeno, Cleanthes and Chrysippus were Greeks, later Stoics like Seneca and Marcus Aurelius were Romans. The Hellenistic Age, as the Stoic period is also called, began with the death of Alexander the Great in the fourth century BCE and lasted until the second century CE and the rise of Christianity. During this time, the Greek city-states became part of the Roman Empire, which absorbed much of Greek philosophy and culture along with its territory.

The name 'Stoicism' comes from the 'Stoa Poikile,' or 'Painted Colonnade,' in the central square in Athens, where men met to listen to Zeno; his followers came to be known as the men from the *stoa* and, later, the Stoics. Not far away was a property belonging to Epicurus known as 'the Garden'; here, he set up his school. His philosophy became known as Epicureanism, and is usually presented in opposition to Stoicism. Both schools were very close to the Academy where Plato and his followers had taught, and where, a century before the Stoics, "the young Aristotle had himself sat at the feet of Plato."[33] Thus, the roots of Stoicism are firmly planted in the Greek tradition, but its branches reach into the world of the Romans and the early Christians.

Because it extends over such a long period and covers the ideas of many different philosophers, Stoicism cannot be described as a homogeneous philosophy. It can be seen, however, as a philosophy of nature in a general sense, and it can be called a system—one that covers physics, ethics and logic, presenting them as related aspects of the one reality. "In the course of its five-hundred-year history as an organized movement, some of its leaders devoted themselves mainly to understanding the macrocosm, and others emphasized the ethical, political, and religious life of man the microcosm. But all the Stoics believed that the *fundamental injunction laid on man is to follow the law of nature,* and in the development of Stoicism this injunction acquired a systematic meaning."[34]

This injunction to live in accordance with nature, which will be the guiding thread of our discussion of Stoic philosophy in relation to the body, represents the strongest possible diversion from the Platonic world of Forms, with its attendant idea that the natural world is inferior to the intelligible world. For the Stoics, knowledge, including knowledge of the body and the self, will begin and end principally with knowledge of nature. The Platonic unity of macrocosm and microcosm is still important, but, for the Stoics, this idea is expressed materially. Stoicism rejects the dualism of Plato; as will be explained, Stoicism is a monistic philosophy; everything is one, and it is material.

Like Plato, the early Stoics were influenced by Heraclitus. But while Plato was influenced by Heraclitus' belief in eternal change (which, as we have seen, led Plato to his theory of Forms), the Stoics were more influenced by his notion of reason as creative fire (*pneuma*) and by his idea of the subordination of the individual to the law of nature (*logos*).[35] During its middle period, the centre of Stoic philosophy moved from Athens to Rome and Stoicism became more eclectic, although the emphasis continued to be on universal harmony or living in accordance with nature. The late period of Stoicism, which flourished in Rome in the first and second centuries CE, took on a moralizing tone with its emphasis on ethics, and, although it was not a religion, came to be seen as a rival to the Christian religion.

A challenge to any account of Stoic philosophy is the paucity of original works available to the modern reader. We have only fragments of the writings of the early Stoics, and many of their ideas are set out in the works of other writers. Cicero, for example, wrote about the Stoics, but is not considered to have been one himself. Other information about the Stoics comes from later writers who actually opposed Stoic philosophy (e.g., Plutarch and Sextus Empiricus). In spite of the fact that early Stoics like Zeno, Cleanthes and Chrysippus are known to have written volumes, we are left only fragments of their writings, or interpretations by later writers, some of whom may have been hostile to their beliefs. We do have original texts of Seneca and Marcus Aurelius (two Roman Stoics) and of Epictetus (a Greek slave who spent his youth in Rome), authors who are often taken as the representatives of Stoicism, but their works tend to focus only on the ethical life—something that contributed to the perception of Stoicism as a predominantly moral philosophy. Stoicism was very influential in the development of Christian thought, as it "provided a great deal of material to those members of the Christian church who wished to build up an intellectual structure on their faith. They might absorb it, alter it, or refute it; but in any case they were in part moulded by it."[36]

In looking at the body from a Stoic point of view, we will examine some of the Stoics' principal notions, including monism, *pneuma*, fate and living in accordance with nature, all of which contribute to a theory of the body as a source of knowledge of the self and the world. Before moving on to those aspects of Stoicism that are of central interest to our narrative of the body, however, it is important to deal with certain aspects of Stoic ethics that I believe are often misunderstood, particularly as it is generally seen in opposition to Epicureanism. While happiness for the Epicurean is perceived (since the Renaissance at least) as rooted in pleasures of the body (as witnessed by the modern connotation of the word 'epicurean'), the Stoic is perceived as shunning bodily pleasures and worldly goods and finding happiness in enduring suffering—the more suffering, the better. Neither interpretation is correct, although it must be acknowledged that certain writings of the Stoics (for example, Epictetus and his slogans such as "bear and forbear" or "sustain and abstain") have contributed to the misinterpretation.[37] In reality, however, the Stoic position is more nuanced than this; comfort, pleasure, wealth—all things usually seen as indicative of worldly success—are acceptable to the Stoic (and even to be preferred to their opposites). What is not acceptable is that one should see his or her happiness depending upon such things. For the Stoic, "virtue and vice are the sole constituents of happiness and unhappiness. These states do not in the least depend, they insisted, on the possession or absence of things conventionally regarded as good or bad—health, reputation, wealth, etc."[38] One can be virtuous, and thus happy, without any of these things; there is nothing intrinsic to these things that will bring either virtue or happiness. The Stoics believed that anything that can be used either well or badly cannot be called good in itself. "But wealth and health can be used well and badly. Therefore wealth and health are not something good."[39] These things the Stoics labelled 'indifferents' in the sense that they are 'indifferent to happiness'; one can be happy (or virtuous) with or without them. This does not mean that one should not prefer health over illness, or even wealth over poverty; it does mean, however, that, even if a person is ill or poor, he or she can still be happy and virtuous. Detachment is the watchword of the Stoic.[40] If I have comfort today, along with fine clothing and good food and wine, there is nothing wrong with this, provided that I am happy; but if tomorrow I lose it all, I must still be of such character that I can remain happy in spite of what I have lost. My happiness is *indifferent* to the achievement of these fleeting things. Epictetus would say that I must accept what cannot be changed, keep my will "in harmony with what happens" and "accept all things contentedly."[41]

Stoic Monism

As pointed out above, Stoicism is a system that sees everything as one: logic, physics and ethics are all interconnected and interdependent. This seems very strange to the modern mind, which sees three distinct disciplines and which rejects any suggestion of the normative (ethics) in science (physics). It will be easier to understand if we think back to Plato's idea of the cosmos as an intelligent, living whole directed toward the Good. In this context, the Stoic concept of unity is more comprehensible.[42]

> Some Stoics compared their logic to the wall, their physics to the tree, and their ethics to the fruit of a fertile field.... Stoic logic protects the physics and ethics of Stoicism, laying down rules for the validation of truth claims. Physics, protected by these rules, displays the structure of the cosmos. And ethics, the practice for which the field was cultivated, shows men how to imitate and participate in that structure.[43]

The Stoic notion of physics is much broader than our own and includes what we would call metaphysics, and even what is now studied as psychology. In other words, it does not restrict itself to the physical world that can be seen and/or experimented on, but includes principles that explain the entire universe and its causes, including human life and human knowledge. As Diogenes Laertius explains,

> They [the Stoics] use 'world' [*kosmos*] in three ways: of god himself, the peculiarly qualified individual consisting of all substance, who is indestructible and ingenerable, since he is the manufacturer of the world-order, at set periods of time consuming all substance into himself and reproducing it again from himself; they also describe the world-order as 'world'; and thirdly, what is composed out of both [i.e. god and world-order].[44]

Everything in the world is both God and matter, something that differs from Plato's account in the *Timaeus*, in that both principles are material, and the divine, or active, principle is *immanent* in matter. Plato's god is transcendent; the cosmos is a whole, but it moves (or is drawn) in the direction of Reason and the Good, which are not of the material world. The Stoic cosmos is teleological, like Plato's, but the teleology is, like Aristotle's, immanent and not transcendent. For the Stoics, everything is material. It is a fundamental principle of Stoic physics that only bodies are capable of acting or of being acted upon, and thus, "god and matter must each be corporeal since they are most basically what can act or be acted upon respectively."[45] For the Stoics, it is inconceivable that an immaterial god could act on a material world. An important ramification of these principles is that the soul also is material.

Like Plato's cosmos, the Stoic cosmos is a living, intelligent, ensouled and divine being. In other words, God and cosmos are one, and the divine principle is omnipresent in nature, which is self-generating and self-directing. God is not a detached craftsman, like the platonic demiurge, but a 'designing fire,' acting rationally *in* the world. Nor does the world develop independently of God; the history of creator and creation are identical.[46] Thus, the world is divine and functions according to divine laws, or providence, which are immanent in nature; God and nature are unfolding as one; all change and movement in the universe is rational and determined. Everything that happens in the universe is an expression of the divine order and intelligence. Fate is an ever-present reality in the Stoic universe.

Pneuma and Fate

The notion of God as a designing fire is central to the Stoic conception of the living universe and its unfolding. "Designing fire, which must be distinguished from the fire of ordinary experience, is the necessary consequence of god's constant conjunction with matter. He acts *in the form* of fire, but fire on its own is not sufficient to explain the nature of his activity."[47] This designing fire is the vital principle of all living things, and, as the world's active—or seminal—principle, accounts for the immanence or self-directedness of the world's activity as an intelligent whole. This vital principle is also identified with air in the form of breath (a combination of fire and air), also generally known as *pneuma*.[48] *Pneuma* is a multi-purpose concept for the Stoics, having broad explanatory value and serving as the all-important cosmic connector— providing an explanation not only of how the world holds together or coheres, but how its parts are interconnected and act upon one another. For the Stoics, *pneuma* permeates all matter, in varying degrees, thus accounting for the world as a dynamic continuum. "The *pneuma* explains the cohesion of the particles in a rock, and, at a more complex level, the growth of a plant, the behaviour of an animal, and the rational action of a human being; soul and reason are simply particular manifestations of *pneuma*."[49]

Fire and air are only two of the four elements that make up the Stoic universe, the other two being earth and water. *Pneuma* works to create the dynamic continuum referred to above by blending with the other elements in different proportions, creating different levels of tension, elasticity and movement in things. This explains why different things have different qualities.

> The Stoic conception of 'through-and-through blending' sets no limit to the relative quantities of its constituents; so we may reasonably conjecture that the proportions of air to fire in 'breath' vary in relation to the different qualifications they generate in matter; and matter itself, as constituted by earth and water, must be regarded as a further variable.[50]

In living things, this blending gives rise to soul; at the level of the macrocosm, it accounts for the world-soul. At a more specific level, the degrees of tension (or vibration) of the breath—it is the air aspect of *pneuma* that accounts for the variations in tension or tensional movement of objects and beings—will account for the differences between, for example, animals and plants, or plants and stones. This tension also accounts for differences in human souls: "As breath, the soul is characterized by its tensile motion, a physical property with important bearing on a person's moral condition."[51] Tension also accounts for the death of an organism; when the tension of the *pneuma* slackens, the blending of air and fire ceases and the organism begins to disintegrate.

This unity of God, world and *pneuma* means that everything is interconnected and, ultimately, determined. Every thing is part of the living whole; every soul is part of the world-soul, the designing fire. "Chrysippus says that fate is a certain natural everlasting ordering of the whole: one set of things follows on and succeeds another, and the interconnexion [*sic*] is inviolable."[52] And it is the tension or vibration in the *pneuma* that, "is the basis for the interesting Stoic theory of 'sympathy' or 'fellow-feeling' of the different parts of the universe, earthly and heavenly, for one another."[53] We must not think of causality in the mechanistic sense, which requires some form of contact for one thing or event to be the cause of another. The notion of sympathy or vibration plays this role in Stoic monism and allows for the interconnectedness of all things, as well as for the interaction between microcosm and macrocosm that is evident, for example, in astrology.

The 'designing fire' is also described in Stoicism as a 'seminal principle,' a phrase whose meaning is not immediately obvious to the modern reader, who might want to apply a sexual connotation to the phrase. And so he should (although many commentators on Stoic *pneuma* avoid its sexual origins). John Rist explains how *pneuma* is the instrument of God's plan, which is captured in Stoic cosmic mythology:

> Zeus, remembering Aphrodite and *genesis*, softened himself and relaxed himself, and having quenched much of his light, changed into fiery air (i.e. *pneuma*) of gentler fire. Then having had intercourse with Hera … he ejected the entire seminal fluid of the universe....[54]

This explains the connection between *pneuma* and providence or fate; the design or plan is "the semen-like reason-principles of the universe,"[55] which is an emission of Zeus into the world. One could think of this in genetic terms as the encoding of the living cosmos; "the semen-like reason-principles convey, a little like genes, the encoded messages which are the decrees of God and Reason for the development of the universe."[56] Thus, *pneuma*, while sustaining the world, also determines its course. Everything that happens is an expression of the divine order and intelligence, or, in other words, the order and intelligence of the divine whole. This determinism occurs both at the cosmic level and at the level of the individual; the actions of every individual are determined by fate. This does not undermine moral responsibility, however, since fate and moral responsibility are considered to presuppose each other. This is a difficult concept to grasp for modern readers, since we do not tend to see free will and determinism as compatible. We tend to link personal responsibility (and therefore reward and punishment) to free will; the Stoics did not—or, more precisely, they had a different notion of free will.

Together, the notions discussed above—of *pneuma*, cosmic sympathy and fate—lead to one of the central themes of Stoic ethics, one that is fundamental to the Stoic view of the body: the notion of living in accordance with nature.

Living in Accordance with Nature

Because nature (or the cosmos) is an ordered, unified whole, the human being is part of that whole, body and soul. In other words, human nature is a part of the universal nature and functions according to the cosmic laws of nature. Thus, for the Stoics, the way to knowledge and to happiness for a human being is to live in accordance with nature. Nature, here, means more than the 'natural' world; it should be taken to mean our whole environment, the world that we live in. We can think of it more as "what pertains to us ... in virtue of our being citizens of the world."[57] Humans are capable of living in accordance with nature because they are capable of understanding their own natures, their own natural constitution, their own strengths and weaknesses. Since individual natures vary, what is in accordance with nature for each individual is different and must be learned over a lifetime. We do, however, have an understanding of our connection with nature and a natural impulse to move toward what is good for us. This is encapsulated in the Stoic notion of *oikeiosis*, a notion that can be translated as 'appropriation,' meaning "a recognition of affinity coupled with affection."[58] As explained by Cicero,

> [T]he Stoics believed that right from birth, a living creature feels an attachment for itself, and an impulse to preserve itself and to feel affection for its own constitution and for those things which tend to preserve that constitution; while on the other hand it conceives an antipathy to destruction and to those things which appear to threaten destruction.[59]

The concept embraces the idea of self-consciousness, as well as self-affection or attachment to self, which is prior to any impulse to desire or pleasure. As Cicero explained, "it would be impossible that [infants] should feel desire at all unless they possessed self-consciousness, and consequently felt affection for themselves. This leads to the conclusion that it is love of self which supplies the primary impulse to action."[60] Unlike the Epicureans, who saw pleasure as the first impulse, the Stoics held that any drive to pleasure is not primary but a by-product of self-affection—since much early behaviour of an animal or human (for example, learning to walk) may even entail pain or frustration. For the Stoics, at a very fundamental level, all animals, including humans, have knowledge of what is needed to preserve themselves, to grow and to develop. This is not a simple reference to instinct, but to a form of consciousness and assent, however obscure. As Seneca explains,

> [E]very one of us understands that there is something which stirs his impulses, but he does not know what it is. He knows that he has a sense of striving, although he does not know what it is or its source. Thus even children and animals have a consciousness of their primary element, but it is not very clearly outlined or portrayed.[61]

A. A. Long believes that the concept of *oikeiosis* was unique to the Stoics, and he writes of one second-century Stoic philosopher, Hierocles, who treated the notion in depth but whose work was not discovered until early in the twentieth century:

> In a continuous chain of argument, which occupies some three hundred lines of a Greek papyrus, Hierocles seeks to prove the following thesis: All animals from the moment of birth perceive themselves continuously. Hierocles' animals (which tacitly exclude fish and insects) include birds and reptiles as well as humans and other mammals. Self-perception, he argues, is both their primary and their most basic faculty.[62]

Hierocles' notion of self-perception is similar to what Cicero and Seneca describe, but it is important because it comes from a real Stoic text—his *Principles of Ethics*—which Long describes, and "the closest thing we have to an uncontaminated text-book or series of lectures on mainstream Stoicism by a Stoic philosopher."[63] This is important, given the problem of sources cited earlier. But it is also important because it links the concept to the foundations of Stoic ethics. This assumes a link between our bodily nature and our ethical life, which is, in effect, what living in accordance with nature is all about.

In using the term "self-perception," Hierocles does not imply any kind of introspection such as we would consider when we refer to our self, or to perceiving our self. There is no mind-body dualism here; the Stoics did not see the self as something on a different level from the body, as we are accustomed to think, given our modern (post-Cartesian) concept of self. For Hierocles, the 'self' refers to an animal's particular body parts and their functions: "the self that an animal perceives is the way its body is structured with a view to living its life as a bird or a bull etc."[64] Or a human, one should add.

Long sees an echo of the Stoic conception of *oikeiosis* in the modern idea of proprioception, which can be defined as "that continuous but unconscious sensory flow from the movable parts of our bodies (muscles, tendons, joints), by which their position and tone and motion are continually monitored and adjusted."[65] The two concepts are separated by close to two millennia, not to mention by philosophical, psychological and biological developments that make a direct comparison dangerous (e.g., Hierocles' self-perception does not seem to be limited to moveable parts and includes the ability to perceive powers in other animals), but both concepts attempt to explain animals' and humans' ability to function as well-organized wholes, and to adapt to their environments. Loss of this ability is now recognized as involving a loss of our "sense of self," a fact that suggests a notion of self which is physical rather than mental; in other words, one that is much closer to the Stoics than to the Cartesian disembodied consciousness that we will meet later in our narrative.

For the Stoics, *oikeiosis* is not limited to purely bodily phenomena or to physical explanation. In humans, the early accommodation to nature that is represented by *oikeiosis* is gradually supplanted by reason, as self-perception and concern for self-preservation are replaced by a focus on virtue and the soul. But this does not mean that adult humans, in their search for wisdom, neglect their bodily nature. Cicero's account of *oikeiosis* describes several stages in the development of reason, all of which are in harmony with the primary impulses of nature. We move through the original impulse of self-preservation, then through a stage of learning habits that allow us to retain those things that are in accordance with nature, and finally reach a point of choice fully rationalized and in harmony with nature. But the later stages build on the primary stage, and, in the words of Cicero, "as all 'appropriate acts' are based on the primary impulses of nature, it follows that Wisdom itself is based on them also."[66] Thus, wisdom is always grounded in this early bodily impulse. This can be so because, for the Stoics, nature is both rational and good—and the body is part of nature.[67]

Hierocles' account also refers to an expansion and development of *oikeiosis* as an animal matures, but how he might have explained this development in humans we will never know, as that part of his work has been lost. He does explain, however, the interaction of body and soul and describes the latter as a faculty of perception, which "is capable of responding perceptively to every condition of the animal's body."[68] Long believes that Hierocles likely thought, as Cicero reports, that *oikeiosis* in the animal is simply the embryonic form of a developed sense of self that is both bodily and rational. Humans have the ability to reflect on their nature and, in the Stoic context, "have to decide what their nature, as so constituted, requires."[69] Thus, we are able to choose to live according to nature or not; we are also capable of getting it wrong.

As discussed earlier, the universe, for the Stoics, is providentially ordered, governed by fate and perfectly harmonious. Everything happens as it should. A consequence of this is that, in coming to see the harmony of the universe, the rational human adult comes to see that he himself is part of the harmony. And to understand the cosmic harmony, we have to understand our own place in it; this is something we come to see by reflecting on our *own* nature. We have the choice to move with our nature (and our fate) or to be dragged along by it. Knowledge is, in the end, what will determine how we choose. This knowledge is, at least in part, bodily knowledge. Our bodily self-perception does not end with reason; it is enhanced by it. As expressed by Long, "there is something to think about in the proposal that the 'proprioceptive' capacities, which enable other animals to monitor their lives, are what we, as humans, start from and can shape by reflection and training into ethical dispositions."[70]

The Stoic Body

At this point, there are a number of things we can conclude about the Stoic body, particularly as it compares to the dualistic model of Plato that we have already encountered. As can clearly be seen from the analysis of *oikeiosis* above, the body, far from being an obstacle to knowledge, is a *source* of knowledge. It is a source of knowledge about our own nature, but also about nature as a whole, since adaptation to the environment is an integral part of the self-perception or belonging that is experienced in the early stages of *oikeiosis*. The body is not a container for the soul; it is not a prison or a tomb; the body and soul are an integrated whole (more about this later). It is not necessary to escape the body in order to achieve wisdom and the ethical life, since knowledge of the body is the beginning of the shaping of an ethical life, as shown above. One's bodily needs and desires do not need to be kept in check constantly by a higher part of the divided soul. Good habits must, of course, be developed, but the idea that one is fighting one's baser nature is absent from the Stoic account; it's about shaping one's true nature more than controlling one's base tendencies. In fact, in the Stoic view, given the link between impulse and living in accordance with nature, natural desire is actually the basis of virtue, and evil comes about because of false judgments about what is good, or excessive attachment to fleeting and 'indifferent' things. Even sexual activity has a higher status in the Stoic world, as indicated by the cosmological myth of Zeus and Hera and the insemination of rational order into the world; reason is there given a mythical, sexual connotation that at least precludes the sexual act from being seen as an inherently base desire.

We have seen that Plato believes the body to be the cause of leading the soul into evil, by which he means attachment to the things of the world and the senses, most notably bodily pleasures. But we also saw that the senses lead us astray in other ways, since they are unreliable and cause us to err in our perception of the world; they drag the body down into the "things that are never the same," and the soul becomes "confused and dizzy," as Socrates told us in the *Phaedo*. For Plato, true knowledge comes only from the soul, and from the world of Forms. The Stoic attitude toward the senses is much more down-to-earth. Like Aristotle, the Stoics do not denigrate the senses or the knowledge that senses give us; rather, they see the soul as a blank slate on which a person's conceptions are inscribed through the senses. We have perceptions that result in memories of perceptions, and the piling up of these memories becomes experience. Sense impressions are prior to reason, and reason develops out of them. Further, sense impressions imply that there is an 'impressor': "The cause of an impression is an impressor: e.g., something white or cold or everything capable of activating the soul."[71] This does not mean that the Stoics believed that the senses *never* fail us; but it does mean that they "affirm the *normal* reliability of impressions, treating sensory ones as paradigmatic, without raising questions about problem cases or the differences between certainly reliable impressions and all others."[72] In other words, we can rely on our senses most of the time, and we build knowledge according to what we take in through the senses. Assenting to our impressions—in the sense of grasping reality—leads us to the stage of belief and then knowledge. This is in stark contrast to Plato and to later arguments of Descartes; the latter, in particular, claims that, because the senses deceive us sometimes (e.g., a stick will look bent in a glass of water; the sun appears smaller than the earth, etc.), they cannot be relied upon for true knowledge. Both Plato and Descartes, because of their dualism, must contend with the question about things as they appear to us versus things as they "really" are. The Stoics assume that, if I have an impression of a white object, it is caused by a white object in the world. At the same time, the "claim that every impression has a corresponding impressor does not imply that every impression will be an equally clear and distinct indication of its object."[73] The wiser the person, the clearer the grasp of reality will be. But impressions are easily distinguished from figments of the imagination, and the existence of the latter does not necessitate putting all bodily impressions under suspicion or seeing the senses as an impediment to knowledge. The senses are the first stage of knowledge, and, even for the sage, knowledge is ultimately grounded in the body.[74]

While the Stoics were monists and perceived all aspects of the world, including soul, as material, they were not materialists in the modern sense.

They did not reduce all reality to soul-less matter. All matter is ensouled, for the Stoics, but soul, at whatever level, is material. At the same time, it is important to recognize that distinguishing various levels of soul is a conceptual problem for monists. A dualist can be more or less clear about the ontological distinction between soul and body. Further, dualists can explain how humans are different from animals: they attribute to humans a higher level of soul (as is the case with Plato, where only the rational part of the soul is immortal), or they insist that only humans have a soul (as is the case with Descartes, who denies soul to animals). The dualist, however, runs into difficulty in explaining how an immaterial soul can act on a material body. This is something the Stoics were quite clear about: nothing immaterial can causally interact with something material. Dualists have difficulty getting around this problem. Further, as we will see with Descartes, if only humans have souls, certain aspects of animal behaviour become problematic (e.g., do animals really feel pain?). The monist avoids the problem of interaction between the material and immaterial worlds; because everything is material, body and soul can interact. This being the case, however, finding an adequate explanation for what it is that differentiates humans from animals becomes problematic for the monist. Are there only differences of degree between humans and animals (and vegetables and rocks)? Or is the rationality of humans something qualitatively different, and therefore something that can only be explained by positing a different kind of soul? And if so, is this soul something that survives the death of the body?

In answering these questions, Stoics appear to want to have it both ways. Long points out first that "there is in Stoicism a great chain of being which tolerates no discontinuity or introduction of principles which operate at one level but not at another. The entire universe is a combination of god and matter, and what applies to the whole applies to any one of its identifiable parts."[75] At the same time, he tells us that, "no philosophers have emphasized more strongly than the Stoics did that rationality is *the* determinant of human life, and that it marks human beings off sharply from all other animals.[76]

But it turns out that there is no real contradiction between these two positions; the blending of *pneuma* and the different levels of tension and tensile movement in animals and things can account for different degrees of soul and body. At the most basic material level, *pneuma* works simply to account for the coherence (or holding together) of an object (this the Stoics referred to as *hexis*). At the level of plants, *pneuma* is manifested as growth, which the Stoics referred to as *physis*, which is not soul as such. But in animals and humans, *pneuma* becomes *psyche*, or soul. As explained by Long,

> The unity of any 'unified body', be it a stone, plant, animal, or human being, is explicitly attributed not to the form or arrangement or insepa-rability of its parts, but to one of its corporeal constituents, *pneuma*, and the 'cohesion' of 'tensional movement' this establishes throughout all the rest of the body. More general, all 'unified bodies' are instances of 'complete blending.'[77]

But the Stoics still have to account for the rational soul of humans, and at the same time explain the presence or absence of rationality in animals. What activities of the human soul (or rational mind) can be attributed to animals and what activities are exclusively human? Can those activities that are strictly human be accounted for simply by another, more refined, blending of *pneuma*? The answer to these questions is actually quite sophisticated: what differentiates humans and animals is "the presence or absence of *logos*: the growth and maturity of rationality are conceived *as totally modifying the psychic parts and functions which, in themselves, are common to all animals including humans*."[78] What this means, in effect, is not so much the addition of another level of soul, but a modification of the entire soul. This allows the Stoics to explain human language and thought without depriving animals of such soul activities as imaging and impulses, and even non-verbal understanding. This is important in the context of *oikeiosis*, discussed above. This self-perception of all animals is not simple instinct, but a form of consciousness. It is *bodily* awareness. Humans have this, but all of this is transformed, as it were, with rationality. It would thus appear to be a difference in degree that also allows for a difference in kind, or quality. All animals have impulses that connect them with their environment; the adult human has impulses that he can reflect on and choose to act on or not. The Stoics refer to this as the capacity to *assent*, a capacity that animals have at a non-rational level,[79] but which, in humans, is transformed by *logos*.

Thus, one can see that, in relation to the total blending of *pneuma* in different levels of 'unified bodies,' the human being is at the top of a series that moves from *hexis* to *physis* to soul and then to rational soul, the latter representing a modification of the former levels. All of these classifications can be seen as different levels of the combination of God and matter, with humans being the closest to God due to their rational soul. Further, in spite of their monism and their notion of blending, the Stoics do tend to talk about body and soul as two different things. This raises the question of what happens to the human soul at death. As pointed out earlier, death results when the tension of the *pneuma* slackens and the body no longer holds together or coheres. Since everything is material, there is no immaterial 'place' for the soul to go, and, since God is material and immanent in the world, there is no immaterial god to flee to. If the soul is material, it is difficult to conceive of it as lasting forever in some other kind of state. One would think that the Stoics would be clear on the fact that the soul does not survive the body, since soul and body cannot exist without each other. But there are different points of view on life after death in Stoic philosophy (which may be accounted for by the fact that there are so many different Stoic philosophers). Since the body and soul are both material, but separate, entities united in the living being, it is not contradictory to say that the soul can live on without the body, without necessarily being immortal. The soul could, according to F. H. Sandbach, "hold itself together for a time, contracted into a spherical shape and risen to the upper air: the weaker souls would break up first and only those of the ideal wise men would persist until finally caught up in the conflagration that would end the world-cycle."[80] Marcus Aurelius held that, at death, both soul and body would perish into non-existence, saying that every part of himself, "will be reduced by change into some part of the universe, and that again will change into another part of the universe, and so on forever."[81]

Given the lack of immortality, and thus of any reward or punishment after death, one must ask what is the Stoic goal of the good life. The answer is very simple: living in accordance with nature—one's own nature and nature as a whole. Each 'person' is a part of the whole. There is no concept of a separate self, in either the Platonic sense of a soul that will be born again in another body, or in the Christian sense of an individual soul, living only once, that will receive reward or punishment at the end of time. Even in the earthly life (which is the only life, for the Stoic), living in accordance with nature is not a matter of seeking happiness or satisfaction for oneself. Harmony with the whole is the goal, and this can only be achieved by living in accordance with nature, which is an end in itself. This is the only way to achieve happiness; to be in conflict with nature or one's own nature is to be unhappy. In this sense, virtue is its own reward.

Thus, what happens to an individual might seem to be evil or unjust, but the individual has to look to the wider whole in order to understand his suffering and submit to it. Chrysippus uses the analogy of a foot that must get muddy because the man of whom it is a part must pass through some mud in order to accomplish a task. "If the foot had brains," says Chrysippus, "it would be bent on getting muddy."[82] As our foot is part of our body, so our body is part of the world, and we must accept what happens to us, even though it does not suit our individual purposes. Since living in accordance with nature is our goal, we will be just as bent on living our part as our foot is on getting muddy. Therein lies happiness.

Morality and happiness are grounded in nature and in our bodily nature. We are not separate souls making choices detached from our bodily reality. The body is us. And we are part of nature. We can choose to live our life in accordance with nature, or we can resist and be dragged along by fate—but, whichever we choose, we do it as a body and not as a detached soul, mind or self.

A Note on Neoplatonism

The move away from Plato, demonstrated by the philosophies of Aristotle and the Stoics, did not entail the end of Platonism by any means. Aristotle left the Academy after the death of his master, but the Academy continued under various successors and went through different philosophical phases through the Hellenistic age, including a philosophical school of Scepticism, which existed alongside of the Stoic and Epicurean schools.

What is referred to as Neoplatonism began with the Egyptian-born philosopher known as Plotinus (along with his best-known disciple and biographer, Porphyry) in the third century CE, and lasted through to the sixth century, co-existing with Christianity and influencing many Christian thinkers, in particular Augustine. Long after its demise, its influence spread through the history of Western philosophy, and we will have occasion to note this influence at different points in our story of the body, in particular in the chapter on the naturalism of the Renaissance. For this reason, it is useful to give a brief description of it here.

Plotinus and his followers and successors did not call themselves Neoplatonists, the term being an invention of nineteenth-century scholars who wrote about them, and one about which there is a certain amount of debate. The Neoplatonists simply considered themselves Platonists, and even modern scholars have difficulty separating the elements of the different forms of Platonism from what they have termed Neoplatonism. As Remes points out, "Plotinus' view of Plato is—and this is vitally important—both post-Aristotelian and post-Stoic. That is, he is well informed of the criticisms of Plato's teachings, as well as of the developments and steps made by intervening Peripatetic and Hellenistic philosophers."[83] In fact, according to Pauliina Remes, the natural philosophy of the Neoplatonists is both Aristotelian and Platonic, building on Aristotle's view of the role of soul in nature, but also holding to Plato's idea of a world-soul as expressed in the *Timaeus*. This Neoplatonic world-soul is called the Soul of All, and it "unifies the universe into one, a reified and supreme living being, the parts of which connect to one another and form a unified whole."[84] Its role is similar to the Stoic *pneuma*, but for the fact that the *pneuma* is material.

It is this idea of a unified, living universe, along with a hierarchy of levels of being, that is most relevant to my story of the human body and its connection to the cosmos. In Plotinus the human being finds its place in a hierarchical system of levels comprising, first, material and extended nature, which represents our concrete existence in the spatiotemporal world; second, "bodily life, with endeavours and desires connected to the world human beings perceive and live in,"[85] explainable by the Aristotelian levels of the soul (nutritive, sensitive and rational); third, the Intellect, which empowers the embodied rational soul, but is not itself embodied; fourth, the One, which endows human beings with existence, as well as unity and harmony. In this hierarchy, a human being is "not an outside spectator, nor firmly to be located at any single level," but rather "encompasses, or is fundamentally related to, the metaphysical levels."[86] In other words, we participate in all these levels of being. More precisely, the One generates or unfolds the properties and formations of the different levels in a process referred to as *emanation*. "Emanation refers to the way in which the multiplicity of the beings and properties of the sensible realm unfolds itself in the hierarchy of generation from the One, and has a place within that hierarchy depending on its immediate cause."[87]

Neoplatonism blends elements of Platonic, Aristotelian and Stoic philosophies. Many scholars have compared it to Eastern philosophies, in particular Indian philosophies (which will be of interest to the story of the body that unfolds in the discussion of yoga in Chapter 8 and of alternative medicine in Chapter 9).[88] As such, it can be seen as a Western (as opposed to Eastern) antidote to materialism and mechanism. It is relevant to our modern world, according to Mayer, because it is a "monistic, non-materialistic, mystically inspired, but intelligently developed and cogently presented system of thought."[89] And it is relevant to my story of the body as part of the holistic stream of our Western philosophical tradition, elements of which, as with Stoic philosophy, could usefully be recuperated in any search for a more coherent account of mind and body. Its influence can be seen in the philosophy of Spinoza, which we will meet in Chapter 6, which I have titled "The Road Not Followed."

Notes

1. Jonathan Barnes, *Aristotle* (Oxford and New York: Oxford University Press, 1982), 3.
2. Barnes describes his style as often "rugged" and refers to "abrupt transitions, inelegant repetitions, careless allusions" and even "staccato jottings." Barnes, 3.
3. It should be noted that much of what later philosophers rejected was the Christianized version of Aristotle, and not necessarily his original ideas.
4. Barnes describes the Lyceum as being unlike a formal university and more like "a public leisure centre.... There were no examinations, no degrees, no set syllabus; probably there were no official enrolments—and no fees." Barnes, 5.
5. The death of Alexander caused the Athenians to revolt against the Macedonians, and, although Aristotle was not Macedonian (he was born in Stageira), his family's connections to the Macedonian royal house and his own earlier association with Alexander and his father, Philip of Macedonia, fed rumours and allegations of impiety against him that caused him to flee the city.
6. Richard Tarnas, *The Passion of the Western Mind*, 55.
7. Tarnas, *Western Mind*, 57.
8. Helen S. Lang, *The Order of Nature in Aristotle's Physics: Place and the Elements* (Cambridge and New York: Cambridge University Press, 1998), 3.
9. Lang, 50.
10. Lang, 51.
11. Lang, 52.
12. Lang, 52. Tarnas explains the relation between form and matter quite nicely when he states, "every substance not only possesses a form; one could say that it is also possessed by a form, for it naturally strives to realize its inherent form. It strives to become a perfect specimen of its kind. Every substance seeks to actualize what it already is potentially." Tarnas, *Western Mind*, 58.
13. Lang, 57.

14. Tarnas, *Western Mind*, 59.

15. Material bodies—plants, animals, humans, houses, chairs—are composites of form and matter, and these Aristotle refers to as substances. "All substances thus consist of two 'parts,' stuff and structure, which Aristotle habitually calls 'matter' and 'form.' Matter and form are not physical components of substances: you cannot cut up a bronze statue into two separate bits, its bronze and its shape. Rather, matter and form are *logical* parts of substances: an account of what substances are requires mention both of their stuff and their structure." Barnes, 48.

16. Paolo Biondi, *Aristotle: Posterior Analytics II.19* (Québec: Les Presses de l'Université Laval, 2004), 137.

17. Hugh Lawson-Tancred, ed. and trans., *Aristotle, De Anima (On the Soul)* (London and Toronto: Penguin, 1986), 412b, 158.

18. Biondi, 137. A lifeless body (i.e., a corpse) would not be a 'body' for Aristotle, since it would not have the capacity to live and perform vital functions. "The lifeless body is like the eye which cannot see or the axe which is spoilt for use. We may apply to them the same names as before; but as the nature is not longer the same, the application is irrelevant, misleading and equivocal." R. D. Hicks, ed. and trans., *Aristotle, De Anima* (Cambridge: Cambridge University Press, 1907), xliii.

19. *De Anima*, 402a, 126. And, Aristotle continues, "So just as pupil and sight *are* the eye, so in our case, soul and body *are* the animal."

20. Aristotle includes celestial bodies (and/or their intellects) among living things. Contrary to earthly beings, these are considered immortal.

21. Barnes, 66. See *De Anima*, Book II, Ch. 1, for the first account, and Ch. 2 for the second.

22. Aristotle's notion of potentiality and actuality presupposes a proper nature for each species and for each individual living thing, a presupposition that is not generally accepted today.

23. Hicks, lxi.

24. Tarnas, *Western Mind*, 61. See also Terrell Ward Bynum, "A New Look at Aristotle's Theory of Perception," in Michael Durant, *Aristotle's De Anima in Focus* (London and New York: Routledge, 1993), 92: "The form in question is the perceived quality, which initially is actualized in the object, but not the sense-organ.... Prior to perception, the object has a form which the sense-organ does not have. Afterwards, the organ has taken in the form of the object without its matter."

25. See Biondi, 141: "Since the end of seeing is seeing itself, and, generally, the end of sensing is the act of sensing itself, there is an activity going on of which the sensitive soul is the principle; however, since the soul cannot activate or actualize itself but needs the occasional causality of the sensible object and the instrumental

causality of its bodily organ, the impulse set up in the organ by the sensible quality and its transmission to the sensitive soul is like a motion whose end is the activity of sensation."

26.   Tarnas, *Western Mind*, 59. See Aristotle, *Posterior Analytics*, II, 19, where Aristotle states, "Thus these states [of knowing the principles] are neither innately existing in us in a determinate form, nor do they come to be from other higher states of knowing; instead, they come from (sense-)perception...." Biondi, 7.

27.   Tarnas, *Western Mind*, 61.

28.   Lang, 52.

29.   R. J. Hankinson, "Philosophy of Science," in Jonathan Barnes, ed., *The Cambridge Companion to Aristotle* (Cambridge: Cambridge University Press, 1996), 128.

30.   Hankinson, 128. This wording does suggest design, although Hankinson emphasizes that it is only metaphorical and is simply a reformulation of Nature's goal-directedness.

31.   Hankinson, 120.

32.   It should be noted that there are debates but no agreement about whether or not the rational soul in Aristotle is in some way immortal. Aristotle's discussion in *De Anima* (Book III, Ch. 4 and 5) is famously unclear and open to different interpretations.

33.   A. A. Long and D. N. Sedley, *The Hellenistic Philosophers*, Vol. I (Cambridge University Press, 1987), 3.

34.   Philip P. Halie, "Stoicism," in *Encyclopedia of Philosophy*, Vol. VIII (New York: The Macmillan Company and The Free Press, 1967), 19. Emphasis added.

35.   This is not to say they were not influenced as well by Plato. Sandbach reports that the father of Zeno, the founder of Stoicism, "is said to have brought home from Athens many 'Socratic books,' which fired the young man's imagination." He also tells us that Zeno came under the influence of Plato's views through the Academy, which was "the influence recognised by the scholars of antiquity," and the place one should look for the sources of Zeno's thought. F. H. Sandbach, *The Stoics* (London: Chatto & Windus, 1975), 20–22.

36.   Sandbach, 18. Rist tells us that two of the Church Fathers, Clement of Alexandria and Origen, "knew the Stoics well," and that Philo Judaeus, a major source for the synthesis of ideas by the Church Fathers, "is full of Stoicism." John Rist, *Man, Soul and Body: Essays in Ancient Thought from Plato to Dionysius* (Aldershot, Hampshire, UK: Ashgate, 1996), 27.

37.   The Epicureans and Stoics had one very central disagreement: the Epicureans believed that a human's primary impulse was pleasure; the Stoics disagreed, believing that it was self-preservation, as we will see. For the Stoics, pleasure was a secondary impulse—even an infant must know what is good for it before it can be attracted by the pleasurable.

38. Long and Sedley, 357.

39. Diogenes Laertius, *Lives of Eminent Philosophers*, 7–104–5, quoted in Long and Sedley, 354.

40. Happiness, living in harmony, and virtue are all linked in Stoic ethics.

41. Epictetus, *The Discourses as Reported by Arrian, The Manual, and Fragments*, ed. W. A. Oldfather, Vol. I (Cambridge: Harvard University Press, 1995), 93–95.

42. We also must remember that the question to ask is not whether they were right, but what they were trying to explain. That being said, there are some writers today who look to Stoic physics as being closer to modern physics than the average person might suspect. Even Sandbach, who is sceptical about oversimplifying such similarities, does concede that, "in some ways Stoic views approached modern ones more nearly than did those of other ancient thinkers." See Sandbach, 71.

43. Halie, 20.

44. Diogenes Laertius, 7.137, in Long and Sedley, 270. The idea of god consuming and reproducing the world refers to the Stoics' very strange notion of eternal return. There are periodic conflagrations, where all is absorbed in fire, and then the universe is reconstituted. Interpretations of this are many and controversial, but this notion is not at all central to our discussion of the body.

45. Long and Sedley, 273. The corporeality of the two Stoic principles is not without conceptual difficulties, and these are discussed by Long and Sedley, 274. See also Sandbach, 73–74. Debates about the logical consistency of the Stoic notions of god and matter go beyond the purpose of our narrative; we can acknowledge the Stoic principle as a foundation for an eventual theory of the human body without having to accept, without question, the adequacy of the principle itself.

46. Long and Sedley, 277.

47. Long and Sedley, 278.

48. According to Long and Sedley, the modification from fire to breath was made by Chrysippus, who extended the notion of his predecessors that the animal soul or vital principle was *pneuma* or breath: "Following their analogical reasoning from microcosm to macrocosm, Chrysippus opted for 'breath' rather than heat on its own as the sustaining principle of the world" (279). Aristotle, too, had a notion of *pneuma*, but it was much more limited and less developed than that of Chrysippus. It was in Chrysippus, according to Rist, that "the theory of *pneuma* in its original form reached its fullest development." Rist, 34.

49. Terence Irwin, *Classical Thought* (Oxford: Oxford University Press, 1989), 167.

50. Long and Sedley, 289.

51. Long and Sedley, 320.

52. Aulus Gellius, *Noctes Atticae*, 7.2.3, in Long and Sedley, 336.

53.   Rist, 40. The notion of sympathy will be encountered again, especially in some
       Renaissance natural philosophers; it is a useful notion to account for action at a
       distance.
54.   Rist, 41.
55.   Rist, 45.
56.   Rist, 46.
57.   Genevieve Lloyd, *Providence Lost* (Cambridge: Harvard University Press, 2008),
       90. According to Lloyd, the "vague cliché—'following nature'—does not do
       justice to the richness of Stoic ethical theory. It is often overlooked, for example,
       that the Stoics' version of nature is closely connected with the origins of modern
       ideas of cosmopolitanism. What is natural to human beings is, for the Stoics,
       what pertains to us—not by virtue of our belonging to any particular polis, but
       by virtue of our being citizens of the world. This transcendence of self-interest
       and provincialism is one of the great legacies from their remarkable idea that we
       inhabit a cosmic city—'the world of gods and men.'"
58.   Long and Sedley, 351. This term is also translated as 'affinity,' 'orientation' or
       'belonging.'
59.   Cicero, *De Finibus Bonorum et Malorum*, trans. H. Rackham (Loeb Classical
       Library, 1914), 233.
60.   Cicero, 233.
61.   Seneca, 121.13. *Ad Lucillium Epistulae Morales*, trans. R. M. Gummere (Loeb
       Classical Library, 1962). See also Pembroke, "Oikeiosis," in A. A. Long, *Problems
       in Stoicism* (London: Athlone Press, 1971), 117. Pembroke points out that the
       Stoics differed from other philosophers of antiquity in that "childhood is accorded
       the status of a fully natural phenomenon and that the child himself is treated as
       the chief agent in his own education."
62.   A. A. Long, "Hierocles on *oikeiosis* and self-perception," in *Stoic Studies*
       (Cambridge: Cambridge University Press, 1996), 251.
63.   Long, 252.
64.   Long, 256.
65.   Long, 258. Long is quoting the neurologist Oliver Sacks from his book *The Man
       Who Mistook His Wife for a Hat* (1987, 43). Much of Sacks' work is devoted to
       what happens to a person's sense of self and body when normal proprioception
       is lost. In the case cited by Long, "Sacks' patient had lost the capacity to feel her
       body as something that belonged to her." This sense of our body as *ours*—that
       it *belongs to us*—is what is central to the Stoic concept of *oikeiosis*.
66.   Cicero, 239.
67.   "As rational beings, we appropriate impulse, recognizing with affection our own
       natures. This basic connection between reason and impulse underpins the joyful
       recognition of necessities that is the core of Stoic ethics. All this gives a distinctive

concreteness to the Stoic version of detachment; necessity is embedded in the unpredictable vicissitudes of life." Lloyd, *Providence*, 93.

68. Long, 259.

69. Long, 262.

70. Long, 262.

71. Long and Sedley, 237.

72. Long and Sedley, 240.

73. Long and Sedley, 239.

74. The Stoic theory of perception is not without problems; Sandbach points out that, while the general outline is clear, the details are obscure because of lack of evidence. However, the important point for this analysis is the fact that the Stoics did not turn away from the body in their search for an explanation of how we obtain knowledge of the world, nor did they question the existence of the objects of perception, as would the later empiricists.

75. Long, 228.

76. Long, 244.

77. Long, 230.

78. Long, 244. Emphasis added. Interestingly, the human embryo remains in the state of *physis* until birth, when *physis* becomes soul. But the development of rationality is a gradual process. As we have seen with *oikeiosis*, the human infant and child only gradually develops the capacity to assess and judge what it needs for its proper functioning.

79. Long and Sedley refer to this as a "primitive form of assent—'yielding'—to the appropriate impression. The human form of assent renders both impressions and impulses rational. See Long and Sedley, 322.

80. Sandbach, 83.

81. Quoted in Raymond Martin and John Barresi, *The Rise and Fall of Soul and Self* (New York: Columbia University Press, 2006), 32.

82. Sandbach, 36.

83. Pauliina Remes, *Neoplatonism* (Berkeley and Los Angeles: University of California Press, 2008), 3.

84. Remes, 79.

85. Remes, 102.

86. Remes, 101.

87. Remes, 46.

88. There is speculation in the literature that Plotinus encountered Indian philosophy in his voyages to the East, but it is considered more likely that Eastern and Western scholars developed similar philosophies in isolation from each other.

89. John R. A. Mayer, Introduction to *Neoplatonism and Indian Thought*, ed. R. Baine Harries (Norfolk, VA: International Society For Neoplatonic Studies, 1982), 2.

CHAPTER III

The Resurrection of the Body: Christianity

If it is difficult to generalize about a unified philosophy of the body in Stoic philosophy due to its temporal and geographic spread, it is even more difficult with respect to Christianity, a religion that has spanned two millennia, has been reformed and transformed, and has sprouted multiple branches throughout its long history. At the same time, there are certain fundamental beliefs of Christian philosophy and religion, which have their roots in the first centuries after Jesus Christ, in which the body—human and divine—figures prominently. In fact, the body is the focus of several central mysteries of the Christian faith: the Incarnation, the Eucharist and the Resurrection. These may not all be articles of faith in many contemporary Christian sects, but they were all central to the Christian faith at its beginnings. This chapter will focus on conceptions of, and attitudes toward, the body during the development of the Christian religion from the time of Christ through the Middle Ages.[1] It will also examine the ideas about the body held by two major Christian figures who have been both recognized thinkers in the history of philosophy and the most influential theologians of Roman Catholicism: Augustine and Thomas Aquinas.

The most striking fact about the body in the Christian religion is the ambivalence expressed toward it by the tradition; in spite of the fact that it is central to the main mysteries of the religion, the body tends to be denigrated as the occasion of sin and ultimate damnation. This underlines a central paradox about the body as a source of both sin and salvation—which gives the body itself an air of mystery in the works of many Christian philosophers. Because of the belief in life after death, the Christian view of soul and body is essentially dualist, like Plato's; however, as we will see, the belief in a final resurrection of the body adds another dimension to this dualist metaphysics and deepens an ever-present ambivalence and ambiguity.

Influences on Christian Thought

Christianity is a *revealed* religion based on doctrines of redemption and salvation. Its central tenet is love—the love of God and of one's neighbour. It originated essentially as a practice, not a philosophy; it offers its adherents a way to salvation and to an afterlife with God. While some scholars maintain that Jesus was in fact a philosopher of the Cynic school (because of the similarity of that school's philosophy of virtue as the road to happiness, and its rejection of conventional striving for power, wealth or fame), at least in its beginnings, Christianity did not represent a philosophy. As expressed by Richard Tarnas, "Christianity began and triumphed not as a philosophy but as a religion— eastern and Judaic in character, emphatically communal, salvational, emotional, mystical, depending on revelatory statements of faith and belief, and almost fully independent of Hellenic rationalism."[2]

As it developed as a religion, however, the need for a philosophical framework was recognized and, during its first four centuries, a group of philosophers and theologians known as the Church Fathers cloaked the new religion in a philosophy.[3] In so doing, they drew on many elements from Greek and Roman thought, including Stoicism. This might seem strange given some of the metaphysical positions of the Greeks, such as Plato's Forms or the monism of the Stoics, for example, but the Church Fathers tended to think of the Greeks either as having borrowed their ideas from the Old Testament or as having 'anticipated' Christianity; they were seen, in a sense, as Christians before their time.[4] Further, the language of Platonism was understood by the ancient and medieval mind; this allowed for easier acceptance of Christian ideas as being continuous with past thought.[5] As for the Stoics, as pointed out in the last chapter, they both influenced the Church Fathers and, at the same time, were seen as rivals to the emerging Christian religion. In spite of the differences, the Stoic belief in divine providence, along with their ethical system (emphasized by the Roman Stoics), were easily adapted to the notion of the divine as transcendent rather than immanent. Jesus himself stated that he came not to abolish the laws and the prophets, but to complete them, and

Christians eventually took this to refer not only to the Jewish law and prophets, but to Greek philosophy, as well.[6] In addition, many of the pagan mysteries and deities were subtly absorbed into the new religion and the many myths and descriptions of the divine came to be understood as literal truths that worked their way into the doctrine of the new religion.[7]

Given that the Old Testament forms part of the Christian Bible, it is interesting to look briefly at the meaning attributed to body in early Hebrew thought, since the early Hebrews did not hold a dualistic view of mind and body. They had, rather, three interlinked concepts that can be seen to cover what we generally think of as mind and body. The term *nephesh* is traditionally translated as 'soul,' but this is a narrowed meaning; the term "is designed to be seen together with the whole form of man, and especially with his breath; moreover man does not *have nephesh*, he *is nephesh*, he lives as *nephesh*."[8] But *nephesh* also means 'throat' in the sense of "the organ that takes in nourishment" or as the seat of vital needs.[9] It can also be used to designate the whole person. The term *basar* means 'flesh,' a term that can be applied both to humans and animals, but it can also mean the human body as a whole: "Like *nephesh*, therefore, *basar* points towards man *per se*, but now in his bodily aspect."[10] Further, it means flesh in the sense of what binds people together in relationship or kinship, but can also mean the relationship of all living things. It is also interesting to note that, while in English the term 'body' can be used to indicate a corpse, *basar* is never used in this way. Thus, to the extent that *basar* means body, it can only refer to a living body. The third term, *ruah*, originally meant wind.[11] But it also means the breath of God and the essence of life, with a connotation of the dynamic and creative activity of God. To the extent that *ruah* belongs to humans, it comes from God: "Only when Yahweh infuses the *ruah* as breath into the bones covered with sinews, flesh and skin, will the bodies live."[12] Further, *ruah* can mean both soul and heart, but also vitality, consciousness and even character, somewhat like the Stoic *pneuma*.

It can be seen from the above that the clear distinction between soul/mind and body that has developed in the Western philosophical tradition (much of which has been influenced by Christian thought) is not present in the ancient Hebrew notions of soul and body, which are multi-faceted, inter-mingling elements of both. There does not seem to be a term for a purely material conception of the human body or for a purely immaterial conception of soul or mind.

The Body in the Christian Mysteries

As noted above, all of the central mysteries of the Christian faith are body-based. In other words, the body is at the centre of Christian belief, a fact that raises its ontological status at the outset. The most important and fundamental mystery is the Incarnation, the founding event of the Christian faith. Jesus Christ is believed to have been both fully God and fully human (i.e., in a *human* body). In other words, God became embodied (incarnated) in the person of Jesus Christ. The mystery centres on the question of how the divine nature and human nature can be one, and how Jesus can be God without admitting that there is more than one God.[13] But more important from our point of view, the central and founding dogma of the Christian Church holds that *God took on human flesh.* In other words, the human body is right at the centre of the core beliefs, without which there would be no Christianity. The other most central article of faith is the suffering and crucifixion of Jesus, which further emphasizes real, living flesh over abstract soul or mind. In addition, the notion that Jesus is the *logos* (meaning Reason, but also the Word) is present in some Christian writings, including the Gospel of John, which opens with the words, "In the beginning was the Word, and the Word was with God, and the Word was God."[14] The Church Fathers may have identified Jesus with the *logos* because of the influence of Platonic and Stoic philosophy, which interpreted *logos* as divine Reason. They may simply have wanted to express the Incarnation in terms that would be understood by the Hellenistic world. Whatever their reason, in this synthesis of the Greek idea of a divinely rational cosmos and the Jewish doctrine of the creative Word of God, "Christ, the Logos, became man: the historical and the timeless, the absolute and the personal, the human and the divine became one,"[15] raising the human body to a holier dimension that that of Plato's container or prison.

Like many articles of the Christian faith, the Incarnation was not a belief that was accepted without controversy or argument. Indeed, it was a burning question as late as the fourth century after Christ. Speaking of the Church fathers mentioned above, Margaret Miles points out that the "differing understandings of Christ's corporeality of the Eastern and Western fathers became apparent quite early," so that some, such as Clement of Alexandria, attempted to deny ordinary bodily functions like digestion to Jesus, while others, such as Tertullian, "emphasized Christ's physicality almost to the point of crudity."[16] Ultimately, as we will see in Augustine, the union of the divine and the human in the Incarnation came to be seen as an analogy of the union of the soul and body in humans.[17] Disturbingly, it also came to be seen as an analogy for the relationship between men and women; the long-standing belief that woman is to man as matter is to spirit slipped easily into the interpretation that man signifies the divinity of the Son of God and woman his humanity, something that had an enormous influence on the spirituality of medieval women. While the idea that woman symbolizes matter was often used by male theologians to denigrate women, women saw it differently, putting the emphasis more on Christ's physicality and identifying with that.[18] This resulted in particularly feminine forms of mysticism and devotion, as we will see later in the chapter, but it is not a vision of the feminine or the female body that has worked to women's advantage in the history of the Christian church.

A second important central mystery of the Christian faith is the doctrine of the Eucharist, also referred to as the *transubstantiation*. This entails a belief in the real presence of Christ in the communion host, a transformation brought about by the words and actions of the priest during the Mass. To many Christians, especially Roman Catholics, this is not a symbolic presence, but a real one; in other words, what one receives at communion is the *body of Christ*. In fact, these are the very words that the recipient utters upon receiving the host.[19] Not all branches of Christianity interpret the Eucharist in this way. However, what is of interest to us here is that, at the beginnings of the Christian Church, the belief that the presence of Christ was real was so entrenched that it was taken for granted. Long before transubstantiation became a doctrine of the Church, "most Christians thought that they quite literally ate Christ's body and blood in the sacrament" of the Eucharist.[20] This doctrine emphasizes once again the idea of body and flesh at the core of Christian belief, but it also brings food to the centre of spirituality and worship, as the "reception of food between one's lips remained a uniquely important mode of spiritual encounter," in particular for religious medieval women.[21] Food represents body, and at the moment of the consecration of the bread and wine, God becomes food-that-is-body. Eating the body of Christ was more than symbolic: "to eat was to consume, to take in, to become God."[22] Even though the belief in literally taking in and becoming God has not survived the centuries of Christian reforms, the fact remains that—at least in relation to early Christianity— no other period in the history of the Church "has placed so positive (and therefore so complex and ambiguous) a value on the bodiliness of Christ's humanity."[23]

The final mystery of the Christian religion that brings the body to the centre is the belief in the resurrection of the body. This entails not only belief in the physical resurrection of Christ three days after his crucifixion, but the resurrection of the body of every person at the end of time. The former refers to the Easter mystery and the latter to the Redemption or Final Judgment (which will follow a final conflagration, or end of the world). For the Christian, the term "resurrection" implies the actual resurrection of each and every individual body. More will be said about this later, but it must be emphasized, here, that the idea of the resurrection of the body underlines the resolutely personal nature of the Christian religion; each life and each death is *personal*, pertaining to *this* soul and *this* body. Christianity is not unique in its belief in the immortality of the soul. As we have seen, Plato's doctrine of reincarnation includes the notion of immortality, but not before the soul passes through many different bodies. Buddhism holds a sort of immortality, but it is not personal; it implies the fusion of the soul with the One, but not the survival of an individual. Christianity posits the clear belief in individual salvation; the soul will live on after death, and at some future unknown time it will be joined by the body, the same body that 'housed' it on Earth.[24] Belief in an afterlife can serve to allay the fear of death and resolve questions relating to injustice in the existing world through a heavenly system of reward and punishment. However, these goals could be met without the need to include bodily resurrection. It can be argued that spiritual immortality should be enough; Platonic reincarnation, for example, clearly accounts for reward and punishment. But for a religion that puts the body at its centre as a result of the Incarnation, immortality has to go further; it must deal with the question of the impermanence of the body, as well as its destruction and decomposition after death, which, in Plato, for example, entailed a negative view of the body.

Each central Christian mystery has at its core an expression of body that, at least in principle, elevates the body from a purely material status and makes it an essential part of Christian faith and salvation.[25] At the same time, there is much in the philosophical and theological literature of the Christian world that expresses ambivalence about—if not outright rejection of—the body, which appears surprising and often contradictory. In the rest of this chapter, I will try to unravel some of the knots of ambiguity surrounding the issue of the Christian body, examining in the process the thought of Augustine (354–430 CE) and Aquinas (1225–1274 CE), while taking a closer look at a number of Christian beliefs and practices related to the body.

Augustine

According to Terence Irwin, Augustine's *Confessions* show us, "more clearly than any other literary work of late antiquity, what it was like to approach Christianity through the outlook of Greek philosophy, and more generally from the literary and cultural background of the later Roman Empire."[26] This fact in itself accounts for much of the ambivalence that is built into Augustine's various accounts of body and soul; among other things, he was trying to reconcile the Platonic idea of the body as a container, tomb or prison with Christian theology's need of a body that is reunited with its soul at the end of time. He also had to reconcile Plato's idea that the essence of the person is the soul with the Christian belief that God took on a truly human body in the person of Jesus Christ. To the extent that Augustine succeeded in Christianizing Plato, his success in relation to the body was at best mixed.

Augustine's name dominates the history of Western thought from the fifth to the thirteenth centuries, that is, until the time of Thomas Aquinas. He was born in what is now Algeria (then part of the Roman Empire), had a Roman education, which included Greek philosophy, and was influenced by the ideas of Plato (although he absorbed Plato's thought through the writings of Plotinus and the Neoplatonists, rather than through those of Plato himself). He was raised as a Christian (Christianity being officially accepted in the Roman Empire at that time), but was later "appalled by the ignorant and superstitious views" that he received from his upbringing.[27] This renders his later conversion all the more surprising, since the intellectuals in his environment were the pagans, not the Christians. For an intellectual of Augustine's day, versed in the teachings of Plato, "to accept the Incarnation would have been like a modern European denying the evolution of the species: he would have had to abandon not only the most advanced, rationally based knowledge available to him, but by implication, the whole culture permeated by such achievements."[28] Augustine's *Confessions* reflects the intellectual turmoil that he went through over the years as he moved closer to the Christian religion while continuing to reject it.

As a young man, Augustine studied law and fraternized with the Manicheans, radical dualists who held that the universe was divided into forces of good and forces of evil, a philosophy that he eventually rejected.[29] Although they considered themselves Christians, the Manicheans rejected both baptism and the Eucharist, and held that matter and the physical world were inherently evil; it was only in spirit that goodness and light could be found. At the age of eighteen, Augustine took as a mistress a young woman of Carthage who was not his social equal. However, he lived with her faithfully for fourteen years and had a son with her, a situation that was not unusual for a man of his age and station at that time (and would be described today as a common-law marriage). The woman is never named, and, in spite of his fidelity and his offspring, Augustine later refers (in his *Confessions*) to their relationship as one built solely on lust, something that seems to have influenced his later views of sexuality and marriage. In the interests of his career and professional ambitions, he was urged by family and friends to take a wife, and, at the age of thirty-two, having broken with his concubine, became engaged to a girl of twelve, a situation that required him to wait two years until she was of an age to marry. In the meantime, however, he underwent a dramatic conversion to Christianity (although he had been brought up as a Christian, he had not been baptized) and the marriage never took place. After his conversion, he gave up his career, undertook a life of both religious and philosophical study and, in 396, at the age of forty-two, became Bishop of Hippo, a position he occupied until his death in 430.

In spite of Augustine's limited direct knowledge of Plato and the Greeks, he was the conduit of ancient thought in the West after the sack of Rome. As the Roman Empire was collapsing around him, Augustine seemed to realize that his writings "would provide future generations of Western Christians with much of their intellectual raw material,"[30] a not unmixed blessing when it comes to Christian, and especially Catholic, attitudes to the body over the centuries. Whether this was his intention, "by his stress on 'concupiscence' (uncontrolled desire) he set the West on the path of identifying sin with sex."[31] His *Confessions* is, to the modern reader, somewhat sex-obsessed,[32] focusing on his overactive libido both in his youth and later, but his efforts to come to grips with the body in philosophical terms are much more nuanced. His notions are generally far removed, for example, from the Platonic idea of the body dragging down the soul and leading it into sin. In fact, for him, it is the soul, not the body, that leads to sin. The lust of the eyes, for example, is caused not by the eyes themselves, but by the way in which the eyes are used by the soul. In one of his sermons he speaks of his body as something he wants "to be healed as a whole, for I am one whole. I do not want my flesh to be removed from me for ever, as if it were something alien to me, but that it be healed, a whole with me."[33]

Augustine inherited Plato's mind-body dualism, along with a belief in the superiority of the immaterial, god-like soul, and in some of his earlier writings he refers to the body as a "dark prison" and a "cave" (suggesting shades of both Plato and the Manicheans). In his later writings, however, he attempts to come to grips with the unity of body and soul, referring to the union of soul and body in the *persona*, a term much more suggestive of unity. His driving motivation in relation to the body is to explain both the unity of the human body and soul *and* the unity of the divine and human natures of Christ in the Incarnation. Both the doctrine of the Incarnation and the doctrine of the Resurrection prevented Augustine from holding the body in disdain, and in his own search for God, the body has a "high epistemological status."[34]

Aquinas

The second philosophical giant of the Christian religion is Thomas Aquinas (1225–1274), born in Italy in the region of Naples. He studied at the University of Naples, entered the Dominican Order in his twenties and studied under Albert the Great, an Aristotelian Scholastic philosopher. He also studied at the University of Paris and later taught there in the faculty of theology. He became an intellectual at a time when new Latin translations of Greek works were becoming available and when Christianity, after centuries of exclusion of non-Christian culture, was opening itself up to more secular thinking.[35] In a manner similar to Augustine's Christianizing of Plato, Aquinas accomplished the same task for Aristotle by adapting his work to fit the theological concerns of the Church. He wrote volumes of both theology and philosophy, and is recognized as an important philosopher in the Western tradition. According to Tarnas, the "extraordinary impact Aquinas had on Western thought lay especially in his conviction that the judicious exercise of man's empirical and rational intelligence, which had been developed and empowered by the Greeks, could now marvellously serve the Christian cause."[36] He did not see the natural world or knowledge about the natural world as antithetical to knowledge and love of God, and in fact believed that the study of nature and nature's order can lead one to God, a position that brings him closer to the Stoics than to Plato or even Augustine.

Aquinas held an Aristotelian vision of soul and body, believing that the whole person, not just the soul, is the human agent. He accepted Aristotle's principle of form and matter, and of the soul as the form of the human being. At the same time, in conformity with Christian theology, he holds that the soul is immortal. This is a difficult position to maintain, since, as we have seen in Aristotle, considering the soul as the *form* of a human being puts into question its survival after the death of the body. Aquinas partially solved this difficulty with his ideas about resurrection: after death, the soul lives on, but before the resurrection of the body, it is incomplete and imperfect. It has need of the body in order to be perfect and it will attain this perfection when it is reunited with its body at the end of time. More will be said below about this reunification of body and soul. What is important, here, is the status given to the body in Aquinas' thought: the body is intrinsically necessary to the person, and to knowledge, both in life and after death.

Aquinas did not believe that the person is the immortal soul. The person is composed of an immortal soul *and* an ultimately immortal body. Further, he did not believe that the soul could have knowledge without the body and he rejected Plato's notion of an intellect that has direct knowledge of transcendent Ideas or Forms. Unlike Plato, Aquinas did not think that the body was an obstacle to knowledge. On the contrary, he "denied the human intellect's capacity to know the Ideas directly, asserting the intellect's need for sensory experience to activate an imperfect but meaningful understanding of things in terms of those eternal archetypes."[37] While Plato spoke of the intellect participating in the Forms or Ideas as the ultimate reality (bodily and earthly existence being in essence unreal), Aquinas spoke rather of human beings participating body and soul in God's existence, thus giving to God what Plato gave to the Forms. Man participates in God's being and does not have to flee empirical reality to know God or to participate in his being. In coming to know the world, man comes to know God, to the point that by "expanding his own knowledge, man was becoming more like God, and to be like God was man's true desired end."[38] This view that the body is necessary for knowledge can be seen as approaching the Stoic notion of the body as a source of knowledge.

Between these two giants of Christian thought, there was almost a thousand years of history and much theological and philosophical debate; it would be surprising if there were not major differences between them in relation to the human body. Some of the historical as well as philosophical differences can be seen through an examination of debates surrounding the question of the resurrection of the body, which raise philosophical problems about the ontological status of both body and soul between the moment of death and the time of the final judgment.

Resurrection and Relics

While not all Christians take the notion of the resurrection of the body to mean a literal return of the earthly body, this was the most common interpretation of both early and medieval Christians, and it was considered heretical to think otherwise. For example, the Fourth Lateran Council in 1213 "required Cathars and other heretics to assent to the proposition that 'all rise with their own individual bodies, that is, the bodies which they now wear.'"[39] The current Catholic catechism confirms the dogma of the resurrection in these words: "By death the soul is separated from the body, but in the resurrection God will give incorruptible life to our body, transformed by reunion with our soul. Just as Christ is risen and lives for ever, so all of us will rise at the last day."[40]

It goes without saying that this belief raised certain philosophical problems that did not go unnoticed by Christian thinkers. In fact, there was much debate about how resurrection of the body could actually happen. Practical questions were raised about what would be the age, gender, size and state of health of the risen body, whether it would have the use of the five senses, and especially whether or not it would eat. Augustine "was consistent in holding that we rise with gender; he was uncertain about our age at resurrection although he suggested in one passage that we will all rise aged thirty; he was inconsistent about whether or not we return with the shape—i.e., height and weight—we had on earth."[41] Aquinas believed that we would have our sense of touch, but we would not eat.[42] Further, the belief that we would have our real, earthly body at the Resurrection posed even more difficult problems at a time when Christians were being thrown to the lions: how will the bodies of people who have been eaten, or otherwise dispersed, be resurrected? This resulted in the curious belief in 'regurgitation'; at the end time, the body parts would be regurgitated and reassembled. Nothing is beyond the power of an omnipotent God, as the following inscription on a medieval miniature of a resurrection scene indicates:

> The bodies and members of people once devoured by beasts and fish are brought forth by God's command, because the members of the saints will rise incorrupt ... and they will be presented at God's command.[43]

Medieval paintings are replete with scenes of regurgitation and reassemblage. Moreover, the concern about people who were eaten by animals or by other humans, through cannibalism, was widespread enough that a very dubious explanation about it even has a name: the chain consumption argument. This ingenious argument held that it was impossible for the material of one human body to become part of another human body because such matter could not be digested—it would be excreted. So, if a human were eaten by a fish and the fish then eaten by another human, "the human material that had become part of the flesh of the fish would not become part of the flesh of the humans who ate the fish, but would be excreted by them."[44]

But consumption of human flesh by animals, fish or other humans was only one problem that needed explanation. What about the bodies of saints, which had been dispersed all over the medieval world in the form of relics? How will these bodies be reassembled when the trumpet sounds? This was a larger problem that pitted two deeply held yet contradictory beliefs—the belief in the power of relics and the belief in the resurrection of bodies—against each other.

Relics had great value, since it was believed they could enable miracles. But relics were spread far and wide, so the reassembling would be a task of equal difficulty to that posed by the consumption of humans by animals. Moreover, it was believed that the martyr or saint is wholly present in the smallest fragment of bone or drop of dried blood; it has to be so for the relic to be capable of causing miracles. But how could this belief be reconciled with the belief in the resurrection of the saint's body? Victricius of Rouen believed in the wholeness of the person in every part, insisting that the relics were never drained of their power:

> Let no one, deceived by vulgar error, think that the truth of the whole of their bodily passion is not contained in these fragments.... We proclaim, with all our faith and authority, that there is nothing in these relics that is not complete. For where healing power is present the members are complete.[45]

Initially, Augustine was not interested in relics; he even participated in efforts to downplay practices relating to them. But he became convinced about miracles resulting from the relics of the martyr Stephen, and ordered that miracles attributed to Stephen at Hippo be recorded. Further, his experience with Stephen's relics affected his understanding of resurrection. He came to believe that the whole martyr must be present in the fragments that cured the sick, and, "if this tiny bit was already whole in Hippo, how can we think that any piece will be missing when the trumpet sounds?"[46]

Augustine's notion that the whole of Stephen is present in the smallest fragment of the dead Stephen is certainly an argument against a purely material body or the body as a mere container or tomb in the Platonic sense. Some vital aspect of Stephen—of his soul—must still be present in order for the relic to have the power (either directly or indirectly) to cure the sick or raise the dead. If its power is limited to the power of intercession with the divine, the relic still has to be seen as housing something more than the physical Stephen. That in itself is an interesting issue to explore regarding the Christian view of the body. But in relation to the belief in resurrection, it raises questions about how the body of Stephen will be reassembled on the last day.

In the centuries between Augustine and Aquinas, two rival interpretations regarding the status of the risen body were held at different times by different thinkers and theologians. The first interpretation was organic, based on what is referred to as the 'seed metaphor'; in the same way that seeds die in the ground and are then 'resurrected' as new plants, so we "are seeds, which are cast into the earth bare and rot and then rise again with bodies."[47] This explanation was naturalistic; it helped explain resurrection as something natural rather than supernatural. It was therefore resisted by many who thought that it demonstrated less than total faith in an omnipotent God who was capable of performing any supernatural act and thus of resurrecting the dead in a way that could not be explained in natural terms. This second school of thought saw the resurrection as the reassembling of parts—every bit that was in the tomb, and, in the case of the relics of martyrs and saints, all their parts from wherever they were—into the same body that existed before death. This still raised many explanatory problems, but one problem that it did solve was the problem of identity. The seed metaphor, while able to explain regrowth of the same *type* of plant, could not account for the regrowth of the *same* plant. So the seed metaphor had two problems: it gave an inadequate account of identity, and it allowed resurrection to be seen as something natural, not supernatural. On the other hand, it was more organic and less dualistic in its view of the body, since it saw each person as a mind-body unity. In spite of this, from the second to the fourteenth centuries, "doctrinal pronouncements, miracle stories and popular preaching continued to insist on the resurrection of exactly the material bits that were laid in the tomb."[48] The identity of the body was important; it had to be the *same* person who was rewarded in heaven or punished in hell. Despite its complications, the notion of reassemblage, as it was called, could accommodate this important point.

Whatever the means by which resurrection would be accomplished, it was held that the resurrected body would have qualities that the earthly body does not have. Among these were *claritas*, or brightness; *agilitas*, or the ability to move quickly; *subtilitas*, meaning that the body will be more spiritual and subject to the will of the soul; and *impassibilitas*, meaning it will be incorruptible and will not be subject to feelings such as pain. The particular qualities are less important than the notion that the resurrected body and soul will be more closely united and the resurrected body will be more complete and perfect than the earthly body. It was Aquinas' view that the resurrected body adds qualities that the soul does not have alone; it adds a certain capacity for knowing. The soul needs the body for sensation, so without the body the soul of the dead person has very limited sensory powers. This is an important point in relation to Aquinas' view of the body and to his epistemology, which, as pointed out earlier, is based on knowledge through bodily experience. The person is incomplete without the body. At the resurrection, the body is necessary to complete the person and to complete the soul's capacity for knowing. In Aquinas' view, the soul alone can only grasp universals; it needs its body (and sensation) in order to perceive individual things, as particulars. Whatever its epistemological merits, this view raises the ontological status of the body. In Aquinas, "without bodily expression there is no human being (*homo*), no person, no self."[49]

Sin, Sex and Salvation

We have seen that explaining both the Incarnation and the Resurrection is philosophically problematic; the explanations do, however, present the human body as both philosophically and theologically important. Adding the Eucharist to the equation does not clarify Christian notions of embodiment—either the divine body that is ingested, or the human body that partakes of the divine through swallowing the host—but, like the other two central mysteries, it reinforces the body's importance.

Both Augustine and Aquinas hold that the human being is a union of body and soul. They are not always consistent in how they explain this union, and it is easy to question the coherence of their metaphysical explanations. But their motivation is clear: reconciling their theological beliefs with their philosophical influences, they cannot explain the body away. At the same time, there is the question of sin, much of which is seen as being caused by bodily desires in general and sexual desires in particular. Thus, there is another side to the story of the body, and one way of viewing this dichotomy is to look at Paul, a first-century convert to the teachings of Jesus, whose views strongly influenced Augustine and represent a lasting influence on Christian doctrine.

Body and Flesh: The Influence of Paul

Peter Brown tells us that, in Paul's letters, "we are presented with the human body as in a photograph taken against the sun: it is a jet-black shape whose edges are suffused with light."[50] The darkness, of course, is the body's ever-present weakness and vulnerability to sin; the light is the spirit represented by the resurrection of Jesus. The following is a quote from one of Paul's letters to the Romans, whose Platonic echoes are hard to miss:

> Now the works of the flesh are obvious: immorality, impurity, licentiousness, idolatry, sorcery, hatreds, rivalry, jealousy, outbursts of fury, acts of selfishness, dissensions, factions, occasions of envy, drinking bouts, orgies, and the like. I warn you, as I warned you before, that those who do such things will not inherit the kingdom of God. In contrast, the fruit of the Spirit is love, joy, peace, patience, kindness, generosity, faithfulness, gentleness, self-control. Against such there is no law. Now those who belong to Christ [Jesus] have crucified their flesh with its passions and desires.[51]

Paul can accommodate the dichotomy of the body as good and the body as bad by creating another dichotomy—that between body and flesh. The idea of flesh captures the body's tendency to be led astray into bodily pleasures. Instead of the *body* dragging the soul down, as Plato would have it, it is the *flesh* that drags both body and soul in the wrong direction, the direction of sin. This way of expressing the dualistic nature of body is not unique to Paul, but it helped to imprint the notion of flesh on future generations of Christians. As Brown says, "Paul crammed into the notion of the flesh a superabundance of overlapping notions. The charged opacity of his language faced all later ages like a Rorschach test: it is possible to measure, in the repeated exegesis of a mere hundred words of Paul's letters, the future course of Christian thought on the human person."[52] The body might be essentially good, but the flesh is not, at least at the human level. At the same time, it should be remembered that the word flesh does not carry a negative connotation when it is used in relation to the Incarnation; "the Word was made Flesh" is a common way of expressing the fact that God took on a human body. So Paul's dichotomy is an artificial one, albeit one that endured.

Adam and Eve

Another important influence on the Christian view of the body is the story of the Fall, recounted in Genesis, and common to both Jews and Christians. Adam and Eve sinned. The result of their sin is that human nature entered a fallen state. The depth and extent of this fallen state is subject to different interpretations, but the idea of humanity being in a fallen state and needing redemption adds a further dimension to discussions of the body, especially in relation to sin. One of the most crucial aspects of the story is the fact that the Fall was the fault of Eve, the first woman, and it is Eve the temptress who survives in the Christian psyche. To this is added a large dose of guilt tied to the fact that Jesus' suffering and death on the cross is explained, in large part, as the act that accomplishes the redemption of man for the sin that drove Adam and Eve out of the Garden of Eden into their fallen state. Thus, the death and resurrection of Christ can be seen as a joyful, redemptive event, or as an occasion for guilt about man's original sin and his continuing sinful state—or both, resulting in another of the ambiguities that plague the Christian view of the body and of human nature.

The fact that there was a 'fall' means that there must have been an original 'perfect' state from which humanity had fallen. Tarnas refers to the Fall as "man's primal error bringing the dark knowledge of good and evil, the moral perils of freedom, the experience of alienation and death," an event through which "man had ruined the perfection of creation and divorced himself from the divine unity."[53] The Fall is a central notion of the Judeo-Christian religion and volumes could be, and have been, written about its meaning in relation to different dimensions of earthly life. It is used to explain the existence of evil in the world, and is also the source of the Christian idea of original sin. It was used for centuries as a justification for not probing too deeply into the knowledge of nature's secrets, an attitude that only came to an end with Francis Bacon's Great Instauration early in the seventeenth century.[54]

The existence of evil has also been used throughout the centuries as a justification for the denigration of woman (because Eve seduced Adam into eating the forbidden fruit) and woman's sexuality. These ramifications of the biblical story are well known. A less-discussed question about the story is one that preoccupied Augustine and is connected to our story about the body: What kind of bodies did Adam and Eve have? And a subsequent question arose as well: Did Adam and Eve have sex? One hypothesis, one that Augustine held but later revised, was that Adam and Eve did not have truly material bodies; their bodies were spiritual and only became material when they were chased from the Garden of Eden. John Rist explains this original spiritual body as being a kind of matter, but not flesh. He describes it in Neoplatonic terms as an envelope or bearer of the soul.[55] After the Fall, the body became matter. The body falling into matter is reminiscent of Plato's *Timaeus*, where the soul falls into the material body with the resultant confusion that we saw in Chapter 1. Augustine later changed his view of an original, non-fleshy body when he began thinking about resurrection. The resurrected body, he concludes, will be fleshy but nonetheless perfect: "the flesh itself will become spiritual."[56] Whatever the original state of Adam and Eve's bodies, for Augustine, the earthly body is a corruption of an original perfect body, and at the time of the resurrection, it will become that perfect body again.

As for whether or not Adam and Eve had sex, this was a debated question. The traditional interpretation of early Christian thinkers was that sexual relations, even in a married state (Adam and Eve were presumed to be man and wife), were incompatible with the original state, and had to have come about after the Fall, "the result of a sad decline, by which Adam and Eve had lapsed from an 'angelic' state into physicality, as so into death."[57] So, for them, there was no sex in Eden. But Augustine disagreed with this interpretation—at least in his later writings, once he had accepted that flesh and paradise were not incompatible. However, although he admitted that Adam and Eve would have had sexual intercourse, he maintained this would only have been for the purpose of begetting offspring and would have been secondary to a state of perfect friendship that they enjoyed with each other (an attitude that reflects his ideal of married life). Recall that Augustine himself was unable to achieve that state with a woman, and saw even a long-term relationship in which he was faithful to his mistress as merely an expression of lust. Augustine's ambivalence about sex would seem to be a clear case of theology following personal history:

> Sexual desire still disquieted Augustine. In mankind's present state, the
> sexual drive was a disruptive force. Augustine never found a way, any

more than did any of his Christian contemporaries, of articulating the possibility that sexual pleasure might, in itself, enrich the relations between husband and wife.[58]

When discussions about the body before the Fall are looked at in parallel with discussions about the body after the Resurrection, especially as related by Aquinas, one is faced with an interesting metaphysical conclusion about the body in Christianity: it began in a perfect state in the Garden of Eden, before earthly time, and it will arrive again at that perfect state at the Resurrection, at the end of earthly time. In between these two timeless places is earthly existence, in which the body exists in a fallen state, subject to the sins of the flesh (which, if not avoided or overcome, can threaten the final perfect state and lead instead to an end state of total suffering in hell). There are parallels with Plato, here: the timeless world of Forms, from which the soul comes and to which it will return, after an 'in-between' state in a body whose needs and desires make returning to the final perfect state difficult (the ever-present possibility of returning to Earth as a donkey). But there is one very important difference between the Christian story and the Platonic story: in the timeless, perfect state, whether before the Fall or after the final Resurrection, human beings, in the Christian story, are *embodied*. The body exists in the perfect, timeless realm, and it is good. The body may have its disruptive elements during its earthly life, but *it does not have to be shed* in order to achieve final perfection. It is about one body and one soul and their relation to God. Another major difference has already been pointed out: in Plato's transcendent, perfect realm, the soul participates in the perfect knowledge of the Forms; in the Christian otherworld, body and soul together participate in the perfect love of God.[59] The latter reflects the individual and personal nature of the Christian religion. However, it can be said that, as the Platonic body is an obstacle to perfect knowledge of the Forms, the Christian earthly body (in the form of flesh and especially in its sexuality) is an obstacle to the perfect love of God. The Christian may not have to flee the body to find God, but does have to overcome the flesh.

Woman

The Christian idea of an original perfect state of the body (whatever its degree of spirituality versus physicality) had ramifications for the female body and for the lives of women. Somehow women became the repositories of the mythical perfection of body through their virginity. Virginity is prized above everything "because the virginal body signifies most powerfully the incorruptibility of flesh which was ours in Paradise and will be fully restored in Christ."[60] This laid a heavy burden on women, whose virginity became an object of much male obsession. Ambrose, teacher of Augustine, whom Virginia Burrus refers to as a renowned recruiter and consecrator of virgins and theorist of virginity,[61] extended the symbolism of virginity in his writings to cover more than simple sexual purity. For him, virginity became a symbol for doctrinal purity, resulting in the all-too-frequent juxtaposition of the virgin and the harlot. Over the centuries, this opposition has served to control women's behaviour, especially their sexual behaviour.[62] The obsession with female virginity and the effort to control women's bodies are common to all patriarchal cultures, but one interesting aspect of the phenomenon in the early Christian world was the resistance of some women to this attempt at total bodily control. Many ascetic women chose to remain celibate. For example, Brown refers to the fecundity associated with the virgin state. Some upper-class and well-educated women chose to live as intellectuals, using their creativity for intellectual rather than maternal pursuits; such women actually enjoyed more advantages than many men. For example, Marcella, a fourth-century woman, spoke Greek, had a library well stocked with Greek books and used her home as a meeting place for visiting clergy. "For such a woman, virginal fertility implied a high level of creativity, in the mind, by word of mouth, and through the pen."[63] Again, there are parallels with Plato's discussion in the *Symposium* of intellectual offspring, although in this case it is women purposefully foregoing female fertility to follow the male urge to leave intellectual works, instead of real children, to posterity.

In the Middle Ages, women's resistance to the male obsession with their bodies took on different and dramatic forms, many of which revolved around food and fasting. Bynum explains that, for some late medieval women, "fasting became an obsession so overwhelming that modern historians have sometimes thought their stories preserve the earliest documentable cases of anorexia nervosa."[64] Although certain factors, such as control, provide tempting points of comparison with anorexia, Bynum does not believe that the comparison is appropriate, since the food and fasting experiences of medieval women played themselves out in a much broader cultural and religious context. In our day, women "cultivate not closeness to God but physical attractiveness by food abstinence, which they call *dieting*."[65]

For the most part, extreme fasting by medieval woman was a form of renunciation that was central to their spirituality. Men also practised renunciation, but for women the focus was on food and the body. As Bynum explains it, "each gender renounced and distributed what it most effectively controlled; men gave up money, property and progeny; women gave up food."[66] Marriage was not a happy state for women at this time, and voluntary starvation became a way for a woman to avoid unwanted husbands, brutal sexual relations and the dangers of childbirth. Thus, many of them substituted what we might consider a warped form of piety for the restricted worldly roles that were offered to them.

What is most interesting about the fasting practises of medieval women from the point of view of this narrative on the body is the connection between spirituality and flesh, or eating, which is linked to two of the central tenets of the Christian religion that we have already seen: the crucifixion and the Eucharist. "Late medieval theology emphasized Christ as suffering and Christ's suffering body as food,"[67] and this association seems to have been a preoccupation of women much more than of men. Not only was Christ believed to be food, but also woman herself was seen as food—the lactating virgin being a popular symbol of the time.[68] Further, the breast milk of women was seen as 'transmuted blood,' allowing an analogy between "a God who feeds humankind with his own blood in the eucharist and a human mother whose blood becomes food for her child."[69]

With such rich symbolism surrounding the female body and the idea of food and feeding, it can be seen that food was much more than simple sustenance for medieval women, and that the refusal to eat (or, in many cases, the inability to eat) took on dimensions far beyond modern notions of dieting and ideals of slimness. Fasting, for women, was a way of imitating Christ, fusing themselves with the suffering of Jesus, which, for those whose only food was the communion host, was joined to an ecstatic obsession with the Eucharist as an act of literally "feeding on the body of God."[70] From this point of view, refusing food is not a rejection of body but rather its exaltation; one unites with God not only spiritually but also physically. In Bynum's view, women did not see themselves (as male theologians did) as flesh opposed to spirit, or even as female opposed to male; they saw themselves as both flesh and spirit, male and female, and their bodies as a means of approaching the humanity of God.[71]

Much of the ambiguity and ambivalence surrounding the Christian view of the body is reflected in the stories of fasting medieval women; in the seemingly fantastic explanations of the resurrection of the body; in the speculations of bodily life in Eden and post-resurrection; as well as in the serious theological and philosophical explanations of the Incarnation and its meaning in relation to the human body, which have been discussed in this chapter. These have all left their mark on Western attitudes toward the body through the ages, and, in spite of the raised ontological status that the centrality of the body in Christianity should entail, this status has more often than not been diminished by a preoccupation with the body's role as the occasion of sin and as an impediment to salvation. However, as Bynum points out, it was in those early Christian centuries, in particular during the medieval period, that the body had a status that it would never again attain in Western thought. Our exploration of the body in the following chapters will reflect this, and give occasion to remember Augustine's plea to see himself healed as whole, body and soul. It will also allow us to assess the failure of Western philosophy, psychology and biology to bring an end to the dichotomy of body and soul in any meaningful way to this day.

Notes

1. My analysis is limited to Western Christianity and does not cover the Eastern Christian traditions.
2. Richard Tarnas, *The Passion of the Western Mind*, 100.
3. Some of the better-known Church Fathers were Tertullian, Clement, Justin, Origen and Augustine.
4. For example, Augustine reports a conversation with Simplianus (the 'spiritual father' of Ambrose) in which Simplianus warns Augustine against philosophers "full of fallacies and deceptions," while pointing out that, "in all the Platonic books God and his Word keep slipping in." Augustine, *Confessions*, ed. Henry Chadwick (Oxford: Oxford University Press, 1991), 135.
5. Tarnas, *Western Mind*, 108. Scott has a more down-to-earth view of the eventual acceptance of Christianity in the Roman world, stating that it was an "ideology uniquely suited to serve the needs of the dominant classes of Roman society. It provided a cosmic justification for the existing hierarchical order as rooted in human sinfulness and divine justice, and it encouraged every person to accept her or his place in that order." T. Kermit Scott, *Augustine: His Thought in Context* (Mahwah, NJ: Paulist Press, 1995, 57).
6. Terrence Irwin, *Classical Thought* (Oxford: Oxford University Press, 1989), 202.

7. It should be noted that this absorption of Greek thought and the resulting emergence of a formal Christian doctrine did not happen quickly; it took about four hundred years of conflict and accusations of heresy—and a number of ecclesiastical councils—to settle the many doctrinal disputes around conflicts between the old religious beliefs and practices and the new Christian ones. "The Councils of Nicaea (325CE) and Chalcedon (451CE) more or less define the period of fundamental theological argument and definition." Irwin, 204.

8. Hans Walter Wolff, *Anthropology of the Old Testament* (Philadelphia: Fortress Press, 1974), 10. Wolff attributes the narrowing of the meaning of this and other terms, such as 'heart,' 'flesh' and 'spirit,' to linguistic and cultural misunderstandings: "The question still has to be investigated of how, with the Greek language, a Greek philosophy has here supplanted Semitic biblical views, overwhelming them with foreign influence" (7).

9. Wolff, 13.

10. Wolff, 28.

11. The fact that *ruah* originally meant wind is interesting, since, for the very early Greeks, *pneuma* (breath) also meant wind, and for the ancient Chinese, the term *qi*, which is a term for vital energy as well as for breath, originally meant wind. See Shigehisa Kuriyama, *The Expressiveness of the Body* (New York: Zone Books, 2002), 242ff.

12. Wolff, 33.

13. This raises another important mystery of the Christian faith, the Trinity: God as Father, Son and Holy Spirit—three persons in one God, or one substance (as opposed to three gods), with God the Son being the actual person, Jesus Christ. According to Irwin, a "long series of reflexions, arguments, controversies, schisms, heresies, and persecutions resulted in some measure of agreement, eventually over most of the Christian world, on the doctrine of the Holy Trinity." The Council of Chalcedon in 451 settled the question when it declared that Christ was "one and the same Christ ... acknowledged as of two natures, unconfusedly, unchangeably, indivisibly, inseparably." See Irwin, 212, 213.

14. *New American Bible*, Saint Joseph Edition (New York: Catholic Book Publishing Co., 1987).

15. Tarnas, *Western Mind*, 102.

16. Margaret Ruth Miles, *Augustine on the Body* (Missoula, MT: Scholars Press, 1979), 84. In the case of Tertullian, his belief in a material soul, influenced by the Stoics, allows him easily to accept the union of body and soul in Jesus, but goes against traditional Christian belief in an immaterial soul. The Gnostics, on the other hand, would not even attribute physicality to Christ's *body*, believing that his body was an illusion. They believed that the notion that the Word was made Flesh was purely metaphorical. This belief, known as Docetism, was considered heretical.

17. According to Miles, "Augustine was the first of the fathers to recognize the full conceptual difficulty of the Incarnation because it was only in Augustine that the Stoicism of the earlier fathers and the Platonism of Plotinus and Porphyry came to full rational consciousness, and, therefore consciousness of conflict." Miles, *Augustine*, 92.

18. Caroline Walker Bynum, *Holy Feast and Holy Fast* (Berkeley: University of California Press, 1987), 263. Bynum emphasizes that medieval women did *not* internalize the male idea of their gender as inferior: "Women saw themselves not as flesh opposed to spirit, female opposed to male, nurture opposed to authority; they saw themselves as human beings—fully spirit and fully flesh.... Religious women in the later Middle Ages saw in their own female bodies not only a symbol of the humanness of both genders but also a symbol of—and means of approach to—the humanity of God" (296).

19. Section 1413 of the revised Catholic catechism states, "By the consecration the transubstantiation of the bread and wine into the Body and Blood of Christ is brought about. Under the consecrated species of bread and wine Christ himself, living and glorious, is present in a true, real, and substantial manner: his Body and his Blood, with his soul and his divinity (cf. Council of Trent: DS 1640; 1651." *Catechism of the Catholic Church*. English translation promulgated by Pope John Paul II on 8 September 1997. See www.scborromeo.org/ccc.htm (accessed 30 October 2008).

20. Caroline Walker Bynum, "Fast, Feast, and Flesh: The Religious Significance of Food to Medieval Women," *Representations*, 11 (Summer 1985): 2. However, according to Smith, the Eucharist emerged out of banquet traditions shared by Greeks, Romans, Jews and Egyptians, and only developed later into a "stylized symbolic meal governed by church order traditions that specified the prayers and the appropriate order and hierarchical leadership." Dennis E. Smith, *From Symposium to Eucharist: The Banquet in the Early Christian World* (Minneapolis: Fortress Press, 2003), 285.

21. Bynum, *Holy Feast*, 58.

22. Bynum, *Holy Feast*, 251.

23. Bynum, *Holy Feast*, 252.

24. Before any non-believers scoff at the notion of the resurrection (or at any notion of immortality), they might think about contemporary hopes of resurrection of the body through cryonics—freezing the body in a bath of liquid at -196 degrees. Strictly speaking, the hundred or so persons who have been cryopreserved to date, while legally dead, are not really dead—their 'life' is being preserved. According to Alcor, one of the world leaders in cryonics and cryonics research, these people are being kept alive "with the intent of restoring good health when technology becomes available to do so." Their status is compared that of frozen embryos

and not that of dead persons. The procedure can be performed after cardiac death but not after brain death. See http://www.alcor.org/index.html (accessed 30 July 2010). One might conclude that one does not have to be religious to hope for the resurrection of the body.

25.   I would like to emphasize, here, that these three articles of Christian doctrine are complex, that volumes have been written about them and that people were martyred over them. For purposes of this narrative, what is important relates not to the details, nor to the coherence of the doctrines themselves, but to the simple fact of the centrality of the notion of body to the Christian faith.

26.   Irwin, 214.

27.   Irwin, 215.

28.   Peter Brown, *Augustine of Hippo* (Berkeley: University of California Press, 1967, 2000), 300.

29.   He rejected it, but it left its mark on him in his interpretation of the Fall and of evil in the world, especially in his emphasis on concupiscence and sexuality, in which "the germ of the Neoplatonic and more extreme Manichaean dualism lived on." Tarnas, *Western Mind*, 145.

30.   John M. Rist, *Augustine: Ancient Thought Baptized* (Cambridge: Cambridge University Press, 1994), 18.

31.   Chadwick in the introduction to the *Confessions*, xviii.

32.   According to Miles, "Augustine felt himself to be what twentieth-century people might call a 'sex-addict,' and there are pleasures that addicts must deny themselves in order to maintain equilibrium in their lives. For Augustine, sex was consuming, totalitarian. As an addict, it was not possible for him to enjoy a sexual relationship in freedom. And so his conversion revolved around the resolution of this problem area in his life." Given the huge influence of the *Confessions* in subsequent centuries, his description of his own sexual problem contributed "to the subsequent glorification of the sexless life in Catholic Christianity." Margaret Miles, *Desire and Delight: A New Reading of Augustine's* Confessions (New York: Crossroad, 1992), 38.

33.   Augustine, *Sermon 30.4*, quoted in Rist, 92.

34.   Miles, *Desire*, 62. Miles points out that "Augustine pays the minutest attention to physical movements, feelings, and appearances in order to identify the state of the soul. Emotions, yearnings, even the truth of a human life are described as somatic: the soul's movements are describable only as physical events."

35.   Because much of the Greek corpus was lost at the time of the fall of Rome, only a few Latin translations of Greek works (Plato's *Timaeus* and *Phaedo*, and Aristotle's *De Anima*, for example) were available to the thinkers of the Middle Ages. This changed with the Crusades and the fall of Constantinople, when the original texts stored in the libraries of the East became available, along with

learned commentaries by Arab thinkers. "Medieval Europe's sudden encounter with a sophisticated scientific cosmology, encyclopaedic in breadth and intricately coherent, was dazzling to a culture that had been largely ignorant of these writings and ideas for centuries." Tarnas, *Western Mind*, 176.

36.   Tarnas, *Western Mind*, 188.

37.   Tarnas, *Western Mind*, 185.

38.   Tarnas, *Western Mind*, 188.

39.   Caroline Walker Bynum, *The Resurrection of the Body in Western Christianity, 200–1336* (New York: Columbia University Press, 1995), 155.

40.   *Catechism of the Catholic Church.* English translation promulgated by Pope John Paul II on 8 September 1997. See www.scborromeo.org/ccc.htm (accessed 30 October 2008).

41.   Bynum, *Resurrection*, 98.

42.   Bynum, *Resurrection*, 267, note 17.

43.   Bynum, *Resurrection*, 119. Bynum's text contains thirty-five plates of depictions of the last judgment and resurrection, many of which show scenes of animals regurgitating human body parts.

44.   Raymond Martin and John Barresi, *The Rise and Fall of Soul and Self* (New York: Columbia University Press, 2006), 58. It is not clear how this argument, made by Athenagoras in the second century, applies to the case of humans being eaten by lions or by cannibals, but Bynum (*Holy Feast and Holy Fast*) tells us that the chain consumption argument became increasingly important in the third century (33).

45.   From Victricius of Rouen, *De laude sanctorum*, ed. Jacob Mulders. Quoted in Bynum, *Resurrection*, 107.

46.   Bynum, *Resurrection*, 106.

47.   Bynum, *Resurrection*, 29.

48.   Bynum, *Resurrection*, 10.

49.   Bynum, *Resurrection*, 269.

50.   Peter Brown, *The Body and Society* (New York: Columbia University Press, 1988), 47.

51.   Letter to the Galatians (5:19) in *New American Bible*, 291.

52.   Brown, *Body and Society*, 48.

53.   Tarnas, *Western Mind*, 126.

54.   The influence of Francis Bacon and his Great Instauration will be discussed in Chapter 4.

55.   Rist, 98.

56.   Rist, 99.

57.   Brown, *Body and Society*, 399.

58.   Brown, *Body and Society*, 402.

59. To be fair to Plato's story, or at least one version of it, we should remember the connection between knowledge and love set out in the *Symposium*.

60. Virginia Burrus, "Word and Flesh: The Bodies and Sexuality of Ascetic Women in Christian Antiquity," *Journal of Feminist Studies in Religion*, 10 (1994): 33.

61. The notion of a 'theorist' of virginity certainly raises a few questions about the good Bishop's preoccupations!

62. Burrus, 31. "If the virgin represents a community whose boundaries are intact, the heretical harlot expresses the threatening image of a community whose boundaries are uncontrolled. Just as she allows herself to be sexually penetrated by strange men, so too she listens indiscriminately and babbles forth new theological formulations carelessly and without restraint: all the gateways of her body are unguarded" (36).

63. Brown, *Body and Society*, 370.

64. Bynum, *Holy Feast*, 4.

65. Bynum, *Holy Feast*, 298.

66. Bynum, *Holy Feast*, 193.

67. Bynum, *Holy Feast*, 260.

68. Aside from countless paintings of Mary with Jesus suckling at her breast, a number of paintings of the period portray the legend of Bernard of Claivaux being nursed by the Virgin Mary—a stream of her nurturing milk pouring out from her breast to the kneeling saint.

69. Bynum, *Holy Feast*, 270.

70. Bynum, *Holy Feast*, 200.

71. Bynum, *Holy Feast*, 296.

CHAPTER IV

From Astrology to the
Cult of Dissection:
The Renaissance

One of the threads of the first chapters of this book has been the notion of the macrocosm-microcosm, entailing the belief that a human being is a reflection in miniature of the cosmos and is in some manner connected with it. This is evident in the Platonic myth of creation, where the Demiurge creates the human soul out of the same material as the world-soul. In Plato's dualistic vision, it is the soul that reflects the cosmos, since the body, as an impermanent part of the ever-changing world, will die, and the soul will return again in another body. The Stoic monistic vision, forgoing the notion of immortality, is able to accommodate body and soul as a part of nature and as intimately tied to the cosmos through the *pneuma*. The tempered dualism of Christianity maintains elements of both the Platonic world-soul and the Stoic *pneuma*, while refusing the immanence of the divine so evident in the others. In these different worldviews—however the Earth and human being are conceived as connected to the cosmos, and whether that connection is direct or indirect—human life on Earth is at the centre of the cosmos and is influenced by it.

This chapter looks at the period of the Renaissance, in particular from the point of view of the concept of macrocosm-microcosm. As the name suggests, the Renaissance was a period of revival; it was also a period of tumult in all areas of activity: intellectual, artistic, economic, scientific and religious. "Such a prodigious development of human consciousness and culture had not been seen since the ancient Greek miracle at the very birth of Western civilization. Western man was indeed reborn."[1] Many structures of religion and society were transformed or dismantled in the process. The Protestant Reformation divided Christianity and put the authority of the Roman Church into question, at the same time as it ultimately resulted in a more secular society. Though the Copernican Revolution displaced planet Earth from the centre of the universe, the influence of the Renaissance humanists put man at the centre of earthly life, putting greater focus on life in the here-and-now, as opposed to a future life in paradise.

At the same time, the voyages of discovery to what came to be known as the New World both expanded the known horizons of the Earth and challenged the minds of its European inhabitants. Writing of Amerigo Vespucci's recognition of the enormous impact of the discoveries of the sixteenth-century explorers, Richard Popkin states:

> ...he quickly saw that all previous pictures of the world were false, that previous science and philosophy could not be relied on, and that the newly discovered lands to the west were new in a most radical sense—they had none of the moral and religious traditions and foibles of Christian Europe. The inhabitants of the new lands were people living according to nature and living, in some ways, a better life than that of the "civilized" Europeans.[2]

It is difficult to overestimate the revolutionary change that occurred during this period (usually defined as the years 1450 to 1600) and its impact on the future of Western thought—difficult, as well, to cover all of the thinkers whose ideas shaped the religious, secular, philosophical and scientific ferment of the time. However, the Renaissance represents a turning point with respect to centuries-old beliefs about the connection between man and the cosmos; at its beginnings, through an exalted philosophy of naturalism, the macrocosm-microcosm was front and centre in natural philosophy; at its end, the concept broke down, as the intellectual world moved to the mechanism of the scientific revolution and the beginnings of modernity. This chapter traces the evolution of perceptions of the human body through this dramatic philosophical shift from naturalism to mechanism, in particular through a discussion of three of the many influential thinkers of the time: Marsilio Ficino (1433–1499), Andreas Vesalius (1514–1564) and Michel de Montaigne (1533–1592).[3]

Renaissance Naturalism

The terms 'nature' and 'naturalism' have many different meanings, depending on both the context and the historical period. In this chapter, 'naturalism' is meant to describe philosophies of the Renaissance, which, by reviving certain Platonic and Neoplatonic views of nature, relied on explanations of the cosmos that were principally holistic and, to varying degrees, animistic. While it is difficult to encompass all Renaissance philosophers within one definition, the following captures the essence of the naturalism of this period:

> The universe of most of the philosophers of nature, like that of the Neoplatonists, was an enchanted world of ensouled objects linked together and joined to a higher realm of spirit and absolute being. A universal world-soul pervades all creation and makes all creatures, even rocks and stones, alive and sentient in some degree.[4]

Although the animism inherent in this view is difficult to reconcile with the Christian view of a transcendent God, Renaissance naturalism represented what Dupré refers to as the "retheologising" of nature. It was a reaction to the weakened link between the Creator and the world order evident in the philosophy of the Middle Ages, and it attempted to reaffirm that link through an emphasis on immanence as opposed to transcendence.[5]

Naturalism represents a philosophy of nature that embraces cosmology and metaphysics. But it also has its anthropological dimension in which the human person is part of nature, often at a given level in the hierarchy of being. Thus, the cosmological and metaphysical transformations that mark the move from naturalism to mechanism in science have an anthropological counterpart that will be played out in Descartes' approach to the human body (which will be examined in Chapter 5). Naturalistic explanations of the body (seen as a living part of living nature) are quite different from mechanistic ones (where both the human body and nature itself are explained by laws governing inert matter). The result of the move from naturalism to mechanism is a transformed notion of the human body and the human person.

One of the crucial aspects of the move from naturalism to mechanism concerns the relation of consciousness (mind or soul) and nature, and whether or not these two must be separated in any scientific explanation of the world. For the naturalistic philosophies of the Renaissance, the answer is a definitive no; all of nature is in some way alive, and to some extent conscious, and any explanation of the world must accommodate this fact. In relation to the body, this means that there are direct links with the living cosmos, which can be demonstrated, for example, through astrology and magic. It also means, in relation to the soul, that there is a closer link between God and his creation than Christian theology could comfortably accommodate. That this was not problematic at the time might be seen by modern eyes as strange, but it is an indication of what is often called the *syncretism* of the Renaissance: many apparently contradictory elements found their place in an approach to truth that was very inclusive. Thus, explains Richard Tarnas, "the Mother Church, mediatrix between God and man, matrix of Western culture, now assembled and integrated all her diverse elements: Judaism and Hellenism, Scholasticism and Humanism, Platonism and Aristotelianism, pagan myth and biblical revelation."[6]

There were many reasons for this syncretism, a predominant one being the recovery and translation of original works of Plato and other Greek writers. The original works of the Greeks, which had been lost to the Christian world, had been preserved in the Byzantine world; they became available to Western scholars at the time of the fall of Constantinople. Thus, scholars now had access to the original Plato and other ancient writers, which resulted in a revival of pre-Christian thought, especially Platonism. Although Christian thinkers knew of Plato, this had been the Christianized Plato of Augustine, who had, as we have seen, absorbed his Plato through Plotinus and knew little of the original. Now, thinkers began to assimilate classical myths and ideas with the ideas inherited from the Scholastics and the Church Fathers. "A flexible syncretism was emerging, encompassing diverse traditions and perspectives, with Platonism espoused as a new gospel."[7] This syncretism would not endure, but while it lasted, ideas flourished that were heretical before and would be heretical after the Renaissance, and glorified notions of the human body flourished with them.

The Naturalistic Body: Marsilio Ficino (1433–1499)

The Renaissance naturalists had different ways of explaining the human body, but in most of them human beings are seen as being integrally linked to the cosmos, often through different levels of being. There are higher creatures than humans (e.g., angels) and lower creatures (e.g., animals); the soul may partake in the higher levels, but both soul and body are affected by the heavens. Marsilio Ficino's philosophy of the body is interesting for two reasons: he was one of the few philosophers who wrote specifically and at length about the body and medicine, and his major work on the body (called *De vita*[8]) was extremely influential. It was reprinted thirty times, and the last edition was published in 1647, 148 years after his death and only three years before the death of Descartes.[9]

Ficino was a priest, a doctor and a philosopher who translated the works of both Plato and Plotinus.[10] Like most of his contemporaries, Ficino's approach to philosophy was syncretic; his cosmology is partly Platonic, partly Neoplatonic (particularly in relation to his gradations of being), partly Stoic (he integrates the notion of seminal reasons and a *pneuma*-like world-soul) and, of course, partly Christian (strongly influenced by Augustine). This syncretism is fundamental to Renaissance epistemology and cosmology. In it is expressed the idea that diverse notions and beliefs reflect an underlying unity of being and, therefore, truth. Each of these visions of reality expresses an aspect of the ultimate truth in a different way, and none is rejected. This is a reflection of the Neoplatonic metaphysical assumption that, "there is an ultimate cause and principle, the One, which causes everything in existence and functions as an ultimate explanation for all being."[11] Because of this essential unity, the One and the many are ultimately the same reality, where each level of being reflects every other. The most obvious case, for the Renaissance naturalists, was the notion of the microcosm participating in and reflecting the macrocosm.

Eugenio Garin, writing about Ficino's efforts to define the structures of his planes of reality and their correspondences, states that,

> all the difficulties of his thought are diminished if one grasps the point of the union: what he in fact calls the 'concord of the world' *(concordia mundi)*, and which is expressed as the refraction, slowly moving on different planes, of that living unity which is the cosmos, in which each individualisation in turn is the synthesis of all the others.... And all are 'formal' manifestations of the one living heart of the universe, different signs of that unique living reality which, in its turn, is the same infinite refraction of life.[12]

Like the world of the Stoics, Ficino's universe is a living whole that includes the equivalent of the *pneuma*, which he calls the world-soul. The world-soul contains all things, and, in Ficino's words, "she is equally connected with everything, even with those things which are at a distance from one another, because they are not at a distance from her."[13] As he puts it in *De vita*, the universe is a continuum and it is alive:

> That the cosmos is animate just like any animate thing, and more effectively so, not only Platonic arguments but also the testimony of Arabic astrologers thoroughly proves. In the same works, the Arabic writers also prove that by an application of our spirit to the spirit of the cosmos, achieved by physical science and our affect, celestial goods pass to our soul and body.[14]

For Ficino, reality is comprised of five levels: bodies (which are extended matter, passive and infinitely divisible); qualities (which are powers or material forms that cannot exist apart from matter and can transmit motion without initiating it); souls (which give life to bodies); angels (which guide souls—also called Reason, or the agent intellect); and God (which is pure unity). The five levels represent a living hierarchy, with each degree influencing the one next to it in an ascending or descending manner. Ficino insists on the harmony of all levels of the cosmos and on the presence of one animating principle.

As a doctor and the son of a doctor, Ficino grew up with astrology and practised it as part of his medical training and practice. (That astrology was part of the doctor's repertoire is not surprising, since, in the medical thought of the time, there was a link between the movements of the heavens and changes in bodily humours. Magic, as well, was a physician's tool, used to counteract the fate revealed by the astrological chart). For Ficino, the universe is more than an impersonal system of causes and effects. Human personality intervenes in the causal chain through the celestial powers, using them in "fictitious material representations, talismans and amulets, capable of absorbing and concentrating astral forces."[15]

Thus, Ficino practised both astrology and magic, and *De vita* is devoted to demonstrating how the human body is connected with the heavens and can be influenced and cured by heavenly forces. The third book of *De vita* is titled *On Obtaining Life from the Heavens*, and subtitled *In What, According to Plotinus, the Power of Attracting Favor from the Heavens Consists, Namely, That Well-adapted Physical Forms Can Easily Allure the World-soul and the Souls of the Stars and the Daemons.*[16] While this long title has a magical air, the magic in which Ficino is interested is natural magic, "ways of using plants, stones, musical sounds, and other natural objects as sources of unusual power without any appeal to personal, supernatural agents such as demons or angels."[17]

The concept of world-soul is central to Ficino; it is also called spirit or medical spirit.[18] It is an intermediary in Ficino's world hierarchy, and can be called upon for human benefit:

> You will bend your efforts to insinuate into yourself this spirit of the world above all, for by this as an intermediary you will gain certain natural benefits not only from the world's body but from its soul, and even from the stars and the daemons. For this spirit is an intermediary between the gross body of the world and its soul; and the stars and daemons exist in it and by means of it.[19]

This spirit is available to us through all the things in the universe; we can, according to Ficino, "by way of certain preparations, lay claim to celestial things. For these lower things were made by the heavens, are ruled continually by them, and were prepared from up there for celestial things in the first place."[20] Further, certain things are governed by certain planets. For example, one "obtains things from Venus through ... sapphire, lapis lazuli, brass, coral, and all pretty, multicolored or green colors and flowers, musical harmony and pleasant odors and tastes," while one obtains favours from the Moon through "things that are white, moist, and green and through silver and crystal and pearls and silver marcasite.... To get something from Saturn we use any materials that are somewhat earthy, dusky and leaden.... From Mars, materials which are fiery or red, red brass, all sulphurous things, iron, and bloodstone...."[21] These materials, whose qualities are related to their respective celestial bodies, can draw desired effects from them.

A Renaissance doctor had to bear a number of things in mind before treating a patient, including the patient's astral chart and how it related to his own, the relation between the infected parts of the body and their governing planets, and the position of the stars and planets at the moment of medication! Thus, "you must remember that Aries has power over the head and face; Taurus over the neck; Gemini, the forearms and shoulders; Cancer the breast, lungs, stomach and upper arms."[22] Depending on your ascendant sign, it could be harmful to take medicine when the Moon is in Capricorn (but acceptable when it is in Pisces), or to induce vomiting when the Moon is in Libra; purgatives should only be taken when the Moon is in Cancer, Pisces or Scorpio. The doctor plays the role of mediator between the stars and the patient. Ficino agrees with Galen that, "astrology is necessary for the physician,"[23] and his book is a veritable font of information on how to use it.

De vita provides an epistemological model that includes and links several concepts pivotal to Ficino's astrology and medicine. The first is analogy or sympathy. There are qualities—such as colour, texture or shape—in the microcosm that are analogous to the qualities in the macrocosm (for example, the analogy between the moon and things that are white, moist and green). "Argument from analogy crowds out argument from those material causes and effects which are the staple of modern science ... [moreover, analogy is] the very energy that holds the Neoplatonic cosmos together and hence the basis of those sympathies by which sympathetic magic operates."[24] The ultimate analogous structure is cosmic sympathy manifested in the *musica mundana* and representing the overall harmony of the universe.[25]

The second pivotal concept is mediation—a hierarchy of being where there are no gaps and which allows for the interconnectedness of all things. The world-soul is a mediator, as are the seminal reasons, "the agents of the World-soul's generative activity in matter,"[26] and the medical spirits. The heavenly bodies are alive and act as "a mezzanine between the planes of material and immaterial, man and God."[27] Translated into anthropological terms, the Renaissance theorists held that the human body and soul were connected by a third element, which Raymond Klibansky et al. refers to as "the 'medium', the 'vinculum', or the 'copula', between the other two...." Further, as he explains, "the division of human nature into body, soul and 'spiritus humanus' corresponded to a similar division of the universe into universal matter, universal mind and 'spiritus mundanus.'"[28] In Ficino, as with most Renaissance naturalists, everything is more or less alive; he cannot accept a view that accepts life in the lowliest animal or plant, but not in the heavens or the cosmos, which for Ficino (as for Plato and the Stoics) is a living being.

Both sympathy and mediation are founded on the belief that there is a continuum from form to matter, from thought to sensible beings. Thus, an intelligible cause can produce a sensible effect, or a sensible cause can produce an intelligible effect. At the same time, it must be emphasized that, in Ficino, the human mind escapes the determinism of the stars and can actually will the influence of one star rather than another. As explained by Klibansky, et al.,

> Man as an active and thinking being was fundamentally free, and could
> even, thanks to this freedom, harness the forces of the stars by consciously
> and willingly exposing himself to the influence of a certain star; he

could call such an influence down upon himself not only by employing the manifold outward means, but also (more effectually) by a sort of psychological autotherapy, a deliberate ordering of his own reason and imagination.[29]

Thus, the multiplicity of Ficino's levels of being—so foreign to modernity—is, in fact, a variation on the Renaissance Neoplatonic unity referred to earlier. Since everything reflects the one underlying unity, the role of the philosopher, the doctor or the priest (and Ficino was all three) was to find the similarities in the various levels of being (in particular, between macrocosm and microcosm); to decode the signs and make the links that allow for an understanding of the place of the human being in the cosmic hierarchy; and, particularly in the case of the doctor, to know how to invoke the forces of the different levels to cure the sick and to maintain the healthy.

From the point of view of our modern dualistic and mechanistic thinking, which has difficulty accepting the interaction of mind and matter, the idea of harnessing the forces of the stars falls into the realm of fantasy. We must bear in mind, however, as we did in looking at Plato and the Stoics, what Ficino was trying to explain. In his epistemological framework, mind and matter find themselves on a continuum of being, and from that perspective interaction is neither impossible nor unreasonable. Mechanistic science rejects the idea of a continuum of being, accepting only material causes and mechanistic laws of nature. Even though many believe that credible evidence exists about the possibility of correspondences between the stars and human activity, any such evidence must confront a fundamental question of modern mechanistic science: How can the planets influence events on the Earth if no physical forces have been observed that could cause those events? This question reflects, in Tarnas' view, "the residual strength of materialist and mechanistic assumptions in contemporary scientific thought, even after the conceptual shifts introduced by quantum physics."[30] Tarnas believes that we actually have the philosophical, scientific, technological and psychological tools to take a serious new look at astrology. To do so, however, means questioning the materialist and mechanistic assumptions concerning causality and correlation that have held sway since the scientific revolution:

Instead of the linear causal mechanisms of matter and force assumed in a Newtonian universe, the continuous meaningful coincidence between celestial patterns and human affairs seems rather to reflect a fundamental underlying unity and correspondence between the two realms—macrocosm and microcosm, celestial and terrestrial—and thus the intelligent coherence of a living, fully animate cosmos. The postulation of a systematic correspondence of this kind implies a universe in which mind and matter, psyche and cosmos, are more pervasively related or radically united than has been assumed in the modern world view.[31]

Ficino would be very comfortable with this explanation, and it might not be as unscientific as many might think, as demonstrated by the following description of what quantum physicists refer to as the Zero Point Field:

> The existence of the Zero Point Field implied that all matter in the universe was interconnected by waves, which are spread out through time and space and can carry on to infinity, tying one part of the universe to every other part. The idea of The Field might just offer a scientific explanation for many metaphysical notions, such as the Chinese belief in the life force, of *qi*, described in ancient texts as something akin to an energy field."[32]

It might also offer a scientific explanation for what Ficino was attempting to explain: the interconnection of all things. In the final analysis, the Chinese *qi*, the Stoic *pneuma* and Ficino's medical spirits might be neither more nor less fantastical than the Zero Point Field, which is taken seriously by at least some physicists of our time. For Tarnas and other current thinkers, there is a new vision of reality emerging, one that rejects mechanism and is capable of providing "a general conceptual framework that in many respects [is] not inherently incompatible with the astrological perspective."[33] The *concordia mundi* of the Renaissance might be worth re-examining in light of the emerging paradigm. This is a point that will be emphasized again in the later chapters of this narrative.

Unravelling the Macrocosm-Microcosm: Copernicus and Vesalius

The year 1543 is pivotal in the history of mechanism. This is the date of the publication of two important works, which—while unconnected at the time of their publication—had a double influence on the work of Descartes and, ultimately, on his application of the principles of mechanism to the human body. The first, long recognized for its importance and influence, was Copernicus' *De revolutionibus orbium coelestium*. The second, less well-known but in many ways equally influential, was Vesalius' *De fabrica*, the first scientific work of anatomy. The coincidence of the publication date of these two pivotal works is symbolic in the history of the human body; what Copernicus did to prepare the way for the mechanization of the cosmos, Vesalius did to prepare the way for the mechanization of the human body, the body-machine of Descartes and the development of modern medicine.

This coincidence has not gone unremarked by those whose concern is the human body. The French anthropologist David Le Breton writes that the publication of *De Fabrica* and *De Revolutionibus* in the same year marks the beginning of the invention of the body in Western thought.[34] Hans Jonas has also remarked that the appearance of these two works in the same year "is symbolic of the two sides of the scientific revolution as it eventually took shape: the macrocosmic and the microcosmic, the abstract and the concrete, the mathematical and the empirical...."[35]

Neither Copernicus nor Vesalius made the link between their revolutionary works and the development of mechanistic science, but each played a role in the withdrawal of the cosmic soul and the human soul from natural philosophy. They also provided the basis for a reconceptualization of matter—both natural and human—which would hereafter be interpreted as inert. The major implication of Copernicus' notion of Earth revolving around the sun (along with the subsequent realization that Earth was a planet like all the others) was nothing less than the rupture of the cosmic hierarchy. The notion of macrocosm and microcosm, of the sublunar world as a reflection of the cosmos, would have to give way.[36] The ramifications of Copernicus' theory were not immediately evident to religious authorities, and it was not the Catholic Church but the Protestant reformers (with their focus on Scripture as absolute authority) who initially objected to the heliocentric theory. After 1600, however, the threat to Christian cosmology, theology and even morality became evident, and the Catholic Church, already traumatized by the conflict and heresy of the Reformation, "mustered its considerable powers of suppression and condemned in no uncertain terms the heliocentric hypothesis...."[37] If the Earth moved, it could not be the fixed centre of the universe as the Scriptures maintained, and this called into question the creation of the world and the ultimate salvation of its earthly inhabitants. This was true heresy, even atheism.

Galileo: Sunspots and Inclined Planes

It was Galileo's observations and experiments that signalled the demise of the ancient cosmology and brought about the real Copernican Revolution, along with the wrath of the Church and its Inquisition. As we have seen, one of the pillars of both classical thought and the naturalism of the Renaissance was the idea of the macrocosm and the microcosm, and—whatever the number of levels posited within the cosmic hierarchy—it was held that what was above (the heavenly realm) was perfect and immutable, while what was below (the earthly realm) was imperfect and always changing. Further, the heavenly matter was believed to be essentially different from earthly matter. While the latter was made up of the four elements—earth, air, fire and water—celestial matter was supposed to be made up of a fifth element: the ether or the quintessence. Steven Shapin describes the quintessence as incorruptible matter subject to different principles than the other elements: "So while earth tends to fall until it reaches the center of the universe, and air and fire tend to rise, the heavens and heavenly bodies naturally tend to move in perfect circles, and the stuff of which they are made is itself perfect and immutable."[38] Further, the notion of a world-soul (from Plato to the Renaissance) entails the idea that a spark of the heavenly perfection, the quintessence, permeates the earthly realm, and, through the notion of a final cause or *telos*, directs its workings.

Along with proving that the Earth revolved around the sun (not vice versa) and was thus neither the centre of the universe nor, in fact, below the heavens, Galileo's telescope offered evidence against both the presumed perfection and immutability of the heavenly realm and its influence on earthly objects and events. Evidence of the former came in the form of sunspots, what Galileo referred to as "these importunate spots which have come to disturb the heavens, and worse still, the Peripatetic philosophy."[39] Galileo's discovery that sunspots were actually *on* the sun (and not revolving around it, as had been speculated) showed two things: that the sun was not a perfectly luminous body, but contained impurities or imperfections in the form of spots; and that the apparent movement of the spots was actually due to the movement of the sun on its own axis—a movement similar to the rotation of the Earth on its axis.

The results of Galileo's observations were both metaphysical and epistemological; they changed perceptions of what the natural world is, as well as how we can have knowledge of it. Moreover, states Shapin, "by asserting the similarity of heavenly and terrestrial bodies, Galileo implied that studying the properties and motions of ordinary earthly bodies could afford understanding of what nature was like universally."[40] This, in effect, turned the macrocosmic/microcosmic paradigm on its head. Instead of the Earth being perceived as an imperfect reflection of the celestial world, the heavens came to be perceived as being composed of bodies similar to earthly bodies and subject to the same laws. This is what made the discoveries of Galileo's telescope so threatening to the established epistemological and theological order.

Thus, Galileo set about studying the properties and motions of ordinary earthly objects in order to obtain an understanding of the order of the universe. Among the earthly objects he used to describe experiments were stones rolling on inclined planes.[41] These experiments ultimately led him to the theory that there are no forces inherent in objects which cause them to move, and that an object will either remain at rest or in motion until some external force causes it either to accelerate or decelerate. This is the principle of the conservation of motion that is fundamental to the principle of inertia. That Galileo did not arrive at a fully elaborated principle of inertia[42] does not lessen the importance of his work or the radical nature of his contribution to the development of mechanistic science. His inferences from the experiments with inclined planes contradicted the long-standing position that the state of rest was the natural state for earthly objects, and negated the idea of immanent movement caused either by the formal or material qualities of the object or by the existence of a world-soul permeating earthly matter. The idea that matter is inert was born, and movement was now open to explanation solely by efficient causes. The death-blow was thus rendered to explanation by final causes and, ultimately, to the Aristotelian doctrine of the four causes.[43] Through Copernicus and then Galileo, the way to the mechanization of the 'world picture' had begun.[44]

Vesalius and the Culture of Dissection

The move to the mechanization of the 'body picture' came from another direction—one unrelated, on the surface, to the Copernican or Galilean projects. It was the anatomical work of Vesalius that initiated the practice of dissection as an acceptable scientific enterprise for the study of the body. Until that time, the writings of the Roman physician/philosopher Galen had guided medical study and practice, even though Galen's anatomical investigations never included the dissection of humans.[45] Galen was the recognized authority on the functioning of the human body, and any dissection that took place before

Vesalius was carried out with the object of confirming, not questioning, his writings. However, as Galileo questioned the authority of Aristotle, Vesalius questioned the authority of Galen by recognizing only the higher authority of empirical observation. If there was a contradiction between what he observed in his dissections and what Galen wrote in his books, then it was Galen who stood corrected, not Vesalius.

In the history of anatomy, Vesalius is rightly considered a revolutionary. At a time when the lesser-ranking surgeon or barber wielded the dissection knife, while the doctor explicated from medical texts, Vesalius the doctor held the knife himself. He was the expert; it was up to him to push the limits of anatomical knowledge and to contradict, if necessary, the ancient authority. He approached the cadaver as an object of science. At the same time, his work remains situated within the Renaissance context where the human body was still conceived as an integral part of nature. His drawings of the skeleton or of the *écorché* are always placed in a natural setting—standing in a field surrounded by trees and bushes, seated on a bench, and even, in one often-seen drawing of a skeleton, leaning on a tomb. The body remains contextualized in a life-like pose in a life-like setting; its objectification has begun, but is not yet complete. Vesalius' cadaver is partly object and partly subject. In some drawings, it holds up its own flayed skin, which is no longer part of itself. In Le Breton's words, it has become a caricature of the microcosm, but the latter has not yet disappeared completely.[46] This is the beginning of the body as an object of knowledge. Vesalius did not invent the practice of dissection of human cadavers, far from it—but he presided over the beginnings of the activity as a normal scientific practice. Throughout the entire period of the Middle Ages, the Church either forbade or strictly controlled the practice. For some Christian thinkers, the person was still present as long as the flesh was on the cadaver, so dissection was seen as interfering with the work of nature and the dying person. This idea may not resonate with the modern scientific spirit (although beliefs about the residue of soul or self in the dead body are strong in modern Japan, for example, where death is not final until the family has declared it so), but it was the result of the ambiguity that surrounded the connection between body and soul. In the pre-Cartesian world, and particularly within the context of the Christian belief in the resurrection of the body, precise boundaries between the mind and body, the living and the dead were less easy to draw, and respect for the dead body was paramount. Even as dissection became a more regular practice, the availability of corpses was strictly controlled by the religious authorities, and the only bodies given up to the practice were those of executed criminals, for whom a sentence of hanging followed by dissection brought double humiliation to the victim and his or her family.[47]

The practice of dissection in the Renaissance aroused both fascination and revulsion. The body was considered to house the secrets of the self, so opening it up to explore its insides was seen as a way of unveiling these secrets. Helkiah Crooke, an anatomical writer of the time, wrote: "anatomy is as it were a most certaine and sure guide to the admirable and most excellent knowledge of our selves, that is of our owne proper nature."[48] Dissections were carried out in theatres in front of large audiences—students of medicine, as well as society ladies, merchants and ordinary folk—with a definite air of spectacle. At the same time, the corpses available were generally those of criminals. This marriage of spectacle and prohibition symbolizes the ambiguity of the emerging culture of dissection, along with its break with past thought and practice. With Vesalius, the body was not yet the inert matter that it would become with Descartes, and it had not yet lost its value as a mirror of the cosmos. But in the almost one hundred years that separated De fabrica from Descartes' writings on the body, dissections continued, no soul was found in the process, the wrath of God did not descend upon the anatomist, and the search for "our owne proper nature" was abandoned in favour of purely scientific knowledge of the body. As Jonathan Sawday explains, the seventeenth-century anatomist

> no longer stood before the body as though it was a mysterious continent. It had become, instead, a system, a design, a mechanically organised structure, whose rules of operation, though still complex, could, with the aid of reason, be comprehended in the most minute detail.[49]

The body moved from being the incarnation of the cosmos to being an object of science, devoid of mind, soul and self. "Mechanism offered the prospect of a radically reconstituted body"; and this radical reconstitution represented a move "from an interior in which the body seems ... to speak its own part, to the modern conception of a physiological system no more capable of speech than is a hydraulic pump...."[50] The body moved from being a source of knowledge (of the self) to an object of knowledge (for the knowing subject). At the same time, the subject (anatomist, scientist) moved from a position of observation to one of systematic control of, and power over, both nature and the body.

Giving the Body Its Due: Michel de Montaigne

As the Renaissance was coming to a close, one thinker, the French philosopher and essayist Michel de Montaigne (1533–1592), embodied several of the characteristics of the period, in particular its scepticism. The sceptical writings of Sextus Empiricus (160–219 CE) were among the ancient texts that became available during this period, and, combined with the syncretism already referred to, they contributed to a revival of scepticism. The period of tolerance, with its acceptance of the idea that truth is not singular but multiple, was coming to a close, but as it did so, Montaigne "gave modern voice to the ancient epistemological doubts."[51] He also gave voice to a somewhat Stoic appreciation of the human body as a source of knowledge that would be challenged and ultimately obliterated as a result of the objectification of the body initiated by the work of Vesalius and reinforced by Descartes and the scientific revolution.

Montaigne's most famous work is simply titled *Essays*. It is a three-volume work comprising more than a hundred essays dealing with topics ranging from the most intimate and personal observations to sweeping commentaries on human nature and the events of his time. Living during a time of religious strife, he was the opposite of a dogmatist, believing that many of the theoretical and theological questions, over which Catholics and Protestants fought each other and were ready to die, were beyond the scope of human reason. He did not believe that rational argument was adequate to respond to the metaphysical musings of the philosophers (or the theologians); for every opinion, there was at least one contrary opinion, and who could say which is right? "Is it not better to remain in doubt," he asks, "than to get entangled in the many errors produced by human fantasy? Is it not better to postpone one's adherence indefinitely than to intervene in factions, both quarrelling and seditious?"[52] A slogan for which he is well known is: "Que sais-je?" (What do I know?); he lived by this slogan at a time when Protestants and Catholics were killing each other over their beliefs. In spite of his scepticism, Montaigne was a Catholic and a statesman (he served in public offices, including as a member of the Parliament of Bordeaux), retiring to the tower of his chateau to write his essays only in the later years of his life. He was one of the Renaissance humanists, who, according to Stephen Toulmin, "regarded human affairs in a clear-eyed, non-judgmental light that led to honest practical doubt about the value of 'theory' for human experience—whether in theology, natural philosophy, metaphysics, or ethics."[53]

This sceptical cast of Montaigne (and the other humanists) is important in this narrative mostly because of the contrast it represents to the quest for certainty, which will be the hallmark of the next century and, in particular, the philosophy of Descartes. As much as Montaigne thought that only fools have made up their minds and are certain, Descartes thought that the search after certainty was a laudable and necessary objective, one to which he devoted his life.

Anyone who has read even a few of Montaigne's essays knows that they are heavily sprinkled with quotations. The voices of the past, the writings of the ancient philosophers and poets, speak through him. He hears the voice of the past, absorbs it, digests it, transforms it; then he speaks with his own voice—a voice mediated by, and blended with, these voices of the past. At the same time, the *Essays* are a dialogue with himself—as he added to his texts without deleting what he had written earlier, even if the result was contradictory. Partly this was because he believed that he remained responsible for what he had written in the past, even when he was no longer in agreement with it. But he also questioned whether what he thought later was necessarily better than what he had thought earlier, and is well-known for his statement, "'I' now and 'I' then are certainly twain, but which 'I' was better? I know nothing about that."[54] For him, there is no single truth; conforming to the syncretism of the period, truth, for Montaigne, is multiple. In the end, his *Essays* form a kind of tapestry, a "web of multidimensional cultural materials"[55] that encompasses what Montaigne has read, written and experienced.

As much as Montaigne and the humanists absorbed the past, Descartes (in spite of having had a similar education) would reject it. For Montaigne, separating himself from the past was impossible; for Descartes, it would be impossible to do otherwise. As the world moved from the syncretism and scepticism of the Renaissance humanists of the sixteenth century to the quest for certainty of the rationalists of the seventeenth, dogmatism and intolerance would increase. Absorbing the writings, experiences and traditions of the past would cede pride of place to wiping the slate clean; philosophers such as Descartes would claim "that all truly philosophical problems must be stated in terms independent of any historical situation, and solved by methods equally free of all contextual references...."[56] As we will see in Chapter 5, Descartes' preoccupation with certainty and method will be, in large measure, a reaction to the uncertainty induced by Renaissance scepticism.[57]

It is not only Montaigne's scepticism that sets him apart from Descartes; the self-portrait that is cobbled together in the *Essays* is a portrait of the man, body and soul:

> Those who wish to take our two principal pieces apart and to sequester one from the other are wrong. We must on the contrary couple and join them closely together. We must command the soul not to withdraw to its quarters, not to entertain itself apart, not to despise and abandon the body....[58]

Often, reading the *Essays*, one has the feeling that Montaigne goes a little too far in recounting the trivialities of his life; from his size and shape to his hairiness, his likes and dislikes, the frustrations of his malady (kidney stones), his sex life, no detail is too small or too personal to include in his portrait, which is for him a work of self-knowledge. For him, introspection cannot be limited to examining the mind or soul; knowledge of self is corporeal as well as spiritual and mental. In the *Essays*, he looks at himself body and soul, and, in the process, body functions can be seen to be very central to his self-portrait. His purpose is not to give a picture of 'Man,' but "of a particular one of them who is very badly formed and whom I would truly make very different from what he is if I had to fashion him afresh.... I am not portraying being but becoming...."[59]

Montaigne was born less than a decade before the publication of Vesalius' *De fabrica*, and he must have been well aware, by the time he was writing, of the developing science of anatomy and the changing face of medicine. But he had little use for doctors (a malady he says he inherited, along with his kidney stones, from his father and his grandfather), and less still for the evolving science of anatomy led by the work of Vesalius. According to Jean Starobinski, Montaigne was not impressed with the open-air spectacle of the anatomy theatre:

> Over the long run such careful inventories of the human organism would augment the powers of science whose promises Montaigne held to be illusory. All signs suggest that Montaigne remained indifferent to the corrections that a rejuvenated science of anatomy was making to ancient medieval texts.... While anatomists busied themselves with the refutation of Galen and with bettering Galen's observations, Montaigne was looking back to a stage in the history of medicine well before Galen, to the Socratic

idea that each individual is competent to govern all aspects of his own life, the diet of the body as well as the diet of the soul.[60]

Montaigne was a firm believer in self-knowledge through the body, in the body's own wisdom, and in the knowledge that comes to it through the senses. In his writings, he does not eschew the pleasures of the body, believing instead that the "soul should assist and applaud the body, not refuse to participate in its natural pleasures but delight in it as if it were its husband."[61] He is interested not only in what his mind tells him, but also, and even more so, in what his body tells him. "Abstract concepts and formal arguments, intuitive ideas and propositions are not the only grist for a philosopher's mill: rather, he can attend to the whole of human experience, in varied, concrete detail."[62] Like the Stoics, he writes of living in accordance with nature, which he describes as a gentle, wise and just guide to life, if only we would pay attention:

> I seek her traces everywhere: we have jumbled them together with the tracks of artifice and thereby that sovereign good of the Academics and Peripatetics, which is to live according to Nature, becomes for that very reason hard to delimit and portray; so too that of the Stoics which is a neighbour to it, namely to conform to Nature.[63]

Montaigne's rallying cry to live in accordance with nature would become a faint echo of the past, as the Western world moved on toward the modern age. Because of his interest in the concrete over the abstract, in experience over formal arguments and in nature over artifice, Montaigne is overlooked by modern historians of philosophy—as is, in fact, the entire period of the Renaissance. The mechanization of the 'world picture' had already begun, and, henceforth, when historians of philosophy looked back to the Renaissance, their gaze would fall more on the new methods of science set out in the work of Francis Bacon than on the ancient call to live according to nature expressed in the work of Montaigne.

Francis Bacon and the Death of Nature

One prerequisite for the body-machine to come to the fore was the pre-supposition that nature itself is a machine. The mechanization of the world picture was made possible by the work of Copernicus and Galileo, which over the period of the Renaissance began to put an end to the very important belief in a hierarchical nature and a living cosmos. For the Renaissance naturalists, all of nature was alive to some degree. Just as the belief that the body housed a soul acted as a constraint on the practice of dissection over the centuries, so the belief that the Earth had a soul—and was seen as a nurturing mother—acted as a constraint on certain activities carried out in, and on, the natural world. Metals and minerals, for example, were seen as ripening in the Earth's womb, and mining was seen as a form of rape that needed to be accompanied by strict controls relating to both miners and their work. Rituals and sacrifices were performed in recognition of—and to compensate for—the violation of Mother Earth. However, as Carolyn Merchant points out, "controlling images operate as ethical restraints," and when the images change, so do the restraints.[64] This is what happened as the image of nature was transformed from that of a nurturing mother to that of a machine—one that could be controlled by humans and placed at the service of human needs and interests.

Many factors were involved in this transition, but a very important role was played by Francis Bacon, often seen as the father of the modern scientific method, whose life project was the development of a method for obtaining knowledge, not for its own sake but for its usefulness in the development of new works and inventions for the benefit of mankind.[65] Bacon believed that achievement of this goal required that human dominion over nature, which had been lost as a result of the Fall, be restored. He referred to his project as the Great Instauration, a project of scientific investigation that would restore the rightful power of man over nature: "By the Fall, man fell from both his state of innocence and from his dominion over creation. But even in this life both of those losses can be made good; the former by religion and faith, the latter by arts and sciences."[66] Nature, Bacon believed, was given to man by God to be controlled, dominated and used for human ends; "the pursuit of natural science was therefore a religious obligation."[67] And it is by finding out how nature works and replicating it in the new natural philosophy that nature can be brought to work in the service of mankind. In effect, nature has to be conquered. Summarizing from Bacon's *The Great Instauration*, Merchant writes:

> The new man of science must not think that the 'inquisition of nature
> is in any part interdicted or forbidden.' Nature must be 'bound into
> service' and made a 'slave,' put 'in constraint' and 'molded' [*sic*] by the

mechanical arts. The 'searchers and spies of nature' are to discover her plots and secrets.[68]

No longer would nature be seen as a goddess or as a nurturing mother whose secrets must be respected and, as much as possible, left intact. No longer would the human pursuit of knowledge be seen as recalling Adam's sin. Exploitation of nature would become a fundamental requirement for the new practical knowledge that Bacon sought, and that knowledge would give man complete power over nature's secrets—which, like nature herself, would henceforth yield to human needs and fantasies. More precisely, mechanical science would *extract* the secrets from mechanical nature. Bacon is rightly appreciated for what Tarnas calls his "forceful advocacy of experience as the only legitimate source of true knowledge [which] effectively redirected the European mind toward the empirical world...."[69] At the same time, his rejection of knowledge for its own sake as well as his zealous focus on nature, not as a value in itself, but valuable only as a means to human ends, set the stage for technological progress without limits, the legacy of which is only too apparent in our day. Bacon's work effectively closed the door on nature the organism, and opened the door to nature the machine. Descartes would complete the picture by giving the mechanized 'world picture' its metaphysical underpinning and bringing into clear focus the body machine.

Notes

1. Tarnas, 224.
2. Richard H. Popkin, ed., *The Philosophy of the 16th and 17th Centuries* (New York: The Free Press, 1966), 2.
3. If it is difficult to overestimate the impact of the Renaissance, it is very easy to underestimate the importance of its philosophical thinkers. Of the three I have chosen because of their writings on the human body, only Montaigne warrants a chapter in Popkin's book. There were many Renaissance philosophers who remain unknown to students and practitioners of philosophy because the history of philosophy usually skips from the Middle Ages to Descartes, ignoring such notable thinkers as Marsilio Ficino, Giovanni Pico della Mirandola, Pietro Pomponazzi, Bernardino Telesio, Tommaso Campanella and Giordano Bruno. This lack of recognition is being corrected through recent scholarship. See, in particular, Paul Richard Blum, ed., *Philosophers of the Renaissance*

(Washington, DC: Catholic University of America Press, 2010), where all of the above-mentioned philosophers and many others are introduced and their ideas summarized in individual chapters.

4.   Brian P. Copenhaver and Charles B. Schmitt, *Renaissance Philosophy* (Oxford: Oxford University Press, 1992), 288.

5.   Louis Dupré, *Passage to Modernity* (New Haven and London: Yale University Press, 1993), 58. See also Stephen Menn's discussion of naturalism in *The Cambridge History of Seventeenth-Century Philosophy* (Cambridge: Cambridge University Press, 1998), 63ff. Menn thinks that too many philosophers are often included under the label 'naturalism,' although he admits that there was "a real tendency of thought which understood God's nature and relation to the world in a way incompatible with Christianity, and we call this 'naturalism' rather than 'atheism.'"

6.   Tarnas, *Western Mind*, 229.

7.   Tarnas, *Western Mind*, 216.

8.   Carole Kaske and John R. Clark, eds. and trans., *Marsilio Ficino: Three Books on Life* (Binghampton: Center for Medieval and Renaissance Studies, SUNY at Binghampton, 1989), hereinafter referred to as *De vita*.

9.   Although, as we will see, Descartes often did not reveal his sources, it is unlikely that he had *not* read *De vita*, given its influence.

10.   Copenhaver and Schmitt refer to Ficino as "the moving spirit of the Platonic revival" (127).

11.   Pauliina Remes, *Neoplatonism* (Berkeley and Los Angeles: University of California Press, 2008), 39.

12.   Eugenio Garin, *Astrology in the Renaissance* (London: Routledge & Kegan Paul, 1988), 73.

13.   *De vita*, 243. Naturalism did not shy away from the idea of action at a distance as did the mechanism which followed it. That one level of being can act on another is implicit in the idea of a continuum, but also, and more importantly, in the idea of the macrocosm and microcosm. Sympathy, resonance and analogy are causal categories that will be banned from the mechanistic view of the world, where only efficient causes operated and where causal activity necessitates physical proximity.

14.   *De vita*, 255.

15.   Garin, 46.

16.   Since Ficino was both a doctor and a philosopher, the book offers an insight as to how the human body was perceived in the interconnected world of Renaissance naturalism. As Kaske and Clark point out, Book 3 is both "more philosophical and more occult," and in it, "Ficino eloquently defends the naturalness of his magic by appeal to his cherished belief that the heavenly bodies are animated with an impersonal spirit which in turn pervades all men." *De vita*, 4.

17. Copenhaver and Schmitt, 160.

18. "The most important mediator in the entire work is the medical spirit.... In medical writers the philosophical function of the medical spirit was as a *tertium quid* to bridge the gap between man's body and soul—the function now filled in modern science by electro-chemical nervous transmission.... Ficino greatly extended the importance of the medical spirits by attributing them (or rather it) also to the cosmos, envisioning a *spiritus mundanus* or world spirit between the world's soul and its body." *De vita*, 43.

19. *De vita*, 259.

20. *De vita*, 249.

21. *De vita*, 253.

22. *De vita*, 287.

23. *De vita*, 289.

24. *De vita*, 40.

25. See Garin, 76: "Music, the harmony of the world, the universal harmony, the eternal poem, the theatre of the world: these are all dominant themes from the fifteenth century onwards, and scientists and philosophers were to write and speak about them from Galileo to Kepler, from Descartes to Mersenne."

26. *De vita*, 43. See Chapter 2 regarding the notion of seminal reasons in Stoic cosmology.

27. *De vita*, 43.

28. Raymond Klibansky, Erwin Panofsky and Fritz Saxl, *Saturn and Melancholy* (London: Nelson, 1964), 265.

29. Klibansky, Panofsky and Saxl, 270.

30. Richard Tarnas, *Cosmos and Psyche: Intimations of a New World View* (London: Viking Penguin, 2006), 76.

31. Tarnas, *Cosmos*, 77. Part of the new understanding of cosmic correspondences comes from the psychology of Carl Jung—in particular, his notion of archetypes and of synchronicity. According to Tarnas, Jung's later work "intimated the ancient understanding of an ensouled world, of an *anima mundi* in which the human psyche participates and with which it shares the same ordering principles of meaning. Jung noted parallels between synchronistic phenomena and the Chinese understanding of the Tao, the ancient Greek conception of the cosmic sympathy of all things, the Hermetic doctrine of microcosm and macrocosm, the medieval and Renaissance theory of correspondences, and the medieval concept of the pre-existent ultimate unity of all existence, the *unus munus* (the unitary world)" (57). Tarnas refers to the emergence of the "archetypal perspective" in other discplines, as well, such as anthropology, philosophy of science, linguistic analysis and others. He believes that the idea of archetypes has come full circle, "arriving now in its post-synchronicity development at a place very closely resembling its

ancient origins as cosmic *archai* but with its many inflections and potentialities, as well as new dimensions altogether, having been unfolded and explored" (84). Taking a new and serious look at astrology has also been made possible by the progress of computer technology, which has allowed for the calculation of planetary positions over long periods of time. Tarnas "was gradually able to gain access to precise astronomical data for all the planets extending for many centuries into the past ... the sudden availability of such extensive accurate planetary data permitted [Tarnas and other researchers] to investigate many significant cultural figures and historical events that had long been inaccessible to such analysis" (108).

32.   Lynne McTaggart, *The Field: The Quest for the Secret Force of the Universe* (New York: HarperCollins, 2008), 24. Many physicists might not agree with McTaggart's metaphysical interpretation, but it provides an interesting parallel and is worthy of consideration. (Questions of energy, life force and *qi* will be explored in Chapters 8 and 9).

33.   Tarnas, *Cosmos*, 63.

34.   David Le Breton, *La Chair à vif* (Paris: Éditions A. M. Métaillé, 1993), 74.

35.   Hans Jonas, *Philosophical Essays* (Englewood Cliffs, NJ: Prentice-Hall, 1974), 52.

36.   We will see in Chapters 8 and 9, however, that in Eastern philosophy the notion of macrocosm-microcosm survived in spite of the discovery that the Earth moves. In the holistic metaphysics of the East, the notion refers more to the relation of part to whole than to that of lunar and sublunar realms.

37.   Tarnas, *Western Mind*, 254.

38.   Steven Shapin, *The Scientific Revolution* (Chicago and London: University of Chicago Press, 1996), 23. Shapin further explains that although this vision of the Earth with the cosmos spinning around it was truly anthropocentric, the special place of the Earth "did not necessarily connote special virtue. Although human beings, and their earthly environment, were understood to be the unique creations of the Judeo-Christian God, compared with the heavens and a heavenly afterlife the earth and earthly existence were regarded as miserable and corrupt, and the actual center of the cosmos was hell" (24).

39.   Galileo Galilei, *Dialogue Concerning the Two Chief World Systems*, trans. Stillman Drake (Berkeley and Los Angeles: University of California Press, 1953), 53. (Note that "Peripatetic" means Aristotelian in this context).

40.   Shapin, 18.

41.   It is not clear whether or not Galileo actually conducted the experiments about which he writes or "whether they are best regarded as 'thought experiments,' imaginative rehearsals in Galileo's mind of what *would* happen were certain manipulations to be carried out, given what we already securely know about the physical world." See Shapin, 82.

42. It was only with the work of Beeckman and Descartes that this important principle found its full elaboration. See Wallace Hooper, "Inertial Problems in Galileo's Preinertial Framework," in *The Cambridge Companion to Galileo*, edited by Peter Machamer (Cambridge: Cambridge University Press, 1998), 170–71.

43. See Chapter 2 on Aristotle's teleology and the four causes.

44. The term "mechanization of the world picture" comes from E. J. Dijksterhuis, *The Mechanization of the World Picture* (Oxford: Oxford University Press, 1961).

45. While Hippocrates is known as the "Father of Medicine," it was Galen (Claudius Galenus, also known as Galen of Pergamum) who, six hundred years after Hippocrates (Galen lived from 131 to approximately 210 CE), synthesized the medical knowledge of the Greeks, which was transmitted through later centuries under the name of Galenism. Galen was a philosopher as well as a physician who wrote widely about anatomy, physiology and logic. His philosophy of the body was based on a theory of elements, or qualities, (hot, cold, wet and dry), relating to ancient ideas about individual elements of the universe (air, fire, water and earth), as well as a theory of bodily humours (phlegm, blood, black bile, yellow bile), which result in 'mixtures' that differ with different body types but that must be kept in balance in a healthy individual. In Galen's holistic view of body and soul, these mixtures form the basis for the faculties of the soul, and here the influence of Plato on his ideas is evident: "…we derive a good bodily mixture from our food and drink and other daily activities, and … this mixture is the basis on which we then build the virtue of the soul." P. N. Singer, *Galen: Selected Works* (Oxford: Oxford University Press, 1997), 150. Galen practised dissection on animals, including live animals (but not humans), and thereby contributed considerably to the advancement of the science of anatomy. In the same way that the teachings of Aristotle represented the supreme authority in natural science and philosophy up to the time of Descartes, so the teachings of Galen were the supreme authority in medicine, and his influence can be seen in the medical writings of Ficino, discussed in this chapter. Ideas such as Galen's have been rejected by modern medicine, but Singer points out that they are of interest to many of us today, "interested as we are in the nature of 'holistic' systems of medicine, and in the greater importance that our predecessors gave 'to the soul'" (xxxvi).

46. Le Breton, 57. "Objectivement scindé de lui-même, réduit à l'état de corps, l'écorché de Vésale ne cesse de manifester par l'humanité de ses postures le refus de cet état de fait … objectivement coupé du cosmos, il baigne dans un paysage naturel, caricature du microcosme, mais preuve que Vésale ne peut encore le faire disparaître totalement. L'homme de Vésale annonce la naissance d'un concept moderne. celui de corps, mais il demeure à certains égards sous la dépendance de la conception antérieure de l'homme comme microcosme." (Objectively

separated from himself and reduced to the status of body, Vesalius' flayed man does not cease to manifest, by the humanity of his postures, his rejection of this fact … objectively severed from the cosmos, he bathes in a natural landscape, a caricature of the microcosm, but proof that Vesalius cannot make him disappear entirely. The Vesalian man heralds the birth of a modern concept: the cóncept of body, but he remains in some respects subordinated to the former concept of man as microcosm). (translated by Guy Gagnon)

47.   There is a parallel in China today with respect to the "donation" of human organs for transplant. Because of religious beliefs governing the notions of death and the dead, people do not easily volunteer their organs for transplant, and recourse is made to the bodies of criminals, where organs are taken with or without their permission, both before and after execution (in the former case, the removal of both kidneys before the execution renders the latter redundant!). For a discussion of the situation of prisoners with respect to organ transplants, see Harry Wu, *Retour au laogai* (Paris: Belfond, 1997).

48.   David Hillman and Carla Mazzio, eds., *The Body in Parts* (New York and London: Routledge, 1997), 84.

49.   Jonathan Sawday, *The Body Emblazoned: Dissection and the Human Body in Renaissance Culture* (London: Routledge, 1996), 31. Sawday points out the parallels between the language of colonialism and the language of dissection during the Renaissance, as the body was seen as "a territory, an (as yet) undiscovered country, a location which demanded from its explorers skills which seemed analogous to those displayed by the heroic voyagers across the terrestrial globe…. Eustachius mapped the ear, Fallopius the female reproductive organs…. Like the Columbian explorers, these early discoverers dotted their names, like place-names on a map, over the terrain which they encountered" (23).

50.   Sawday, 29. This also represents a de-linking of knowledge and wisdom. For the latter, some 'secrets' are beyond human knowing; for the former, in the context of the new science, all reality—including the interior of the body—is to be laid bare.

51.   Tarnas, *Western Mind*, 276.

52.   Michel de Montaigne, *Essays*, trans. M. A. Screech (London: Penguin, 1987, 1991), II, xii, 562.

53.   Stephen Toulmin, *Cosmopolis* (Chicago: University of Chicago Press, 1990), 25. Renaissance humanism should not be confused with what, in our time, is referred to as "secular humanism," a term that has very negative connotations in some (notably religious fundamentalist) circles. As Toulmin points out, most Renaissance humanists "saw themselves by their own conscientious lights as sincerely religious," and Montaigne, in particular, "saw himself as being a good Catholic."

54. Montaigne, *Essays*, III.9, 1091.

55. Dudley Marchi, *Montaigne Among the Moderns* (Providence and Oxford: Berghahn Books, 1994), 6.

56. Toulmin, 36. Toulmin points out that this claim is "typical of modern philosophy from 1640 to 1950, rather than of philosophy in either its medieval or its post-Wittgensteinian form."

57. There is a historical dimension to the perceived threat of uncertainty related to the religious wars that the tolerance and lack of firm principles were seen to foster. "If uncertainty, ambiguity, and the acceptance of pluralism led, in practice, only to an intensification of the religious war, the time had come to discover some *rational method* for demonstrating the essential correctness or incorrectness of philosophical, scientific, or theological doctrines" (Toulmin, 55).

58. Montaigne, *Essays*, II, 17, 727.

59. Montaigne, *Essays*, III, 2, 907.

60. Jean Starobinski, *Montaigne in Motion*, trans. Arthur Goldhammer (Chicago and London: University of Chicago Press, 1985), 162.

61. Montaigne, *Essays*, III.13, 1262.

62. Toulmin, 41.

63. Montaigne, *Essays*, III, 13, 1266.

64. Carolyn Merchant, *The Death of Nature: Women, Ecology and the Scientific Revolution* (San Francisco: Harper & Row, 1980, 1990), 44.

65. Gaukroger points out that there was a great concern with practical knowledge and practical benefits in Bacon's time. "Scholastic disputation was rejected in part because it was considered to be of no benefit to anyone, and there was a tendency among the English humanists of the sixteenth century to consider the practical sciences superior to theoretical knowledge." Stephen Gaukroger, *Francis Bacon and the Transformation of Early-Modern Philosophy* (Cambridge: Cambridge University Press, 2001), p. 14.

66. Francis Bacon, *Valerius Terminus: On the Interpretation of Nature*, cited in Gaukroger, 78. It was believed that God had given Adam complete philosophical knowledge and that most of it disappeared when Adam and Eve were expelled from the Garden of Eden.

67. Tarnas, *Western Mind*, 273.

68. Merchant, 169.

69. Tarnas, *Western Mind*, 275.

CHAPTER V

THE BODY-MACHINE: DESCARTES

René Descartes is a pivotal figure in the history of philosophy. He was born in 1596, just as the Renaissance was drawing to a close. He was educated at the Jesuit college of La Flèche at a time when the Jesuits were called upon to counter the Protestant Reformation through the education of young Catholic minds. From the age of ten, Descartes received a classical humanistic education, but he was particularly impressed by the precision and certainty of mathematics. Although he was a product of the scepticism of his age epitomized by Montaigne, he resisted it, and some of his writings, in particular his *Discourse on Method*, are seen by scholars as a direct attack on Montaigne and the uncertainty arising from scepticism. According to Richard Tarnas, there was a sceptical crisis in French philosophy, which Descartes experienced directly and acutely:

> Pressed by the residual confusions of his education, by the contra-
> dictions between different philosophical perspectives, and by the lessening
> relevance of religious revelation for understanding the empirical world,
> Descartes set out to discover an irrefutable basis for certain knowledge.[1]

This chapter will trace his quest for certainty and, more particularly, outline how that quest for certainty led him to the three prongs of his philosophy that bequeathed to the modern age the body-machine: method, dualism and mechanism.

That Descartes' legacy to modernity was a dualistic metaphysics of mind and body—and, as a consequence of that fundamental principle, a concept of the human body as a machine—is a fact generally recognized by all who write about the body today. But most writers simply refer to his famous statement, "I think, therefore I am," with its obvious neglect of the body, as what led him, and us, to the body-machine; few take time to analyze the source of his dualism and his mechanism, or their importance to modernity's ready acceptance of the body-machine as a premise of modern medicine. The purpose of this book is to tell a story about how and why the body-machine came to be, what was lost in the process and what might ultimately be recovered. In relation to Descartes, I want to ask the same question asked in earlier chapters: What was Descartes trying to explain and why? This is particularly important in the case of Descartes, since, while most of the science on which he based his mechanistic conception of the body was ultimately rejected, the paradigm of the body-machine endured. In addition, as we will see in this chapter and the next, Descartes' dualistic conception of the body was highly criticized in his own time—by Hobbes and Gassendi, among others, as well as by his rationalist successor, Spinoza, who rejected dualism out of hand. Further, as John Cottingham points out, "contemporary onslaughts on the puzzle of consciousness ... have all but eliminated Cartesian dualism as a serious contender for an account of the nature and workings of the mind...."[2] This raises a further question, then, in relation to the body: Why has the Cartesian body-machine paradigm endured for almost four centuries?

Method

From his earliest writings to his last, Descartes was concerned with the proper method for arriving at certain knowledge, and he was convinced that, once elucidated, the proper method could be applied to any branch of science and learning. Finding this method became his life's mission, and his commitment to it was confirmed very early in his life and work. Right at the beginning of his earliest work, *Rules for the Direction of the Mind*, Descartes states:

> For the sciences as a whole are nothing other than human wisdom, which always remains one and the same, however different the subjects to which it is applied, it being no more altered by them than sunlight is by the variety of the things it shines on.[3]

This simple statement of what was, in fact, a radically new idea belies the importance that the notion had in Descartes' work and the fact that it "contains within itself the germ of the whole Cartesian revolution."[4] His principle contains assumptions (choices) about knowledge, the mind and man's relation to the cosmos that are not discussed, argued or proven. In other words, it was for him an *a priori* principle that was present from the beginnings of his thought and that governed his approach to all science, including his science of the human body. While his method did not find public expression until the *Discourse on Method* was published in 1637, it was developed much earlier. In 1619, when he was only twenty-three years old, he wrote to his friend Isaac Beeckman: "What I want to produce is … a completely new science, which would provide a general solution of all possible equations involving any sort of quantity, whether continuous or discrete, each according to its nature."[5] Later in the same year, Descartes had a series of dreams that left him full of enthusiasm for the unity of science. He referred to the dreams in a small notebook of early writings seen by his biographer, Baillet, but never published (and now lost). In the third of the dreams appeared a dictionary and a book of poetry containing a poem with the words: "Quod vitae sectabor iter?" (What path shall I take in life?). In what appears to be a rather freewheeling interpretation of the dream, Descartes took the dictionary to mean the unity of all the sciences, and the book of poetry the union of philosophy and wisdom. In the question about what path to follow, Descartes saw a message from God, and the answer, for him, was to follow the path of establishing the foundations of a marvellous new science: the unity of all knowledge. Thus, the dreams served to confirm his life's mission—which remained unfailing and constant. In the *Principles of Philosophy*, published four years before his death, he reiterated his commitment to the principle of the unity of science, and compared philosophy to a tree, the roots being metaphysics, the trunk physics and the branches emerging from the trunk all the other sciences.[6]

Descartes' clear statement of the principle of the unity of knowledge in his earliest writings is notable, first, because it is a clear break with past thinking about human knowledge. Without any explanation or justification, Descartes has put the knowing subject front and centre in the relation between the human mind and the world of which it is (or was until that time considered to be) a part. The epistemological categories of the naturalists (analogy, sympathy and mediation) referred to in Chapter 4, presuppose a continuum of being as well as of knowing; thus, there were different kinds of knowable objects, and therefore different kinds of knowing, as well as different degrees of certainty. Henceforth, there would be "a single kind of knowledge, an identical order of abstraction, one level of intelligibility, one kind of certainty, and one single method to obtain this certainty...."[7]

Second, Descartes holds that knowledge is an activity of the mind alone; the power of knowing is distinct from the body and does not depend on it. Here, Descartes is falling back on Platonic dualism with its suspicion of knowledge gained through the senses. But, as we shall see, Descartes' dualism would be a dualism with a difference; unlike Plato, Descartes would attribute no life-sustaining function to the soul, nor would he attribute rationality to the universe. The essence of the Cartesian soul—as mind—is pure thought;[8] and the human mind, rather than the universe, becomes the seat of reason. Mind, reason and method become a Cartesian trinity for the establishment of knowledge. In effect, "method is itself the mind at work, the unravelling of the processes of thought."[9] Descartes believed that the mind naturally knows how to reason; we need only direct it properly toward the objects for it to know them. It becomes clear that Descartes' mind-body dualism was a new kind of dualism, and that it was already at work in the early development of his method. The mind alone is involved in the discovery of knowledge and in the determination of certainty. The unity of the cosmos has given way to the unity of human knowledge. Human consciousness would henceforth look upon the cosmos with detachment, transforming it into a series of objects for science. At the same time, it should be pointed out that Descartes says very little in these early writings regarding the separation of mind and body, nor about why he is so certain that knowledge is strictly an affair of the mind; nor, for that matter, about why he can be so certain that the 'natural light of reason' is, like the sun, unaffected by the objects upon which it shines.

The Discourse on Method

Descartes' first published elaboration of his method occurs in his *Discourse on Method*,[10] released in 1637, long after the early writings discussed above. Here he sets out an analytic method that can be applied to any subject matter whatsoever and yield certain results. He summarized its four main rules as follows:

> The first was never to accept anything as true if I did not have evident
> knowledge of its truth: that is, carefully to avoid precipitate conclusions

and preconceptions, and to include nothing more in my judgements than what presented itself to my mind so clearly and so distinctly that I had no occasion to doubt it.

The second, to divide each of the difficulties I examined into as many parts as possible and as may be required in order to resolve them better.

The third, to direct my thoughts in an orderly manner, by beginning with the simplest and most easily known objects in order to ascend little by little, step by step, to knowledge of the most complex, and by supposing some order even among objects that have no natural order of precedence.

And the last, throughout to make enumerations so complete, and reviews so comprehensive, that I could be sure of leaving nothing out.[11]

These four rules capture Descartes' double-pronged approach to knowledge using intuition and deduction. The first two deal with intuition, the latter two with deduction. For Descartes, intuition refers to the clear and instantaneous seizing of an idea that arises from the light of reason, and deduction to what can be inferred from what we already know.[12] He is convinced that we cannot make a mistaken inference in deduction—we can make mistakes because of faulty or unclear first principles, but the process of deduction is, for him, something we do by the natural light of reason, and, properly used, cannot be mistaken. As for intuition, for Descartes it is a function neither of the senses nor of the imagination; it is a totally rational act of the mind.[13]

It is important to understand that Descartes' method and his belief in its application to all areas of knowledge depended on another belief: that he could find the simplest constituents of all topics. It was his presumption that all subject matter could be broken down in this way, into the simplest of ideas that can be seized immediately by the intuition, and then combined through deduction to give us certain knowledge of the matter at hand. This is why mechanism is so important to method in Descartes, something that we will see clearly later in this chapter.

The point of the *Discourse* was to set out the method and then to show how it could be applied to various fields of knowledge. A number of appendices to the main work showed the application of the method to such topics as optics and geometry, but Part V of the main work itself demonstrates how it can be applied to the study of the human body. As he tells us in his introduction, this latter section covers "the order of the questions in physics that [the author] has investigated, particularly the explanation of the movement of the heart and of some other difficulties pertaining to medicine, and also the difference between our soul and that of the beasts...."[14]

Part V is actually a summary of another work (referred to by Descartes as his 'Physics' but which includes his treatise on the human body), which was already completed but remained unpublished at the time of publication of the *Discourse*, principally because of the condemnation of Galileo. The laws of nature that Descartes has discovered assume a heliocentric view of the universe, something that was both controversial and dangerous, as Descartes makes clear at the beginning of his discussion in Part V:

> I would gladly go on and reveal the whole chain of other truths that I deduced from these first ones. But in order to do this I would have to discuss many questions that are being debated among the learned, and I do not wish to quarrel with them. So it will be better, I think, for me not to do this, and merely to say in general what these questions are, so as to let those who are wiser decide whether it would be useful for the public to be informed more specifically about them.[15]

After reiterating the basic principles of his method and pointing to the success he has had with it to date ("I venture to say that I have found a way to satisfy myself within a short time about all the principal difficulties usually discussed in philosophy"[16]), he goes on to discuss certain functions of the human body, and how they follow from the laws established by God in nature. In particular, he discusses the functioning of the heart, along with other details regarding the human body, following his method and the laws of nature he has discovered—all of which will be discussed later in this chapter. In the meantime, we will turn to the second prong of Descartes' mechanistic physiology: dualism.

Dualism: *Cogito ergo sum*

As pointed out above, the first rule of Descartes' method was to accept nothing as true unless it presented itself to his mind so clearly and so distinctly that he could not doubt it. In the *Discourse on Method*, and in his later *Meditations*, Descartes attempts to find the one absolutely indubitable principle that can serve as the foundation for the metaphysics, which, in turn, will serve as the roots of the tree of knowledge. "Montaigne claimed in the *Apology* that 'unless one thing is found of which we are completely certain, we can be certain about nothing'…. Descartes answered Montaigne's gambit by setting himself the task of locating the 'one thing' for which certainty is needed. He found this in the *cogito*…."[17]

He arrives at his famous *cogito* (which is short for *cogito ergo sum*, or "I think therefore I am") by means of the rigorous application of the first rule of his method. Ironically, given his concern with uncertainty and the scepticism of Montaigne, he uses the tool of the sceptic, doubt, to arrive at his fundamental certainty. He will doubt everything—but this will be a methodical doubt, not a true scepticism. He will doubt only to the point where he finds one thing absolutely certain. Doubt, for him, is a tool, not a philosophical position. It is a function of his method of suspending judgment on what he has previously believed to be true.

Sitting down in front of the fire, he contemplates what he knows about himself, and, after lengthy meditation, concludes that he cannot know for certain that he is really sitting there in front of the fire: his senses could be deceiving him or he might be dreaming. The senses are capable of deceiving us at least some of the time, so how can he be certain they are not deceiving him at this moment? Experiences when dreaming can be as vivid as experiences when awake, so he cannot be absolutely certain that he is not dreaming. But, he asks, even if I am dreaming, surely the world of thought, the world of mathematics, for example, the truth that $3 + 2 = 5$, must be certain. Even this cannot be known for sure, however, since he can suppose the existence of a deceiving God or a powerful evil genius able to convince him of mathematical truths that are actually false. Finally, he concludes, even if this were the case, he cannot doubt the fact that he is doubting:

> [If] I convinced myself of something then I certainly existed. But there is a deceiver of supreme power and cunning who is deliberately and constantly deceiving me. In that case I too undoubtedly exist, if he is deceiving me; and let him deceive me as much as he can, he will never bring it about that I am nothing so long as I think that I am something. So after considering everything very thoroughly, I must finally conclude

that this proposition, I am, I exist, is necessarily true, whenever it is put forward by me or conceived in my mind.[18]

Descartes might have been content to leave the matter there—as an answer to the epistemological question, What do I know for certain? Hobbes points out in a critique of the *Meditations*, for example, that the most his doubting allows him to say is that thinking (doubting) is going on. It proves nothing about what or who is thinking—there is no 'I' contained in this fundamental certainty (and nothing that proves that whatever is thinking is not a body). But Descartes does not stop at this point; he concludes that, if there is thinking, there has to be something doing the thinking, and he goes on to ask, What is this 'I' that is thinking? This is where he slides from his epistemological investigation into a metaphysical one:

> At last I have discovered it—thought; this alone is inseparable from me.
> I am, I exist—that is certain.... At present I am not admitting anything
> except what is necessarily true. I am, then, in the strict sense only a thing
> that thinks; that is, I am a mind, or intelligence, or intellect, or reason—
> words whose meaning I have been ignorant of until now. But for all that
> I am a thing which is real and which truly exists. But what kind of thing?
> As I have just said—a thinking thing.[19]

Descartes holds that the 'I' cannot be his body, since he can imagine himself without a body and still think. He also says he is no kind of material soul (breath, fire, etc.), "for I have supposed these things to be nothing."[20] His conclusion is, in effect, that the 'I' is a substance that has no need of a body, and that this 'thinking thing' is, in fact, his essence. It is his shift from the question of *how* to the question of *what* that moves him to his metaphysical dualism—and, as they say, the rest is history.

Further, Descartes holds that, even if he allows that our senses (and thus our bodies) give us information about the world, they do not give us true knowledge, which can only come through the mind. He demonstrates this using what has become known as the analogy of the wax. Taking a piece of wax, he points out that the senses can tell us, for example, that the wax is hard, has a certain texture, smell and taste, and when put next to a flame manifests different qualities as it changes shape, temperature and texture. But the senses cannot reveal anything about the nature of the wax, nor can they even assure us that the first set of sense perceptions and the second set refer to the same object. It is only the mind that can tell us that what we are sensing is the 'same' wax. Descartes' conclusion from this is that believing it is the appearance of the wax that gives us knowledge is mistaken. It is our intellect that provides this knowledge. Thus, not only do we have knowledge of ourselves (our minds) without recourse to the senses, but we gain more knowledge about the world outside of us from our intellect than from our senses.

The ramifications for modernity of Descartes' simple act of doubting (and the conclusions he drew from it) are considerable, not just because the *cogito* establishes the metaphysical basis for mind-body dualism, but more importantly because it represents the beginnings of the modern 'self,' detached from its body and from nature. More will be said about this later, but the new relationship of man and the universe that Descartes ushers in with his *cogito* is succinctly described by Tarnas:

> Thus *res cogitans*—thinking substance, subjective experience, spirit, consciousness, that which man perceives as within—was understood as fundamentally different and separate from *res extensa*—extended substance, the objective world, matter, the physical body, plants and animals, stones and stars, the entire physical universe, everything that man perceives as outside his mind.[21]

The thinking self becomes supreme in the Cartesian universe; what begins as an epistemological exercise of determining what *could be known* becomes a metaphysical premise about *what is*, what exists. An enormous leap of logic and faith arises from the simple utterance of the *cogito*.

Mechanism

The third prong of Descartes' philosophy leading to the body-machine is mechanism, a new approach to the philosophy of nature, which he wholeheartedly accepted and applied to his description of the human body.

Descartes did not concern himself with the study of the human body until about 1629, and he had no formal training in anatomy or medicine. In fact, in this area as in many others, Descartes was a self-taught man. "I am now studying chemistry and anatomy simultaneously," he wrote to Mersenne in April 1630, and "every day I learn something that I cannot find in any book."[22] Even though he lived in Amsterdam and Leiden at a time when public dissections were popular, there is no evidence in his writings that he participated in any of these events.[23] He was undertaking his own dissections, in his rooms, of carcasses garnered from local butchers. "I am now dissecting the heads of various animals, so that I can explain what imagination, memory, etc. consist in,"[24] he wrote to Mersenne in 1633, when he had nearly completed his work on what would become his *Treatise on Man*. His anatomical and medical studies were based largely on his reading of others, and on his dissections of animals, both dead and alive. According to his own testimony, he read Vesalius and other medical writers, including Caspar Bauhin, an avid follower of Vesalius.[25] Since Descartes was notoriously silent about the sources of many of his ideas and assumptions, it is impossible to know all the influences on his thought. What is important is that he was not breaking new ground from the point of view of anatomy. In fact, the physiology of the *Treatise* is based on Hippocrates and Galen, as well as on previous biological and medical writers from the mid-sixteenth century onwards.[26] Since Ficino's *De vita* was still current during Descartes' lifetime, it is highly probable that he was influenced by that work, as well—but that influence would have been negative and, perhaps, the target of many of his comments against occult forces in explanations of bodily functions. What Descartes is attempting is a reconstruction of traditional views about the body to fit his dualistic and mechanistic view of the world and to conform to his universal method. This is important since it indicates that his work was less about new discoveries than about redefining the body to fit his mechanistic picture of the world. He was turning the body into a scientific construction and an object of knowledge.

Mechanical Nature

The body-machine is a direct result of Descartes' mechanism, the principles of which he sets out in his work *The World*, which was originally entitled *By what Laws and by what Means the parts of this World will extricate themselves, by themselves, from the Chaos and Confusion they were in.* His chapter on the body is often referred to as the *Treatise on Man*, and is sometimes published as a separate work;[27] but it is important to understand that it was initially an integral part of the larger work, since, for Descartes, explanations of the body follow the same laws that govern nature in general (that is, the laws of physics).

Descartes refers to the Laws of Nature that God has imposed on the world and clarifies his meaning of the word 'Nature':

> [B]y 'Nature' here I do not mean some deity or other sort of imaginary power. Rather, I use the word to signify matter itself, in so far as I am considering it taken together with the totality of qualities I have attributed to it, and the condition that God continues to preserve it in the same way that He created it.[28]

Nature is matter, and matter is made up of simple particles (not the elements of the ancients). There is no void, and the particles "all touch one another on all sides" so that "from the time they begin to move, they also begin to change and diversify their motions by colliding with one another."[29] All change is motion, brought about by the size, shape and speed of the particles, following three laws of nature that Descartes elaborated. The first of these states that each particle continues in the same state unless and until it collides with others. Included in this law of nature is the new idea that rest is also a form of motion, not privation of motion, as had been thought by earlier philosophers. This law represents Descartes' articulation of what has become known as the principle of inertia, which is fundamental to the mechanical view of the universe. There is no natural state of rest, as the Aristotelians thought; further, in the heliocentric view of the universe there is no natural centre of the world. Objects or particles move only because of being moved by other objects (as one billiard ball moves another) and will continue moving until impeded by other objects. Most importantly, they do not move because of any inherent 'occult' qualities.

The second law of nature, for Descartes, holds that when one body pushes another, "it cannot give the other any motion except by losing as much of its own motion at the same time; nor can it take away any of the other's motion unless its own is increased by the same amount."[30] This law, along with the first, deals with the conservation and distribution of motion. The third, the principle of rectilinear motion, deals with its direction: "when a body is moving, even if its motion most often takes place along a curved line ... each of its parts individually tends always to continue moving along a straight line."[31]

These are the three basic laws of nature upon which Descartes will base both his description of the world and his description of the human body. The object of these laws is to explain all change within the universe in terms that are quantifiable and measurable, devoid of occult qualities within matter, or anything over and above matter, like soul or spirit. All change whatsoever (in nature or the human body) can be explained solely in terms of changes in motion. It is not the qualities of particular bodies that explain their behaviour, but the motion of the particles of which they are composed. Before Descartes (and in accordance with Aristotle), different substances were seen to have different essences, depending on their qualities. For Descartes, on the other hand, there are but two substances: mind and matter. The essence of mind is thought; the essence of matter is extension (in space). Descartes is eliminating qualitative explanation and replacing it with a purely quantitative explanation of material substance.

Mechanical Body

In the *Treatise on Man*, Descartes takes on the task of describing the human body as a machine that conforms to the laws of nature already set out. He supposes "the body to be just a statue or a machine made of earth, which God forms with the explicit intention of making it as much as possible like us."[32] Like machines that function solely based on the disposition of their parts, the functions of the body depend solely on the disposition of its organs in the same way that clocks, artificial fountains and other machines function according to the arrangements of their parts:

> And the nerves of *the machine* that I am describing can indeed be compared to the pipes in the mechanical parts of these fountains, its muscles and tendons to various other engines and springs which serve to work these mechanical parts, its animal spirits to the water that drives them, the heart to the source of the water and the brain's cavities with the apertures. Moreover, respiration and similar actions which are normal and *natural to this machine*, and which depend on the flow of spirits, are like the movements of a clock or mill, which the normal flow of water can make continuous.[33]

Descartes provides a description of the body-machine and its functions, like movement, vision and memory, and his explanations of the various functions are made in terms of the size, speed and direction of particles, using the same principles that he had outlined in his physics. For Descartes, all functions of the body are the result of the disposition of its organs just as "the movements of a clock or other automaton follow from the disposition of its counterweights and wheels."[34]

In order to conform to the principles of mechanism, as well as to his dualistic metaphysics whereby only humans have souls, it is important that Descartes' description of the body be made solely on the basis of physical principles, except where conscious human action is involved. Just as he explains fire by the different sizes of particles that descend as ashes (the larger ones) or rise as smoke (the more refined ones), so in his physiology the process of digestion, for example, can be explained by the rise and fall of particles: the "agitation which is induced in the small particles of food when they are heated, together with the agitation of the stomach and the bowels in which they are contained" causes the coarser particles to descend for elimination and the more refined particles to rise to the liver where they are transformed into blood. The agitation and separation that take place in digestion are similar to what takes place "when one shakes meal in a sieve, the purest parts flow out and it is only the small size of the holes through which it passes that prevents the bran from following after them."[35] In the liver, this finer fluid "is refined and transformed, taking on the colour and form of blood, just as the white juice of black grapes is converted into light-red wine when it is allowed to ferment on the vine stock."[36] The blood itself circulates through the body in a similar fashion, finding its way to the spleen, kidneys, bladder, etc., by the same process of separation:

> And through whichever of these places it passes, either the *position, shape*, or *smallness* of the pores through which they pass is what alone makes some go through and not others, and keeps the rest of the blood from following, just as you see in various sieves which, being pierced in different ways, serve to separate different grains from one another.[37]

But the most energetic, strongest and finest parts of the blood go directly from the heart to the brain "inasmuch as the arteries bearing them there are in the *most direct line from the heart*; and as you know, *all moving bodies tend as much as they are able to continue their motion in a straight line*."[38] In this way, the particles of blood conform to the law of rectilinear motion.

The Principle of Life and the Heat of the Heart

In Descartes' conception of the body, the principle of life is the heat of the heart, which he also refers to as the 'fire without light.' The question of the heat of the heart is very important to Descartes because of his efforts to do away with any non-mechanical account of movement in the body. Earlier accounts described the heat of the heart in terms of some form of cosmic fire or spirit that connected all life to the cosmos or world-soul. In the framework of the macrocosm-microcosm, the heart is like the sun, and in some systems, partakes in the essence of the sun. In Descartes' description, the heat of the heart is a purely physical phenomenon. It does not come from soul or from any cosmic fire, although he does refer to it as fire:

> And note that the flesh of the heart contains in its pores one of those fires without light which I have spoken about earlier and which makes it so fiery and hot that, to the extent that the blood enters either of its two chambers or cavities, it is promptly inflated and expanded.... And the fire in the heart of this machine that I am describing to you has as its sole purpose to expand, warm, and refine the blood....[39]

It is the fire of the heart (the fire without light) that allows Descartes to explain the functions of the body without recourse to any idea of soul, be it rational, animal or vegetative. There is no other explanation needed to account for the principle of life other than the fire of the heart.

It is the heat of the heart that Descartes uses to counter William Harvey's theory about the circulation of the blood. Harvey is credited with being the first to explain the action of the heart with respect to the circulation of the blood, and his account differs from Descartes' in one very important respect: for Harvey, the heart acts as a pump, and it is the pumping action of the heart that accounts for the blood entering and leaving the heart. Descartes accepted Harvey's idea of blood circulation, but rejected the notion of the pumping action of the heart for the very simple reason that Harvey's explanation requires the supposition of some unknown occult force that could cause the heart to pump. With Descartes' theory, we need suppose no unknown or extraneous faculties, since the fire without light, through a process of fermentation, can explain the pumping action of the heart. "For what better and swifter arrangement can we imagine than that which is brought about by fire, which is the most powerful agent we know in nature[?]"[40]

The fire in the heart heats the blood, and it is the heat of the blood that alone causes the heart to expand as the blood enters the heart and to contract as it leaves. The expansion and contraction are purely internal *processes*; there is no need for any other principle to account for this life-giving and life-sustaining movement of the heart. Further, this heat is no different in nature "from that which is caused by the addition of some fluid, or yeast, which causes the body with which it is mixed to expand."[41] This is very different from the 'innate heat' of Galen, for example, which is a *quality* of the individual body; Galen insists that

> each body possesses some particularity of mixture which belongs to its own
> specific nature but differs from any other specific nature; further, that if
> the body transforms some familiar or proper substance into its own nature,
> it will thus increase the amount of substance of the heat within it....[42]

Descartes wishes to rid the body of qualities in the same way as, in his physics, he rid the world of qualities in order to explain everything in terms of quantities: of matter and movement, the size of particles and the speed at which they move. More importantly, the heat of the heart, the 'fire without light,' is like any other fire in the world: it is subject to the laws of nature and not, as with Galen, to the qualities of the body in which it finds itself.[43] Descartes was wrong about the action of the heart and Harvey was right, but the fact that Descartes was wrong about this fundamental premise of his mechanism of the body did not lessen his influence on future conceptions of the body-machine.

Movement of the Body

Just as a process of agitation similar to what takes place in a sieve causes nourishment to be transformed into grosser and more refined liquids, including blood, so blood undergoes a similar process of agitation when it flows to the brain, where the more refined particles "without any preparation or alteration, *except being separated from the larger parts and retaining the extreme speed that the heat of the heart has given them* ... cease to have the form of blood and are called animal spirits."[44]

The concept of animal spirits was not an invention of Cartesian physiology; it had been used in various ways since Galen, and we saw one variation of it in Ficino's medical spirits. What is new, here, is Descartes' utilization of this ancient concept to support his mechanistic physiology. Their production is purely mechanical (the process of agitation and separation as through a sieve) and so is their function (which Descartes normally describes in terms of their size, position and speed or motion). Animal spirits can be compared to the water that drives the mechanical parts of the machines in the grottoes and fountains in the royal gardens, as described earlier.

Animal spirits have the power to cause movements "in all bodily parts in which the nerves terminate," including the heart, the liver, the spleen, etc.[45] The animal spirits flow through the nerves, which are tiny tubes that contain "a kind of marrow made up from several very fine fibres which come from the brain's own substance," and which, not completely filling the tubes, leave "sufficient room for the animal spirits to flow easily through them from the brain into the muscles" thus causing the muscles to move.[46] The nerves also contain membranes that act like doors, letting the animal spirits in and out (reacting according to the force of the spirits entering or leaving) and preventing the spirits from returning. All of this action is purely mechanical and operates according to the laws of nature that govern all movement in the universe:

> For you will readily recognise that these spirits, being like a wind or a very fine flame, must flow promptly from one muscle to another as soon as they find a passage, *even though they are propelled by no other power than the inclination that they have to continue their motion in accord with the laws of nature.*[47]

It is the action of animal spirits that accounts for respiration, expanding and contracting the muscles of the lungs, as in a bellows; it accounts for swallowing through the opening and closing action of the throat; it also accounts for the muscular action that controls "how this machine is able to sneeze, yawn, cough, and make the motions needed to expel various excretions."[48] Animal spirits also account for how the body reacts to external stimulation through the senses. For example, if the foot is placed too near to a fire, the heat of the fire touching the skin pulls the tiny fibre (the nerve) which causes the membrane at the end of the nerve (in the brain) to open ("just as when you pull on one end of a cord you cause a bell hanging at the other end to ring at the same time"[49]) and the animal spirits to flow through the tiny tube of the nerve to the muscles of the foot which pull the foot away from the fire. Some animal spirits also go elsewhere, "to the muscles that make the hands move and the whole body turn in order to protect itself."[50]

The movements that are described above are both mechanical and involuntary, that is, they are performed without thought and therefore without any action of the will, which involves the soul. Movements that do involve the will, in other words, voluntary movements, will not become less mechanical because of the implication of the soul. In fact, to return to Descartes' analogy of the fountains, "when a rational soul is present in this machine it will have its principal seat in the brain and will reside there like the fountaineer, who must be stationed at the tanks to which the fountain's pipes return if he wants to initiate, impede, or in some way alter their movements."[51] The movements are just as mechanical, the only difference being that the mechanic is there to initiate or impede the movements.[52]

Vision

The most important fact about vision for Descartes is found not in his *Treatise on Man*, but in the first chapter of *The World*, and is contained in the subtitle: *On the difference between our sensations and the things that produce them.*[53] Descartes is going to make a clear departure from the Aristotelian account of perception as a form of alteration of the sense faculty. In the Aristotelian account, "the sense faculty is like the actual sense-object—it is affected as being unlike but on being affected it becomes like and is such as what acts on it."[54] In vision, the eye takes on the form (without the matter) of the object that is seen; something is transmitted from the object to the eye and the eye is transformed in the process. For Descartes, however, "although everyone is commonly convinced that the ideas that we have in our thought are completely like the objects from which they proceed, I know of no compelling argument for this."[55] As he accounts for both heat and light simply in terms of motion and our perception of light in terms of effects on the sense organ of those motions, so his account of visual perception will rely on the same mechanistic principles. Having denied that real qualities exist in objects, he must also reject the belief that any quality can be transferred from the object to the sense organ.[56] In addition, in the Aristotelian account, sense perception is a function of the sensitive or animal soul, but Descartes, having dismissed the notion of gradations of soul, must account for it in terms of his mind-body dualism and his belief that animals do not have souls.

Of particular interest is Descartes' account of distance perception, which involves the participation of the soul. When the eye is turned toward an object, "the soul will be able to tell the position of this object inasmuch as the nerves from this eye are disposed in a different way than they would be if it were turned toward some other object."[57] The soul's ability to judge size and direction is the result, according to Descartes, of a kind of natural geometry, although the soul can often be deceived, in particular in relation to distance and size.

Like Descartes' description of animal spirits, his description of vision appears somewhat mysterious, and Gary Hatfield points out that it raises serious metaphysical difficulties: "In particular, it raises the question of how extended matter can act upon a non-extended mind, and can do so over an extended area ... and it also raises the question of how a non-extended mind can 'contain' an imagistic representation (as opposed to a mere conceptual understanding) of extension and its modes."[58] Further, given the dependence of this form of visual perception on the soul, one cannot help but wonder whether or not animals can have perception of distance, shape or size. Do animals, too, have a natural geometry?[59] Descartes' statements about the soul judging distance would seem to indicate that this type of perception is unique to humans; however, as with much of his description of the body-machine, he is not consistent and his descriptions often raise more questions than they answer. The account of the natural geometry is one that "represents the height of Descartes' attempt to mechanise the office of the sensitive soul, in this case, of the estimative power."[60]

Both the difficulty of interpreting what Descartes says about perception of distance, shape, pleasure, pain, etc., and the need to give the widest interpretation possible to his position in order not to see Cartesian animals as purely insentient machines are troublesome. Stephen Gaukroger holds that the assumption that animals have no souls or no thoughts is misleading, since "Descartes' claim is that their thoughts and experiences are not like ours, not that they do not have any thoughts and experiences at all."[61] He admits that Descartes can be criticized for carelessness and ambiguity about what he means when he says animals have no thoughts *like ours*, but "so far as I can tell he never (when context is taken into account) unambiguously claims that they have no thoughts at all."[62]

However, Descartes is never ambiguous about whether or not animals have souls. Nor is he ambiguous about the fact that soul and mind are identical, nor that the essence of mind is thought and that thought includes such activities as willing, judging, imagining, etc. Thus, it seems reasonable, following Descartes' own account, to conclude that an animal, which has no soul, cannot have the experiences that are dependent upon having a soul. In addition, Descartes is clear that certain perceptions, such as pain, pleasure, thirst, hunger, colours, sound, taste, smell, heat, cold, and the like, require the interaction of a soul and body. If animals do not have souls, how can they have perceptions, which only the interaction of soul and body can provide?

The ambiguity surrounding the question of animal perception brings to the fore the difficulty of Descartes' goal of a purely mechanistic account of animal physiology. Attributing a degree of thought or sensation to animals, even one that is not like ours, comes precariously close to pre-Cartesian notions of the 'sensitive' soul, where animals share in certain levels of awareness that humans have. Trying to account for aspects of what had been the sensitive soul in purely mechanistic terms is a major cause of much ambiguity in Descartes' account. The difficulty was well articulated by Henry More, who wrote to Descartes:

> Please tell me, Sir, since your demonstration leads you necessarily either to deprive the beasts of all feeling or to give them immortality, why you prefer to make of them inanimate machines rather than bodies endowed with immortal souls....[63]

Problems with the Body-Machine

This chapter has outlined several of Descartes' efforts to apply the principles of mechanism to the human body. These principles are based on assumptions relating to the homogenization of matter and the predominance of the general, abstract and quantifiable over the particular, concrete and qualitative in the new science. The Renaissance idea of body, which emphasized the dignity of each being (or type of being) in a hierarchy of qualitative organization and mutual influence (as described in the previous chapter), had to be discarded to make room for the mechanistic body, devoid of the individual qualities and subsumed under the laws of physics. The homogenization of matter and its distinctness from mind allowed the application of the Cartesian dream of the unity of science; it also transformed the human body into one knowable object among others.

As we have seen, much of Descartes' description of the human body is based on principles regarding the size, speed and direction of particles, which are all that is needed, in his view, to explain the operation of the machine that is the body. Descartes went to great lengths to describe the body in such a way as to prove that the soul (or mind) has no role to play in its operations.

All movement or biological activity that humans share with animals (which is everything except rational thought) is accounted for in strictly mechanistic terms. Even the addition of the soul does not change the mechanistic nature of the human body, since the role of the soul—in willed action, for example—is limited to changing the direction of the animal spirits. Descartes' analogy of the mechanical fountains is clear: the body is the fountain, the soul the fountaineer. The latter can control the switch, but the range of operation is determined solely by the arrangement of the parts of the machine.

At the same time, this application of the principles of mechanism to the human body is not without problems. Ambiguities and confusions arise regarding the precise role of the soul in activities such as perception, which leave the reader perplexed with regard to Descartes' meaning or sceptical with regard to his objective. Those who allow a charitable interpretation to Descartes in regard to his efforts of mechanization tend to smooth over the difficulties of accounting for human and animal behaviour without reference to mind or soul, or even ignore some of his unambiguous statements about what activities of perception, for example, require a soul. Others, relying heavily on Descartes' later efforts to link body and soul, go so far as to question whether or not Descartes was really a dualist, or to suggest that, if he was, he was not really comfortable with it. Cottingham, for example, tells us: "The truth, perhaps, is that Descartes was never completely comfortable with strict dualism, however emphatically he affirmed it."[64] Similar debates have taken place around whether or not Descartes really believed that animals feel no pain, a position that leaves open the question of how he could perform vivisection so enthusiastically if he thought they did. It would seem more generous to Descartes to presume that, when he cut a rabbit open to check the temperature of its heart or the circulation of the blood, he was acting out of ignorance and not out of cruelty.[65]

In the same article where he questions Descartes' true commitment to dualism, Cottingham writes about the "strange fuzziness" surrounding his position on animal feeling and consciousness, and states very aptly: "It is evident that Descartes is in a philosophical mess here,"[66] suggesting that his efforts to mechanize the human body were not an unmitigated success. This may account for why so few people today read either his physics or his physiology, but it does not account for why the mechanistic principles that he defended in relation to the human body endured, nor why they had such a strong influence on the development of modern biology and psychology, both of which have grown out of the assumption of the separation of mind and body.

The fuzziness referred to above extends to other aspects of Descartes' attempt to mechanize the body, as he kept the names but modified the meaning of previously understood concepts. He appears to have been quite aware of this strategy. For example, in January 1642 he wrote Regius regarding public disputations about the question of Aristotelian substantial forms. "I should like it best if you never put forward any new opinions," he wrote, "but retained all the old ones in name, and merely brought forward new arguments." Then he advised Regius that, to avoid conflicts in the future, "you should say that fundamentally you agree with the others and that your disagreement with them was merely verbal."[67]

Descartes put his own advice into practice when he revised the meaning of soul, reducing it to mind without any argument or justification. Responding to Gassendi, who had criticized his use of the word *soul* in the *Meditations*, saying that it was ambiguous, Descartes simply replied:

> it is generally the ignorant who have given things their names, and so the names do not always fit the things with sufficient accuracy. Our job, however, is not to change the names after they have been adopted into ordinary usage; we may merely emend their meanings when we notice that they are misunderstood by others.[68]

For Descartes, the soul (reduced to mind) is thought alone, while for Gassendi (like most pre-Cartesian thinkers) the soul represented an active principle of life, attuned to the cosmos, uniting different levels of being and accounting for change and movement in both humans and animals. With a simple declaration that the mind is not *part* of the soul but the soul in its entirety (a direct result of the *cogito*), Descartes transformed the principle of life while maintaining that he was simply avoiding ambiguous terminology.

Reduction can be defined broadly as "a habit of thought for dealing with complex situations by forgetting some structure in order to arrive at a more manageable and yet still significant remnant. Its advantage is conceptual streamlining; its disadvantage is forgetfulness."[69] In the case of the reduction of the meaning of soul, Descartes has achieved some conceptual streamlining for his mechanistic physiology, but the result is forgetfulness of the principle that held things together in the body and in nature.[70] We have already seen how Descartes accomplished similar streamlining in relation to the principle of life by explaining it solely on the basis of the heat of the heart. His 'fire without light' reduced a metaphysical explanation of cosmic heat to a physical and mechanical one of ordinary earthly fire. Given the problems we have seen in relation to his description of the movement of the heart, it can reasonably be claimed that his reduction was not up to the task he set for it.

His most interesting reduction, however, concerns animal spirits. It is somewhat surprising, given Descartes' reliance on method and mechanism, as well as his laborious study of physiology through the dissection of animal carcasses, that his system has any place for animal spirits, even in what one writer calls their "resolutely corporealized" form.[71] As resolutely corporealized as they were, there was no empirical evidence for their existence nor for their mode of operation, and accounting for them at all appears to go against Descartes' own statement to Mersenne that, after years of dissecting animals, he could find nothing in the body that did not conform to the principles of his physics. In fact, he did not *find* animal spirits at all; he presupposed their existence, in spite of the fact that they were downplayed or ignored by anatomists like Vesalius. Surprisingly, "there was a seventeenth-century shift *toward* animal spirit explanations, revealing simultaneously both increased explanatory ambition and wild speculation."[72]

In Descartes' case, the increased explanatory ambition is rooted in his original dream of the unity of science and his determination to explain animal and human physiology purely on mechanistic principles. To do so, he must reduce all causal explanation to physical, efficient causes, and must explain all change and movement (since change is equivalent to movement) in terms of the size, speed and direction of particles. Animal spirits serve a pivotal role in this system. They act as intermediaries or messengers between the brain and other body parts. The brain is the activity centre of the machine (both animal and human) and the animal spirits are its messengers, directing muscle movement, sense perception, memory and all the other activity anywhere in the body. They are defined in purely physical and mechanistic terms in both animals and humans, the only difference being that in the latter case the soul, acting from its seat in the pineal gland, has the power to change the *direction* of the animal spirits (by inclining that gland in one direction rather than another, a fact that Descartes uses to explain willed action or movement).[73] It is clear that he needed the notion of animal spirits in order to explain the function of the brain and how it controlled bodily processes. He had to accommodate action at a distance from the brain within the explanatory framework of efficient causality, that is, through direct contact. He needed a connector between brain centre and bodily movement (and in the human animal between soul and brain/ body) that was not spiritual or in any way occult. Animal spirits were firmly rooted in medical theory at that time, and Descartes continued to make use of them while adapting their role to his mechanistic theories. For him, they were connectors, but they were not mediators in the sense of Ficino's medical spirits, and their Cartesian adaptation cannot be described as a smooth reduction.

There is one overarching problem regarding the action of the soul on the animal spirits: if mind cannot causally interact with matter, how can it causally interact with animal spirits, which are material?[74] How can it move the pineal gland? Is Descartes not mistaken in supposing that, because the animal spirits are more subtle or rarefied, they are less material? His refusal to admit qualities in matter should preclude such a supposition. This raises the most important problem of all in relation to Descartes' physiology: his dualism.

No one was more aware of the difficulties inherent in Descartes' separation of mind and body and his mechanistic physiology than the young Princess Elisabeth, with whom Descartes carried on an intense correspondence during the last decade of his life. In her first letter to him in May 1643, she asked him to answer the following question:

> How can the soul of a man determine the spirits of his body so as to produce voluntary actions (given that the soul is only a thinking substance)? For it seems that all determination of movement is made by the pushing of a thing moved, either that it is pushed by the thing which moves it or it is affected by the quality or shape of the surface of that thing. For the first two conditions, touching is necessary, for the third extension. For touching, you exclude entirely the notion that you have of the soul; extension seems to me incompatible with an immaterial thing.[75]

Descartes responds to Elisabeth by agreeing that her question "seems to me the one which can most properly be put to me in view of my published writings." He explains to her that, while there are two things about the soul— that it thinks and that it interacts with the body—he has not so far tried to explain the latter because "my principal aim was to prove the distinction between the soul and the body, and to this end only the first was useful, and the second might have been harmful."[76]

Elisabeth has put her finger on the crux of the matter of Descartes' two-substance theory: mind cannot causally act on matter, because the two substances have nothing in common. Secondly, mind cannot act on matter because if it could it would be adding movement into the physical realm, while by Descartes' own mechanistic principles (the principle of the conservation of motion and the principle of inertia), the amount of motion in the physical sphere is constant, and the mind, being immaterial, cannot be supposed to contain or transmit motion. This is a serious problem that Descartes was never able adequately to overcome.

Descartes does attempt to account for mind-body union in his Sixth Meditation, in which he states that he is not lodged in his body as a pilot in his ship. He also took up the question in his final work, *The Passions of the Soul*, in large part as a result of the correspondence with Elisabeth. But his explanation in the latter work, relying on the concept of animal spirits, is inconsistent with his mechanistic physics, as has already been pointed out; and the explanation in the Sixth Meditation is less than convincing, in part because it goes against what he so clearly stated in his Second Meditation about the mind being pure thought. Not all scholars agree on this point, of course. L. J. Beck, while admitting that the question of mind-body unity is "one of the most difficult and controversial points in the whole Cartesian doctrine," nonetheless concludes that Descartes has been misunderstood on this question, that he "was perfectly clear in his own mind and there is no obscurity, wilful or otherwise, in his exposition of his views."[77] In fact, for Beck there is even a "curious gap between the attitude of Descartes, who seems to consider the problem one of the second order, and the vast importance it assumed in the subsequent history of Cartesianism and its presence with us today...."[78] This may be an understatement, and it is a question that will be addressed in particular in the following chapter on Spinoza, since it was this 'error' of his predecessor that Spinoza strove to correct.

The Modern 'Self'

The British philosopher Mary Midgley is a fierce critic of Descartes' dualism and the impact that it has had on Western civilization. She refers to the Westerner's "sense of complacent independence from the earth," an attitude that, though strongly influenced by the Christian idea of immortality of the soul, survives in spite of the fading of the Christian vision. The Christian view of the human soul was replaced with a Cartesian view of the human mind as a detached observer and manipulator of an objectified world: "So when they stopped venerating God, they began instead to venerate themselves as in some sense the supreme beings in the universe—intellectual marvels whose production must have been the real purpose of evolution."[79] With Descartes, as we have seen, the soul became reduced to the human mind, and, in the time since Descartes, we have followed him in disinheriting the world around us "of the attributes of life, soul and purpose which had infused it since the speculation of Pythagoras and Plato, Aristotle and Galen."[80]

It is not an exaggeration to say that part of what was disinherited has been the human body itself, and that the veneration of the intellect has become the veneration of the 'self,' a powerful force and focus of Western autonomy and individualism through which we see ourselves as separate from our bodies and from nature. Following Descartes' method and the principle of the unity of all knowledge, the world, the cosmos and the reasoning subject's body itself are all objects for the mind. As expressed by Hans Jonas,

> The discovery of 'self' ... had a curiously polarizing effect on the general picture of reality: the very possibility of the notion of an 'inanimate universe' emerged as the counterpart to the increasingly exclusive stress laid on the *human* soul, on its inner life and its incommensurability with anything in nature.... As the retreating soul drew about itself all spiritual significance and metaphysical dignity ... it left the world divested of all such claims....[81]

Jonas refers to the physical realm (including the body) as being drained of spiritual elements, leaving the body as the 'tomb' of the soul—which might be seen as a reversion to Plato (or Augustine, in his more anti-body moments), but the comparison is not totally apt. Plato's soul was part of the world-soul— something that has disappeared in Descartes' dualistic explanation. The soul-mind is not connected to anything beyond itself. This, as we will see, has had important ramifications for our view of the self and the human person.

How did what Jonas refers to as the *discovery* of the self come about? A quick examination of Charles Taylor's book, revealingly titled *Sources of the Self: The Making of the Modern Identity*, shows us that the process has a long and complex history. Taylor also provides an insight into the impact of this discovered self on the Western psyche. In fact, as the title suggests, it has shaped our modern lives to the point that, in his view, we "cannot understand ourselves without coming to grips with this history."[82]

While the history of the modern self began before Descartes—for example, Augustine can be credited with making the "first-person standpoint fundamental to our search for the truth"[83]—it was Descartes' dualism (and mechanism) that provided the modern self with its metaphysical and epistemological roots. With Descartes came a new direction that Taylor refers to as epoch-making; unlike either Plato or Augustine, "Descartes situates the moral sources within us."[84] In the Platonic universe, the Ideas (or Forms) were part of the cosmic order (they were not ideas in one's head!): "To be ruled by reason was to be turned towards the Ideas and hence moved by love of them. The locus of our sources of moral strength resides outside. To have access to the higher is to be turned towards and in tune with the cosmic order, which is shaped by the Good."[85] In Descartes' world, on the other hand, reason (no longer Reason) is internalized—reason becomes a question of method. In fact, as we have already seen, reason *is* method for Descartes. Reason becomes an activity of the mind, and ideas are not something external (as in Plato's Ideas), but things in the mind. "So the order of ideas ceases to be something we *find*, and becomes something we *build*."[86] Building requires a builder—a role into which the modern self inserts itself quite easily (since everything outside of it has already been objectified into a mechanistic universe). "We have to objectify the world, including our own bodies, and that means to come to see them mechanistically and functionally, in the same way that an uninvolved external observer would."[87]

Having separated the self from the world around it (including the body), the self becomes an agent of instrumental control. But it is not only the objective world that becomes subject to instrumental control; our own lives become something that we treat in an instrumental fashion, shaping them to the will of the self/agent: "If rational control is a matter of mind dominating a disenchanted world of matter, then the sense of the superiority of the good life, and the inspiration to attain it, must come from the agent's sense of his own dignity as a rational being."[88] Taylor sees this as the root of the modern theme of the dignity of the person (and, one could add, the contemporary obsession with self-esteem and the centrality of the individual). We are no longer attuned to the cosmos—we are each the centre of our own cosmos, and are encouraged to be so. More and more, this means that we must construct our own reality, detached from any encumbrance of family history, social status, geography or political reality. We shape our own destinies—something that entails an enormous responsibility: if we are constructing our own lives, we can get it wrong, which might explain Western society's addiction to self-improvement. Writing about the current trend toward surgical shaping (to correct or enhance body parts), Arthur Frank (echoing Taylor) refers to the idea of the body as a *project*, and of a life as raw material that people somehow expect to shape to their desires and choices: "Many of us moderns," he says, "include doing things with our bodies among the ways to seek the unique point of our lives. At the extreme, the point of one's life can be the modification of one's body."[89] We will examine the phenomenon of extreme body modification in a later chapter. What I wish to underline here is the radical separation of the self and the body, in which the body becomes an instrument for constructing the unique and separate self, a notion the Stoics would have found rather strange.

This radical separation of self and body is one variation on the theme of mind-body separation in Descartes, but there are a number of other dichotomies that resulted from dualistic and mechanistic thinking, which have developed over the centuries and influence our thought and actions even today. One of these is the distinction between reason and emotion, and the predominance of the former (representing mind) over the latter (representing body). Reason (knowledge) is also opposed to sensation, with reason and rational knowledge overvalued at the expense of intuition and knowledge through the body and the senses. As we have seen in Descartes, knowledge from the senses is unreliable and, in the final analysis, is not considered to be knowledge at all. Most influential of all, however, has been the association of maleness with mind and reason, and the association of femaleness with emotion, intuition, body and nature. These oppositions have been relied on regularly to justify male superiority over, and domination of, the female, just as they have been relied on, from Bacon on, as a rationalization for the dominance of the human mind over nature and the manipulation and subjugation of the natural world to human needs and desires. Susan Bordo refers to the "seventeenth-century flight from the feminine," as both empirical science and rationalism took on the project the taming of the female universe.[90] It is no wonder that Descartes is no friend of modern feminist thinkers.

The foregoing is an abbreviated account of Descartes' physiology and its dependence on his metaphysical dualism and his mechanistic science. As has already been pointed out, the details of this account were later ignored or rejected, but the metaphysical structure of a mind-soul-self separated from an objective world, from others in the world and from its own body, remained as the governing framework of science and, in particular, medical science. In the second part of this book, we will see just how much this framework has shaped our individual lives, as well—to a point that seriously impedes our development as whole human beings. The disengaged self has proved useful to the Western concept of the person, and has perhaps served to curtail much political and social abuse of individuals and their dignity. But it has brought with it a serious disadvantage, not the least part of which is the fact that it does not conform to reality, or to the everyday experience of ordinary people. We are not disconnected from this world, from others, or from nature, and we all know it; yet everything around us encourages us to think that we are. In fact, some of our most creative minds are devoting themselves to figuring out how this disconnected mind-self can actually be separated from its physical body and downloaded into a computer or robot (the ultimate body-machine). And many think these new body-machines will be able to find a more suitable home on another planet! "The vision of ourselves as essentially invulnerable minds, independent of earthly support, colonists here whose intellects will always find them a new home whatever may go wrong, is still amazingly strong."[91] It is ironic, however, that the modern, separated self that Western society has spent four centuries developing, nurturing and protecting is the very thing that Eastern philosophies such as yoga tell us we must let go if we truly want to reach self-fulfilment.[92] Our journey through the philosophical story of the body will take us through these differing perspectives.

Before heading there, however, we will take a detour in the following chapter as we examine a very different approach to mind, body and the world from one of Descartes' immediate successors—an approach which, I believe, harks back to the Stoics and across the world to the East. It is what I have referred to as the road not followed: the road of Spinoza and mind-body unity.

Notes

1.   Richard Tarnas, *Western Mind*, 276.

2.   John Cottingham, *Cartesian Reflections: Essays on Descartes' Philosophy* (Oxford: Oxford University Press, 2008), 76.

3.   John Cottingham, Robert Stoothoff and Dugald Murdoch, eds., *The Philosophical Writings of Descartes, Volume I* (Cambridge: Cambridge University Press, 1984), 9. Future references to volumes I and II of this translation of Descartes' works will be cited as CSM I or CSM II.

4.   L. J. Beck, *The Method of Descartes* (Oxford: Clarendon Press, 1952), 21.

5.   John Cottingham, Robert Stoothoff, Dugald Murdoch and Anthony Kenny, eds., *The Philosophical Writings of Descartes, Volume III, The Correspondence* (Cambridge: Cambridge University Press, 1991), 2. (AT X, 156). Volume III of these translations is hereafter referred to as CMSK.

6.   *Principles of Philosophy*, in CSM I, 184, preface to the French edition.

7.   Beck, 16.

8.   Descartes' reduction of the soul to pure mind will be discussed later. Here it is important to point out only that this is a major shift, and one that he *presumes* (and does not prove) from his earliest writings.

9.   Beck, 21.

10.   While the *Rules for the Direction of the Mind* is a detailed work on method, it was not published in Descartes' lifetime.

11.   CSM I, 120.

12.   See Rule Three, CSM I, 120–121.

13.   Descartes' concern here is metaphysical—that is, he is dealing with the establishment of clear and certain first principles. This is his main epistemological concern. It should be emphasized, however, that his application of first principles to branches of science such as physiology or medicine involved more than intuition and deduction. As we will see later in the chapter, Descartes conducted experiments—e.g., dissection of animals—in order to establish hypotheses about the functioning of the human body. But, as we will also see, his hypotheses were designed to fit his established first principles (the laws of nature that will be discussed later in this chapter. As expressed by Desmond Clarke: "He assumed that we can, and ought, to construct our metaphysics first, and that we should subsequently consider physical theories which are consistent with our metaphysical foundation. Thus there must be available independent criteria for deciding which metaphysics to adopt." Desmond C. Clarke, "Decartes' Philosophy of Science and the Scientific Revolution," in *The Cambridge Companion to Descartes*, edited by John Cottingham (Cambridge: Cambridge University Press, 1992), 272.

14.   CSM I, 111.

15.   CSM I, 131. Descartes published the *Discourse on Method* anonymously, specifically because of the "questions that are being debated" which related to the Copernican view of the universe.

16.   CSM I, 131.

17.   Stephen Toulmin, *Cosmopolis* (Chicago: University of Chicago Press, 1990), 42. The *Apology* refers to the "Apology of Raymond Sebond," the longest of Montaigne's *Essays*.

18.   CSM II, 17.

19.   CSM II, 18.

20.   CSM II, 18.

21.   Tarnas, *Western Mind,* 278.

22.   Letter to Mersenne, 15 April 1630, CMSK, 21.

23.   There is a reference in a letter of Regius in May 1640 regarding attendance at a dissection, but at a much later date: "Three years ago at Leiden, when I wanted to see it [the conarium] in a woman who was being autopsied, I found it impossible to recognize it, even though I looked very thoroughly, and knew well where it should be, being accustomed to find it without difficulty in freshly killed animals." CMSK, 146.

24.   Letter to Mersenne, November or December 1633, CMSK, 40.

25.   In addition, Sawday tells us that "[e]ven by the mid-seventeenth century, Vesalius' images in the *Fabrica* still provided the standard record of dissection." See Jonathan Sawday, *The Body Emblazoned: Dissection and the Human Body in Renaissance Culture* (London: Routledge, 1996), 155.

26.   Stephen Gaukroger, *Descartes: An Intellectual Biography* (Oxford: Clarendon Press, 1995), 271.

27.   Neither *The World* nor the *Treatise* was published during Descartes' lifetime because of the controversy over Galileo and the heliocentric view of the universe. As already pointed out, he did summarize parts of the *Treatise* in his *Discourse on Method* (published anonymously for the same reason). In addition, his last philosophical work, *The Passions of the Soul,* published in 1649 not long before his death, provides an account of the body and its functions, which summarizes briefly what is set out in the *Treatise.* In this latter work, however, he attempts to give a clearer understanding of the interaction of body and soul, providing explanations of the function of the pineal gland and animal spirits, which do not fundamentally alter his mechanistic account of the body set out in the *Treatise.* For this reason, my account of his mechanistic physiology in this chapter is based solely on the *Treatise.* The issue of Descartes' use (and reduction) of the idea of animal spirits is discussed later in the chapter.

28.   Stephen Gaukroger, ed., *Descartes: The World and Other Writings* (Cambridge: Cambridge University Press, 1998), 25 (hereinafter referred to as *World*). The idea that "God continues to preserve it in the same way that He created it" is the principle of continuous creation, a principle that explained God's connection with the world He created. Descartes preserves the concept, but modifies it to fit his mechanistic conception of nature. Descartes' comment on 'Nature,' here, is a direct reference to the notion that nature is ensouled or in any other way alive—a view held by the naturalists whose views Cartesian mechanism was to counter.

29.   *World,* 25.

30. *World*, 27.

31. *World*, 29.

32. *World*, 99. As with his description of the natural world, Descartes' description of the human body is written as a 'fable' for reasons of caution. That is why he refers to God forming the bodies "as much as possible like us." The *Treatise* was not published during Descartes' lifetime, again for reasons of caution and fear of reprisal from the religious authorities.

33. *World*, 107, emphasis added. That Descartes includes something as 'occult' as animal spirits in his explanation of the human body is a problematic element of his physiology that will be discussed later in the chapter.

34. *World*, 169.

35. *World*, 100.

36. *World*, 101. Gaukroger points out that this comparison "between the processes of sanguinification and fermentation was traditional, and can be found in Galen … but Descartes' account of the nature of the process involved, which offers a corpuscularian reduction, is very different from the traditional account" (101, n 8).

37. *World*, 104 (emphasis added).

38. *World*, 104 (emphasis added).

39. *World*, 101.

40. *World*, 182.

41. *World*, 102.

42. Singer, 284.

43. Bitbol-Hespériès points out the difference between Descartes and Aristotle or Galen: "…this conception is contrary to Aristotle's, as well as Galen's, although both of them use the metaphor of fire within the heart, a metaphor widely reused in medical works. Thus, according to Aristotle, it is indeed the heart that is the source and seat of animal heat, but this animal heat is explicitly differentiated from the heat generated by 'ordinary fire'…. Descartes' conception of heat as a mechanical process is contrary to the views of both Aristotle and Galen for whom such heat is a mode of being." Annie Bitbol-Hespériès, *Le principe de vie chez Descartes* (Paris: Librairie philosophique J. Vrin, 1990), 71. (Translated by Guy Gagnon)

44. *World*, 106 (emphasis added).

45. *World*, 114. Including the heart in this list seems to contradict Descartes' theory of the heart being moved by the fermentation of the blood, since, as Gaukroger points out, "it seems to imply that animal spirits, acting through the nerves to the heart, cause its motion—which is in effect to say that its motion is due to muscular action"—the very point on which Descartes was in disagreement with Harvey (Gaukroger, 114, n 22).

46.   *World*, 109.
47.   *World*, 112.
48.   *World*, 116.
49.   *World*, 117.
50.   *World*, 117.
51.   *World*, 107.
52.   On this point see Gary Hatfield, "Descartes' Physiology and its Relation to his Psychology," in *The Cambridge Companion to Descartes*, ed. John Cottingham (Cambridge: Cambridge University Press, 1992), 348, where he makes the point that Descartes' position in the *Treatise on Man* suggests that "all motions of the limbs result from a specific mechanical contrivance that is activated solely by the direction of the spirits leaving the pineal gland, which would mean that those motions governed by the soul must be effected solely by influencing the direction of the motion of the spirits."
53.   *World*, 3.
54.   *De Anima*, 171.
55.   *World*, 3. See Gaukroger, *Descartes*, 282ff for an account of why the Aristotelian notions of perception, where our perceptual image of the world resembles how the world is, began to fall apart in the seventeenth century, in part because of Kepler's discovery of the inverted retinal image.
56.   Unfortunately, Descartes' language is often misleading, as when he states, "The change of shape that occurs in the crystalline humour allows objects lying at different distances *to paint their images distinctly on the back of the eye*," *World*, 128.
57.   *World*, 132.
58.   Hatfield, 355.
59.   Anyone who has ever watched a cat stalk and successfully pounce on a squirrel or a bird has to be impressed with its perceptual accuracy, including judging distance.
60.   Hatfield, 357.
61.   Gaukroger, *Descartes*, 288.
62.   Gaukroger, *Descartes*, 454, n 165.
63.   See Geneviève Lewis, ed., *Descartes: Correspondance avec Arnauld et Morus* (Paris: Librairie philosophique J. Vrin, 1953), 107. "Mais dites-moi, je vous prie, monsieur, puisque votre démonstration vous conduit nécessairement, ou à priver les bêtes de tout sentiment, ou à leur donner l'immortalité, pourquoi aimez-vous mieux en faire des machines inanimées, que des corps remués par des âmes immortelles...."

64. See John Cottingham, "A Brute to the Brutes? Descartes's Treatment of Animals," in *René Descartes, Critical Assessments, Vol. IV*, ed. Georges J. D. Moyal (London: Routledge), 329.

65. For Descartes' own description of this event, see his letter to Plempius, CMSK, 81.

66. Cottingham, "Brute," 328.

67. CMSK, 206.

68. CSM II, 246.

69. Emily Grosholz, *Cartesian Method and the Problem of Reduction* (Oxford: Clarendon Press, 1991), 12.

70. Descartes' reductions were fairly early examples of a process that is now entrenched in biology. Birke reports that, a century ago, "reductionism battled against more descriptive accounts within biology. But reductionism was seen as 'more scientific,' in that it assumed experimental approaches and sought explanations in physicochemical processes. Thus it eventually won out." See Lynda Birke, *Feminism and the Biological Body* (New Brunswick, NJ: Rutgers University Press, 2000), 140.

71. John Sutton, *Philosophy and Memory Traces* (Cambridge: Cambridge University Press, 1999), 44.

72. Sutton, 32. Sutton adds, "the use of spirits in alchemy and chemistry is not as surprising as their continued presence in supposedly austere mechanical philosophies."

73. Changing only the *direction* of the animal spirits does not interfere with the principle of the conservation of movement.

74. While there are different grades of matter in Descartes, there are only two grades of being: matter and mind. And while animal spirits are the most refined and subtle type of matter, they are, nevertheless, purely material.

75. Andrea Nye, *The Princess and the Philosopher* (Lanham, MD: Rowman & Littlefield, 1999), 9.

76. CMSK, 218 (AT III, 665).

77. L. J. Beck, *The Metaphysics of Descartes: A Study of the Meditations* (Oxford: Clarendon Press, 1965), 262, 276.

78. Beck, 269. It should be emphasized that the resolution of the mind-body problem is not the objective of this book, and the question of whether or not Descartes adequately addressed the mind-body union is secondary to my main concern, the body-machine. Descartes did not waver in his mechanistic conception of the human body, no matter what explanations he provided for its union with the soul or mind.

79. Mary Midgley, "Souls, Minds, Bodies & Planets," *Philosophy Now*, 48:5 (2004), www.philosophynow.org/issue48/48midgley.htm (accessed January 20, 2007).

We will see in a later chapter how many scientists in the world of genetics and robotics think they understand the real purpose of evolution—something that would surprise Darwin, were he alive today, and that reflects a religious, rather than scientific, attitude.

80.   Midgley, 5.

81.   Hans Jonas, *The Phenomenon of Life* (Evanston, IL: Northwestern University Press, 2001), 14.

82.   Charles Taylor, *Sources of the Self: The Making of the Modern Identity* (Cambridge: Harvard University Press, 1989), ix. In fact, Taylor observes, it has also shaped philosophical and scientific thought, and even though such domains are believed to be free of such influences, they "reflect much more than we realize the ideals that have helped constitute this identity of ours" (ix).

83.   Taylor, 133. Jonas actually sees the discovery of self as going back to the Greeks and early Christians.

84.   Taylor, 143.

85.   Taylor, 143.

86.   Taylor, 144.

87.   Taylor, 145.

88.   Taylor, 152.

89.   Arthur Frank, "Emily's Scars: Surgical Shapings, Technoluxe, and Bioethics," in *Hastings Center Report* 34:2 (2004), 20.

90.   Susan Bordo, *The Flight to Objectivity: Essays on Cartesianism and Culture* (Albany: SUNY Press, 1987), 111. The flight from the feminine is not an idea invented by twentieth-century feminists—nor was it limited to Descartes. Bordo quotes Bacon, for example, who believed he was inaugurating "a truly masculine birth of time," and Henry Oldenburg of the Royal Society (a society dedicated to the advancement of science), proclaiming that the business of that society was to raise a "masculine philosophy." As Bordo states: "The founders of modern science consciously and explicitly proclaimed the 'masculinity' of science as inaugurating a new era. And they associated that masculinity with a cleaner, purer, more objective and more disciplined epistemological relation to the world" (105). The masculinization of science went hand in hand with the mechanization of nature, and both are related, in Bordo's view, to "what now appears as a virtual obsession with the untamed natural power of female generativity, and a dedication to bringing it under forceful cultural control" (109).

91.   Midgley, 5.

92.   I would emphasize that the Eastern idea of self-fulfilment is quite different from the Western idea of self-improvement; this will become clear in the latter part of the book.

CHAPTER VI

THE ROAD NOT FOLLOWED: SPINOZA

As we have seen in Chapter 5, in spite of the radical nature of his metaphysics, Descartes was what we might today consider a mainstream thinker. He occupied the same conceptual space as his predecessors, and, while he transformed many ancient concepts and ideas, he took pains to remain within the confines of religious orthodoxy. He would not publish his important work on physics because of the controversy over Galileo and the heliocentric universe. He did his best not to offend the religious authorities—and even to solicit their approval—as can be seen in the Introduction to his *Meditations*, which he dedicated to the good doctors of the Sorbonne. In fact, his need to accommodate Christian belief in an immortal soul in his new mechanistic philosophy was at the root of many of the ambiguities in his dualism; he chose orthodoxy at the price of philosophical clarity.

By contrast, Spinoza took few of Descartes' precautions and became the most notable renegade of the seventeenth century. His philosophy fits into my story of the body as the road not followed largely because of this simple fact: he was a heretic. He was excommunicated from the Synagogue of Amsterdam in 1656 with the following words:

> Cursed be he by day and cursed be he by night; cursed be he when he lies
> down, and cursed be he when he rises up; cursed be he when he goes out,
> and cursed be he when he comes in. The Lord will not pardon him; the
> anger and wrath of the Lord will rage against this man, and bring upon

him all the curses which are written in the Book of the Law, and the Lord will destroy his name from under the Heavens....

We ordain that no one may communicate with him verbally or in writing, nor show him any favour, nor stay under the same roof with him, nor be within four cubits of him, nor read anything composed or written by him.[1]

In addition, his major work, the *Ethics*, was put on the *Index Librorum Prohibitorum*, the Catholic Church's list of forbidden readings, and remained there until well into the twentieth century, when the *Index* was abolished. If Spinoza's road was not followed, it is at least in part because of the enduring perception of him as a renegade (not to mention an atheist). Today, his philosophy is enjoying a renaissance, and from our perspective it appears that his ideas might have been misunderstood in his time. It has even been suggested that he really did not want his work to be understood—except by the few who were capable of grasping his meaning and his method.[2]

Baruch Spinoza was born in 1632 into a family of formerly Spanish Jews who had settled in Portugal after having been expelled from Spain during the Inquisition. These transplanted Spanish Jews were referred to as Marranos;[3] most of them continued to practise their Jewish faith in secret, even though they had been forced to convert to Christianity. As pressure on them increased in Portugal, many fled to more tolerant countries, one of which was the new Republic of the Netherlands. As a result, a fairly large number settled in Amsterdam, among them Spinoza's parents, who had lived in Portugal as Catholics. As an exiled religious group returning to its practice, however, the Amsterdam Jewish community was very strict in its adherence to orthodox religion, and new arrivals were expected to conform. This is the community into which Spinoza was born, and its history of persecution, flight and orthodoxy is important in understanding why the community later expelled "as unworthy of its protection, the greatest genius who had grown within its care."[4]

Spinoza attended Jewish school and the synagogue, where he studied Hebrew and the works of Jewish and Arab theologians. His father hoped he would become a rabbi, but he began to move in another direction when certain teachers introduced him to the scholastics and then to the new philosophy of Descartes. As a result, he became more interested in natural science and Latin than in Jewish theology, much to the consternation of the rabbis. He was already showing himself to be unorthodox within his community as he immersed himself in a philosophical world of secular and naturalistic concerns that threatened both Jewish and Christian orthodoxy. In 1656, at the age of twenty-three, Spinoza was judged to be incorrigible by the rabbis and was cast out of the synagogue with the words cited above. He left Amsterdam, eventually settling in The Hague for the rest of his life. In spite of the terms of the excommunication order, which at any rate applied only to Jews but did include his family, Spinoza did not live an isolated existence. He was surrounded by "a small circle of devoted friends, freethinking Christians from various Protestant circles, who regarded [him] as their master and closely studied, and guarded, his thoughts."[5]

An interesting fact about Spinoza's life was that he was not a full-time philosopher or teacher—he was a grinder and polisher of lenses (for spectacles, microscopes, telescopes), an occupation he took up more for scientific than economic reasons, following his interest in optics. So, along with writing philosophy, he produced high-quality lenses that were much appreciated by scientists of the time. It is probably this occupation that brought him to an early death at the age of forty-four, since breathing the dust from the lens polishing was rather risky for one whose mother and brother both died of tuberculosis.

Spinoza and Descartes

The philosophy of Descartes played a major role in the development of Spinoza's thought. Descartes' philosophy had caused much controversy when it hit the Dutch universities, but eventually it became very influential, and Spinoza came to maturity in an intellectual environment steeped in Cartesian philosophy. So, his philosophical thinking could not but have been influenced by the ideas of Descartes. At the same time, much of his metaphysical thinking was directed toward correcting what he perceived as the errors of Descartes, in particular the latter's notion of two substances created by a transcendent God. Using Descartes' own principles, he contradicted Cartesian dualism and replaced it with a one-substance theory (which rejected both the notion of creation and that of a transcendent God), a theory that could only attract the ire and the condemnation of both Christian and Jewish authorities. Spinoza's *Ethics* may be "one of the most remarkable metaphysical systems in the entire history of philosophy [that] makes the work of Descartes and Leibniz look feeble by comparison,"[6] but in the eyes of the Jewish and Christian intellectual and religious world, Spinoza was a heretic and remained so for three centuries.

Today, Spinoza is seen by many as a hero, a philosopher ahead of his time, and his work is admired for its anticipation of the metaphysical foundations of quantum physics and contemporary neuroscience, for example. As Stuart Hampshire puts it, Spinoza was "less incomplete in his anticipations than any other philosopher; certainly he was less incomplete in his anticipations than Descartes."[7] As Descartes and his influence are now being rethought and his dualism rejected in many circles, Spinoza is coming into his own in the world of philosophy and philosophers of the twenty-first century. Even feminist philosophers are finding in Spinoza an alternative to the dualistic tendencies of modernity. In the introduction to her book, *Feminist Interpretations of Benedict Spinoza*, Moira Gatens explains Spinoza's appeal, in part, "by his commitment to an immanent, naturalistic worldview that is amenable to the human understanding through 'scientific' explanation."[8]

Dualism versus Monism

We have seen the contrast between dualistic and monistic metaphysics before, especially in relation to the dualism of Plato and the monism of the Stoics. For a dualist (and Descartes was a more radical dualist than Plato), mind (or soul) and matter are considered to be two different substances (Descartes), or at least to belong to two different realms of being (Plato). For the Stoics and Spinoza, on the other hand, whatever mind and matter (or, to speak in language more appropriate to the Stoics, soul and nature) are, they are of the same order of being; in Spinoza's case, they are the same substance, expressing itself in two different ways. We have seen that, for the Stoics, this meant that human beings are part of nature and that everything in nature is, to different degrees, ensouled. Similarly, for Spinoza, human beings are part of nature and everything in nature is alive to some degree.

For Spinoza, Descartes' major error was to posit the existence of two substances: mind and matter. He then had to account for how two substances, which had nothing in common, could interact. This, we have seen, he was never able to do with any degree of success. In Descartes' metaphysics, God created mind and matter and transcended both. Thus, Descartes had to explain not only the interaction of mind and matter, but the causal connection between God and creation—another question that posed problems for his mechanism. One of Spinoza's goals was correcting what he perceived as these Cartesian errors.

Spinoza posits a single substance, and that substance is God or Nature (in Spinoza's Latin, *Deus sive Natura*). These two terms can be used interchangeably, since God *is* Nature, or the totality of all that exists. This is the one substance, or, as Spinoza states it in Proposition 14 of the *Ethics*, "There can be, or be conceived, no other substance but God."[9] For Spinoza, mind and matter, or thought and extension, are not substances; they are two different *attributes* of the one substance, and they are the only two attributes that we are able to comprehend, although God, or the one substance, may have attributes that go beyond our ability to conceive of them.[10] We perceive substance only through its attributes and modes, never as a thing in itself. In fact, we cannot actually perceive the attributes of thought and extension either, but only their different modes, such as individual thoughts, ideas or imaginings, on the one hand, or material objects and bodies, on the other. Trees, for example, are modes of the attribute of extension or matter; the thoughts you have as you read this book are modes of the attribute of thought or mind. Ultimately, all things mental and physical are modifications of the one substance: God or Nature. The result of this is expressed by Spinoza in Part II of the *Ethics*, as follows:

Pr. 1: "Thought is an attribute of God; i.e., God is a thinking thing."

Pr. 2: "Extension is an attribute of God; i.e., God is an extended thing."[11]

It can be immediately seen how these two propositions would rankle the religious authorities, but for Spinoza they follow logically from the definition of substance, which, like Descartes, he defines as that which has no need of anything else in order to exist. Spinoza simply takes Descartes' definition to its logical conclusion, the result of which is expressed by Hampshire, as follows:

There can be only one substance so defined, and nothing can exist independently of, or distinct from, this single substance; everything which exists must be conceived as an attribute or modification of, or as in some way inherent in, this single substance; this substance is therefore to be identified with Nature conceived as an intelligible whole.... Thus Spinoza's logic leads remorselessly to the phrase, which shocked the pious, *Deus sive Natura*, as the inevitable name of the unique, infinite and all-inclusive Substance.[12]

The reader might be forgiven for feeling somewhat confused, at this point, wondering if what Spinoza is saying is *really* that different from what Descartes said. After all, whether you call it substance or attribute, you can't perceive it directly anyway, so maybe Descartes' way of defining the world is really much clearer and closer to our experience than Spinoza's way. I will argue, however, that there is a great deal of difference between these two philosophers, and that this difference is fundamental to understanding Spinoza's conception of the human body, a conception that is more relevant to us today than Descartes' dualism and mechanism. But before arriving at that point, we must backtrack a bit and look at Spinoza's philosophy in more detail, a little bit at a time.

Parts and Wholes: The Analogy of the Worm

First, a story by way of analogy, which gives a glimpse of the meaning of Spinoza's entire metaphysics. This is the 'analogy of the worm,' and it is one of the very rare occasions when Spinoza descended from the heights of abstraction for which he is famous to present a concrete vision of his monism—and of the interconnectedness of all things that follow from it. It was in reply to his friend Henry Oldenburg, who, quite simply, asked Spinoza to explain "how we know the way in which each part of Nature agrees with the whole, and the manner of its coherence with the other parts."[13]

Spinoza's reply to Oldenburg's question provides a very important explanation, and it is worth quoting in its entirety:

> Now let us imagine, if you please, a tiny worm living in the blood, capable of distinguishing by sight the particles of the blood—lymph, etc.—and of intelligently observing how each particle, on colliding with another, either rebounds or communicates some degree of its motion, and so forth. That worm would be living in the blood as we are living in our part of the universe, and it would regard each individual particle as a whole not a part, and it would have no idea as to how all the parts are modified by the overall nature of the blood and compelled to mutual adaptation as the overall nature of the blood requires, so as to agree with one another in a definite relation. For if we imagine that there are no causes external to the blood which would communicate new motions to the blood, nor any space external to the blood, nor any other bodies to which the particles of blood could transfer their motions, it is beyond doubt that the blood will remain indefinitely in its present state and that its particles will undergo no changes other than those which can be conceived as resulting from

the existing relation between the motion of the blood and that of the lymph, chyle, etc. Thus the blood would always have to be regarded as a whole, not a part. But since there are many other causes which do in fact modify the laws of the nature of the blood and are reciprocally modified by the blood, it follows that there occur in the blood other motions and other changes, resulting not solely from the reciprocal relations of its particles but from the relation between the motion of the blood on the one hand and external causes on the other. In this perspective the blood is accounted as a part, not a whole. So much, then, for the question of whole and part.

Now all the bodies in Nature can and should be conceived in the same way as we have here conceived the blood; for all bodies are surrounded by others and are reciprocally determined to exist and to act in a fixed and determinate way, the same ratio of motion to rest being preserved in them taken all together, that is, in the universe as a whole. Hence it follows that every body, in so far as it exists as modified in a definite way, must be considered as a part of the whole universe and must agree with the whole and cohere with the other parts.[14]

Thus, if we perceive ourselves and the people and things around us as wholes, we are making the same mistake as the worm in the blood. It is not even enough to see separate things as adding up to a whole; one has to first grasp an idea of the whole of nature, and then see the parts in relation to the whole, which, in effect, determines them. In other words, the whole comes first. If we do not understand this, we will tend to see the system of nature like the worm sees the system of blood, imagining that we and everything around us are wholes that we might or might not interact with. For Spinoza, however, we are part of a wider system: the entire universe; we are interconnected parts, not wholes, and our actions influence and are influenced by the actions of all the other parts.

Several implications of this vision of parts and wholes will be discussed later. Suffice it to say for the moment that, with the mutual interaction of parts and wholes and the idea of moving from whole to part, all individuals are part of a web of interaction and are determined by that web. Spinoza did not believe in free will. More importantly, as will be discussed later, for Spinoza there is no Cartesian self separated from matter and from nature. There is a self, but it is an interconnected self, as we will see.

The *Ethics* and Spinoza's Geometric Method

Two aspects of reading Spinoza are initially confusing for those who are new to his philosophy. The first is that his major work, which is really a philosophical discussion of mind, body and nature, is entitled the *Ethics*. The second is the fact that this book is set out in what Spinoza describes as his geometrical method. It is written as a series of propositions and proofs that are themselves built on the definitions and axioms, which open each of the five parts of the work. We will look at each of these peculiar aspects of Spinoza's work in turn.

Spinoza's *Ethics*

While Spinoza's best-known work is called *Ethics*, not one of its five sections contains the word. Part I is titled "Concerning God"; Part II is titled "Concerning the Nature and Origin of the Human Mind"; Parts III and IV are called, respectively, "Concerning the Origin and Nature of the Emotions" and "On Human Servitude, or the Strength of the Emotions"; and Part V is called "Concerning the Power of the Intellect, or On Human Freedom." None of these titles contains what we might normally consider ethical words such as good and evil, right and wrong. And certainly the first two parts appear to fall into the category of metaphysics, not ethics. But there is a very good reason for the title of this book, one that the Stoics would have understood very well. Like the Stoics, who saw physics, metaphysics and ethics as a unity, Spinoza's aim was to present an ethical system grounded in metaphysics, nature and mind. In his highly interconnected universe, an understanding of the whole (or as close an understanding as humanly possible) is what constitutes the good, and thus forms the basis of an ethical life.

Thus, Spinoza's first job is to discuss metaphysics, to explain the universe in terms of God, mind and body—along with his particular idea of human freedom—in order to set the stage for the later parts of the work that do speak of ethics in the more accepted sense of the term. But Spinoza's view of ethics is unique; he defines "good," for example, as that which is useful to us, and "virtue" as meaning the same thing as power. As he tells us, "The more every man endeavors and is able to seek his own advantage, that is, to preserve his own being, the more he is endowed with virtue. On the other hand, in so far as he neglects to preserve what is to his advantage, that is, his own being, to that extent he is weak."[15] Overall, in his book, "we are given an account of what is 'good' in the sense of being conducive to survival, stability, health, and clarity of mind (Spinoza argues that these stand or fall together)."[16] So, the book really is about ethics, but, since ethics, for Spinoza, is grounded in metaphysics, we get the metaphysics first. As with the Stoics, Spinoza's ethics follows from his metaphysics.

To achieve happiness in life, we must understand our own selves and the world in which we live. Understanding ourselves entails a deep understanding of our emotions and how they keep us in bondage or servitude (a word found in the title of Part IV) and prevent us from being free. Spinoza takes the emotions very seriously; he understands how powerful they are, and how they have the capacity to enslave us. Further, they continue to enslave us as long as we do not understand their power over us. To understand what is right, we must understand nature and human nature. Thus, much of the *Ethics* is devoted to explaining what, in Spinoza's view, the world and humans are like. The rest is to teach us how to gain power over our emotions through knowledge of nature and knowledge of ourselves. This, for Spinoza, is true virtue. We must understand our nature and the nature of the world in order to find happiness. The Stoic notion of living in accordance with nature shines through Spinoza's text.

Spinoza's Geometric Method

Hampshire points out that, if Descartes was a rationalist, Spinoza was doubly so: "no other philosopher has ever insisted more uncompromisingly that all problems, whether metaphysical, moral or scientific, must be formulated and solved as purely intellectual problems, as if they were theorems in geometry."[17] And Genevieve Lloyd states that, while the use of the geometrical method in philosophical writing was not something new at that time, "Spinoza, in presenting the whole of the *Ethics* in geometrical form, goes further than any of his predecessors."[18] This is certainly a barrier to reading the *Ethics*, as many commentators have pointed out, although Spinoza does facilitate things through elaborations and explanations in what are called *scholia*, as well as in appendices to his chapters. Each chapter begins with a number of definitions and axioms; the propositions in each chapter then refer back to these initial assumptions, and each proposition flows from the one before with strict logical necessity. Like Descartes, Spinoza was on a quest for certainty, and he too believed that knowledge of the world could be presented with as much certainty as mathematics. Both took the certainty of geometry as their model; Spinoza just went further with a geometrical exposition of his arguments, insisting that genuine knowledge comes from logically necessary propositions.

In fact, Spinoza's propositions are mutually supporting; each of his propositions connects with those that come before it and those that come after it, the result being an interconnected whole that mirrors reality. As Spinoza himself says in Part II of the *Ethics*: "The order and connection of ideas is the same as the order and connection of things."[19] Nature has a logical order, and is a deductive system. So the key to understanding Spinoza's text is to read through it and try to grasp it as a whole—and to worry about the connections and interconnections later. As Hampshire says, one "has to travel round the whole circle at least once before one can begin to understand any segment of it."[20] The mutual influence of part and whole, which Spinoza describes in his metaphysics, is reflected in his text.

Mind, Body and Nature

As already mentioned, Spinoza's vision of the world is that of a monist. There is only one substance and that substance is God or Nature—we can call it by either name, the meaning is the same. The one substance is the totality of everything that exists—something that we comprehend only intellectually as an underlying reality. We can analyze it as a physical system or as a system of thoughts and minds, but either perspective is the self-creating universe revealing itself to our limited human intellect.

While the one substance can be known either as a physical system or as a system of thought, neither system can be reduced to the other. Spinoza is neither a materialist, reducing everything to matter, nor an idealist, reducing everything to mind. Nor are his systems to be seen as parallel tracks of reality; they are, in effect, one track seen in two different ways: "Consequently, thinking substance and extended substance are one and the same substance, comprehended now under this attribute, now under that."[21] This is one of the most difficult aspects of Spinoza's metaphysics, and one that is often misunderstood. It is especially difficult for us, accustomed as we are to a dualistic tradition that has shaped our thinking and our worldview. Spinoza redesigned Descartes' two-substance theory into a one-substance theory with two universal characteristics or attributes. More than that, however, Spinoza also redesigned Descartes' theory that only humans have minds; he insists that the two universal attributes, being universal, apply to all beings. What we tend to see as human perception, appetites or interests are shared by non-human animals, as well, although at varying degrees of complexity: "even the more thoughtful human desires can be seen also as elaborations of original appetites."[22] Human life and human thought are part of a continuum; we are not the special creatures that the Christian religion teaches—a belief that Descartes' writings reinforce—that is, beings cut off from nature because of the existence of an immortal soul. We are more as the Stoics imagined—part of a continuum of nature, a continuum of desires and appetites. One can see again the heretical aspects of Spinoza's philosophy, from the religious perspective of his time.

On the other hand, we know that we are thinking beings, and we know that the kind of thought we are capable of is not shared by even the cleverest of animals, as Descartes tried constantly to explain to his critics. So, we are forced to ask: Just what is an individual mind (human or other) in Spinoza's monistic system? How can we account for gradations of mind or soul along Spinoza's continuum?[23]

The Mind as the Idea of the Body

The human mind is a mode of the attribute of thought, which is another way of saying that it is part of what Spinoza refers to as the infinite intellect of God. Any thought that I have is but a mode of the one substance as it is expressed through the attribute of thought. In Spinoza's words, "when we say that the human mind perceives this or that, we are saying nothing else but this: that God ... has this or that idea."[24] Spinoza himself recognizes the difficulty of this statement when he adds: "At this point our readers will no doubt find themselves in some difficulty and will think of many things that will give them pause."[25] The notion that my perceptions are God's ideas is a particularly un-Christian way of speaking, and one that would have shocked Descartes.[26]

We are habituated to thinking that we are bodies that have minds, or, more accurately, given Descartes' view of self, that we are minds that have bodies. When we think about it, we cannot satisfactorily explain where (or if) this mind is situated in the body, nor in just what sense we can say it relates to the body of which it seems both to be and not be a part. For Spinoza, however, the mind is the *idea* of the body. "That which constitutes the actual being of the human mind is basically nothing else but the idea of an individual actually existing thing."[27] The individual actually existing thing that Spinoza here is referring to is the human body. We must remember that both the body and the mind are expressions of the one substance. Whatever happens in the body happens in the mind—but not because of some causal relationship between the two. Mind and body simply *are* the same thing; they are two different aspects of the one reality manifested in one individual, in this case the human person. Just how Spinoza defines an individual will be dealt with later. What is important, here, is that nothing happens in the body that does not also happen in the mind; all modifications of body are, at the same time, modifications of mind—and vice versa. Spinoza does not have to explain any causal relationship between two substances because there are not two substances, there is only one substance, and every modification to the one substance is reflected bodily and mentally. There are not two realities to be explained; there is only one: "Each occurrence (mode) as viewed under the attribute of extension is at the same time, and equivalently, an occurrence viewed under the attribute of thought or consciousness, and vice versa."[28] Further, anything that exists in the physical world has its counterpart in the mental world, or, in Spinoza's words, "there is necessarily in God an idea of each thing whatever...."[29] A corollary of this, which has already been mentioned, is that what applies to human beings applies equally to all other individuals "which are animate, albeit in different degrees."[30] Being "animate," in Spinoza's sense, means being able to affect and be affected by the environment, and this varies according to the complexity of the individual thing: the more complex a thing is, the more interactions it has with its environment. Since humans have greater power to affect and be affected by their environment, they are higher up the scale of complexity than animals, worms or flowers.

It is helpful here not to think of mind or thought in terms of cognition as we understand it, and to conclude that it is quite impossible for worms, for example, to think. The mental component of the dual expression of the one substance is not limited to thought in the human sense. Nor is it conceived of as a separate form of reality in the Cartesian sense. It is, rather, an expression of purpose and meaning shown by the worm or the dog or the flower in relation to its environment. Every action or activity of every creature expresses meaning along with physical or bodily movement as it reacts to, and acts upon, the world around it. "The double aspect of activities as having meaning and as involving physical movement applies to creatures at all levels of development, a crab on the ocean floor and a person dancing in Paris."[31] The person dancing in Paris, however, also has the capacity for reflective thinking, which, for Spinoza, means having ideas of ideas. The mind as the idea of the body represents principally a passive state; it becomes active at the reflective level as we become conscious of our ideas and develop the capacity to order them coherently (more about this later in the chapter). Further, as we will see below, activity is always an indication of a higher and more powerful mind and its capacity to act upon the environment rather than being principally acted upon by it.

Spinoza's Individuals

We are still left with two important questions: how to account for individual minds in Spinoza's interconnected system, and how Spinoza actually defines an individual. Because Spinoza has disposed of the Cartesian notion of individual mind substance (which, as we recall, accounted for the essence of individual persons or selves), many philosophers have accused him of disposing of the idea of individuals. If our minds are ultimately explained as ideas in the mind of God, what is it that explains our existence as persons? Spinoza is far from eliminating individual selves, but explains them in a very un-Cartesian manner.

Spinoza's notion of complexity describes how the human mind fits on the continuum of minds in the universe. The mind (or the mental aspect of any individual body) is the idea of the body; thus, minds will vary in complexity to the same extent that bodies do. As we saw with the analogy of the worm, no individual body—and thus, no individual mind—is a whole; all objects are parts of wider wholes. "Each individual is thus enmeshed in a more comprehensive one, reaching up to the all-encompassing individual—'the whole of nature.'"[32]

Complexity is explained further by another of Spinoza's concepts, the *conatus*, which consists of the ratio of movement and rest that is essential to preserving the identity of any organism as an individual. In the hierarchy of parts and wholes, each individual interacts with its environment in such a way that it strives to maintain a certain ratio of motion and rest, which, in effect determines what it is—in Cartesian language, its essence. But the essence of Spinoza's individual is not a Cartesian soul (which, in Descartes' context, only humans have); the essence of any individual *is* the striving (or endeavour) to preserve itself in the interaction of parts and wholes that make up Spinoza's universe. In Spinoza's words, "Each thing, in so far as it is in itself, endeavors to persist in its own being." And, "the conatus with which each thing endeavors to persist in its own being is nothing but the actual essence of the thing itself."[33] The *conatus* manifests itself in the body as appetite and in the mind as will, and the overall result is different levels of power (physical and mental) in the interaction with any organism's environment and its effort to maintain its existence. And the more an organism develops its own powers, the more complex it becomes, physically and mentally. As it advances in complexity, it becomes more aware of its powers; complexity and awareness grow together, not separately—and not one before the other.

Human beings are the most complex of Spinoza's individuals, having the most complex level of interaction with their environment and the greatest awareness of their powers. This is connected with Spinoza's theory of knowledge: there are degrees of awareness, of complexity and of knowledge along the continuum of humans and other creatures. The more complex the interactions that humans have with their environment, the more complex will be their perceptions, and the more knowledge they will have. This complexity manifests itself physically as greater and more complex brainpower, and mentally (since the mind is the idea of the body), as greater awareness and self-awareness.

The Cartesian self is the thinking thing, the mind, separated from the physical world and from the body. Spinoza's self is the mind-body in its striving to maintain its existence (which, in effect, simply *is* the maintenance of the ratio of motion and rest that makes it the individual it is). It is embedded in the world, in constant interaction with other selves and organisms. It is important to understand that there is not an individual, a body-mind that *does* the striving. The self is not prior to the striving; it *is* the striving. There is no separate soul that is unique to human beings. Plants and animals also have souls in the sense that there is an idea of their bodies that conforms to their complexity. Any soul conforms to the type of body it is, and thus there are degrees of soul according to the complexity and the organization of organisms.

Spinoza' *conatus* is integral to the interconnectedness of things and the relation of parts and wholes, which he demonstrates in the analogy of the worm. The ratio of motion and rest to which he refers relates to the relations among parts and wholes, both internal and external to the system in question, and it is the "*form* of multiple inner relations [that] maintains itself functionally in the interactions of the compound with the outside world, thereby testifying to a common conatus of the whole."[34] As long as the pattern is maintained, the individual remains the individual that it is. The identity of an individual human is not tied up substantially with its parts; parts may change, but the identity of the individual remains.

In the human person, this identity, which is the *conatus*, constitutes the 'self.' Thus, what for Descartes was a spiritual substance distinct from the extended substance of its body is for Spinoza a relation of mind and body in its interaction with the world around it. Every perception, every interaction with the environment, is imprinted (and thus expressed) bodily and mentally. For every thought that I have, there is a corresponding state of body, and for every bodily state, there is a corresponding state of mind. As has already been pointed out, these are not two parallel states: *they are the same state expressed through the two attributes of mind and body*.

Spinoza's Body

We have seen a number of very important differences between Descartes and Spinoza with respect to the relation of mind and body. These differences translate into several striking differences regarding the body itself. One important difference is analyzed by Hans Jonas as the difference between machine and metabolism.

In looking at this difference, Jonas points to one of the ironies of Cartesian dualism and mechanism: with the radical bifurcation of mind and matter and the reliance on mechanistic principles to explain bodily functions, "the fact of life itself became unintelligible at the same time that the explanation of its bodily performance seemed to be assured."[35] In other words, the more we came to know about the function of the body, the less we learned about the life of the body. The principle of life, for Descartes, as we have seen, was the 'fire without light,' heat caused by fermentation in the heart, the moving force of the animal machine. The machine keeps going by taking in food, which becomes fuel for the body through the mechanical processes of the digestive system. Thus, Descartes relies, according to Jonas, on a combustion theory of metabolism and a machine theory of anatomy.

> But metabolism is more than a method of power-generation, or, food is more than fuel: in addition to, and more basic than, providing kinetic energy for the running of the machine (a case anyway not applying to

plants), its role is to build up originally and replace continually the very parts of the machine. Metabolism thus is the constant becoming of the machine itself—and this becoming itself is a performance of the machine: but for such performance there is no analogue in the world of machines.[36]

Metabolism is a process of self-constitution of the organism itself, something that demonstrates the inadequacy of the machine model as Descartes intends it. This self-constitution is a function of the inter-relationships that are internal and external, physical and mental at the same time. Because of this physical and mental unity, the 'machine' is 'minded' or 'ensouled' in a way Descartes' machine could never be.

Instead of the machine analogy (which, we will remember, is somewhat more than an analogy in Descartes), Jonas suggests the analogy of a flame:

> As, in a burning candle, the permanence of the flame is a permanence, not of substance, but of process in which at each moment the 'body' with its 'structure' of inner and outer layers is reconstituted of materials different from the previous and following ones, so the living organism exists as a constant exchange of its own constituents, and has its permanence and identity only in the continuity of this process, not in any persistence of its material parts. This process indeed *is* its life, and in the last resort organic existence means, not to be a definite body composed of definite parts, but to be such a continuity of process with an identity sustained above and through the flux of components.[37]

This explanation is far removed from the Cartesian view. Identity for machines without souls can only come from the arrangement of the physical parts, and, as we know from Descartes' own experiences of dissection, knowledge of the body of any organism comes about through a breaking down of its parts into smaller and simpler parts. Any organism, in the Cartesian view, is ultimately the sum of its parts. As machines with souls, human persons are rendered more than the sum of their parts by the existence of the soul or mind. But mind is a separate existence, without causal connection with the body to which it, in a way never fully explained, 'belongs.' Spinoza's organic explanation of the organism works for all levels of being, with the continuum being explained with reference to the degrees of complexity of the patterns of motion and rest, including the inter-relationships both internal and external to the organism. Metabolism is a function of the *conatus* at the same time as it works to sustain it. Spinoza's theory of body and individual provides a holistic view of mind, body and nature as mutually creating and sustaining, as opposed to the Cartesian view of mechanistic relations among parts isolated both from mind and from nature.

Self and Self-knowledge in Spinoza

We saw in the last chapter the impact of Descartes' dualism and mechanism on the modern concept of the self. I have also referred to Spinoza's philosophy as the road not followed; this pertains not only to his metaphysics and its rejection of dualism, but also to the notion of self that flows from this. As we have seen, there is no isolated self for Spinoza. In fact, I maintain that the modern idea of self would have developed quite differently had his road been followed.[38] For Spinoza, the self is embedded in the body as well as in the world. Here is where the difference between conceiving reality as made up of two substances and conceiving it as made up of only one substance with two (or more) attributes of mind and matter comes to the fore. I pointed out earlier that this difference is not merely semantic; there is a conceptual difference that affects how we perceive ourselves and the world around us. Lloyd points out that Spinoza's self is less vulnerable than Descartes' because it is less cut off from the world:

> If a mind clearly understands that it is a mode, it understands also that it is interconnected with the rest of reality. The Cartesian self is fated to the hopeless attempt to insert itself back into a world from which it has been metaphysically separated…. The Spinozistic self, in contrast, is immersed in the whole of nature, and its self-knowledge consists in becoming ever more deeply and reflectively aware of that truth.[39]

Thus, rather than some kind of substance, Spinoza's self just *is* the relation between body and world (*conatus*), based on the notion that the mind is the idea of the body and the body is a part of nature. An individual body is what it is because of its unique relation with its environment, and an individual mind is what it is because it is the idea of that particular body. As we have seen, minds are more or less complex depending on the number of interactions with their environment—every contact between body and the world around it leaving an impression, or modification, of the body (which is expressed in the mind, as well). In other words, depending on the breadth and depth of interactions with and in the world, a body and mind will be more or less complex (and more or less powerful), and the *conatus* will be stronger or weaker. The human body is "affected by external bodies in a great many ways, and is so structured that it can affect external bodies in a great many ways."[40] These modifications of the body are also modifications of the mind: "any mental apprehension involves a body, specifically an individual's own body, as it is modified by other bodies, the ideas of which are included in the idea of one's own body."[41] Thus, the whole (body-mind) is only what it is (its essence, identity, self) based on its relations and interactions with its environment. There is no isolated body in Spinoza, no isolated mind, no isolated self.

Nor is the world objectified in such a way that the mind can distance itself from it to the point of distrusting what is presented to it through the senses. To know himself, in fact, to discover himself, Descartes passed through the process of doubt in the Second Meditation that allowed him to believe that, whether the world existed or not, his mind was what he could know more intimately than any external object, including his body. Spinoza could not—and would not—pass by the same process in order to discover the mind. The route to knowledge of the mind is through knowledge of the body. Thus, to speak of self in Spinoza is to speak of self-knowledge, and self-knowledge begins with the body. Like the Stoics, Spinoza sees the body (and the world) as a source of knowledge about the self. And a corollary of this is that, for Spinoza, knowledge of the self begins with the senses.

Unlike Descartes and other philosophers such as Plato, who were suspicious of knowledge coming from the senses, Spinoza takes the body and the senses as the starting point of knowledge. What the senses tell us is not mistaken, as Descartes would have us believe. It is rudimentary, even confused, but it is the starting point of everything we can know about the world. Our senses might tell us that the sun is only a short distance from Earth; this is an inadequate idea based on limited knowledge, which can be corrected through more sophisticated common sense notions, and then through expert scientific knowledge. As we move up the different levels of knowledge, our idea of the sun becomes more coherent—becoming, eventually, an adequate idea. But even when we understand the true distance of the sun from the Earth, we will still imagine it in the way that the body is affected by it. The original (inadequate) idea of the sun is a stepping stone to the later (adequate) idea. For Spinoza, sensory experience, directly implicating the body, is central to the development of adequate ideas.

This approach to the senses and knowledge conforms as well to Spinoza's continuum of organisms and their complexity, since some organisms will have only a very basic interaction with and 'understanding' of their environment, while more complex organisms, like humans, will have the ability to use their reason to augment and clarify their perceptions. Since there is no detached and isolated mind-seeking understanding of an objectified world, but only a body interacting with and being modified by that world, what the mind perceives is just the modifications of the body. At the lowest level of knowledge, the body is passively receiving modifications (and the ideas of them). One idea will suggest another, but the association of ideas is passive; it is neither coherent nor logical.

These passively received ideas are *inadequate* because they are not accompanied by an understanding of the causes. To put this in context: perfectly adequate knowledge would require a body that was in interaction with the entire universe (and a mind which reflected that). This could only be the mind of God (or Nature as a whole). But each finite individual is capable of interacting with only a small slice of the universe, and understanding the causes of those interactions to a more or less adequate degree. We can never have adequate ideas of the whole, but we can approach perfection according to the greater complexity of body modifications and the corresponding complexity of mind. The more we understand the causes of things, the less passive we become. We are free to the extent that we can truly reach an understanding of the causes of the body's modifications (including those brought about by the emotions). Remembering Spinoza's premise that the order and connection of ideas is the same as the order and connection of things, understanding nature and its logic leads to knowledge that can be used to increase an individual's power in the world. Like the Stoics, Spinoza tells us that, when we come to an understanding of the necessity of nature and our place in it, we both know that things must be this way and desire that they be so. We can either lead the cart of our life or be dragged along by it; the choice is very Stoic.

Spinoza's theory of knowledge (so briefly outlined here) is not without its critics. One can question how an individual can aspire to higher knowledge when circumstances limit his or her interactions with the environment (Spinoza is a determinist, we must remember). But this need not concern us here. What is important, and what is very different from Descartes, is that the body (through sense perception) is essential to *any* knowledge whatsoever. And the knowledge that comes from sense perception, while initially confused, is not false. It is subject to correction and deeper understanding as one moves up into the reaches of science and philosophy to attain adequate ideas. The body is a source of knowledge both of the self and of the world.

Spinoza the Stoic

A number of references have been made in this chapter to similarities between Spinoza's philosophy and that of the Stoics; this is particularly so in relation to the body. For both Spinoza and the Stoics, human beings are embedded in nature and come to knowledge of themselves through knowledge of nature and vice versa. This is expressed in more modern terms by Spinoza as affecting and being affected by our environment. We are thoroughly embedded in the natural world (as well as the social world). We are not separate wholes relating to other separate wholes; we are all parts of the whole of nature. In both the Stoics and Spinoza, we can only truly become what we are by living in accordance with nature.

For Spinoza, this relationship with nature and our environment plays out through the *conatus*, which simply *is* our essence as individuals (and of all individuals down the line of organic existence). It is an original impulse or striving for our own survival; it is not something we *do*, it is what we *are*. This striving to flourish is a desire to augment an individual's power, which ultimately means achieving greater happiness and freedom. For Spinoza, whatever strengthens the *conatus* brings pleasure; whatever weakens it brings pain. Understanding nature and living according to its unfolding strengthens the *conatus* and thus the survival of an individual. And, as already pointed out, this, for Spinoza, is true virtue.

Spinoza's *conatus* harks back to the Stoic *oikeiosis* discussed in Chapter 2, which is also an impulse to survival and includes the consciousness of what is necessary for that survival. As was pointed out in that chapter, this impulse to self-preservation is primary; it provided the Stoics' answer to the Epicureans, who believed the primary impulse was toward pleasure. Because the Stoic universe is providentially ordered, living in accordance with nature becomes the foundation for a happy and fulfilling life. Virtue means living in accordance with nature.

There are differences, of course, and Spinoza would have no interest in accepting the Stoic idea of a providential universe that is looking out for the health and happiness of its human inhabitants. But he still identifies virtue with living in accordance with nature: "Spinozistic virtue is a matter of agreeing with the environment around me. It is a matter of uniting with the bodies that agree with my nature, insofar as they fortify my individual power of persevering."[42] There is no connotation of the good in Spinoza's notion of virtue, at least as it is usually understood in its moral sense. I do not unite with bodies that agree with my nature *because* they are good; they are good because I unite with them and because they help me persist in being.

Another area of comparison between Spinoza and the Stoics relates to the connection between virtue, knowledge and the emotions. For both Spinoza and the Stoics, becoming virtuous is a matter of coming to know oneself; in effect, it is about coming to be what one is, rather than trying to be something that one is not. What prevents this from happening is an inability to control the passions, which interferes with the ability to know one's proper nature and one's place in nature as a whole. Thus, for both Spinoza and the Stoics, control of the emotions is paramount to knowledge and virtue. Spinoza says that "it is necessary to know the power of our nature and its lack of power so we can determine what reason can and cannot do in controlling the emotions."[43] Because of the importance of the role of emotions, Spinoza devotes a large part of the *Ethics* to a discussion of their nature. To understand them is to overcome them. Hampshire sees Spinoza's account of the transition from a life of passive emotion and confused ideas to one of active emotion and adequate ideas as anticipating modern psychology:

> ...the cure, or method of salvation, consists in making the patient more self-conscious, and in making him perceive the more or less unconscious struggle within himself to preserve his own internal adjustment and balance; he must be brought to realize that it is this continuous struggle which expresses itself in his pleasures and pains, desires and aversions.[44]

For Spinoza, control of the emotions is not a question of will, since there is no free will in his world. Further, while the Stoics hold that the emotions can be completely controlled, Spinoza thinks otherwise; the struggle, as Hampshire suggests above, is continuous. I can never eradicate the impact of the emotions, I can simply grow to understand their causes; the more I understand their causes, the more I am able to rise above them. For Spinoza, "the wisdom that cures the passions entails nothing less than the acceptance that the passions are part of the human condition."[45] This is where Spinoza's analysis of the emotions meets his analysis of the levels of knowledge: the more I understand the causes of all the modifications to my body, including those caused by the emotions, the closer I come to freedom. If I remain at that first level of knowledge, which is passive and confused, I will remain in the grip of my emotions (in Spinoza's terms, in 'bondage'). In Spinoza's determined universe, I must come to an understanding of the causal nexus that determines my emotions and my actions. Once I have accepted that I am part of this web of causation, I achieve happiness and freedom. It is not a question of fate, as the Stoics would have it; nor is it a question of yielding to a providential universe, knowing that the whole is good and thus my role in it is for my own good. As stated above, 'good' does not enter Spinoza's equation. The world simply *is*. Understanding and accepting this strengthens the power of my *conatus*, and ultimately brings joy.

Early in Part V of the *Ethics*, entitled "On Human Freedom," Spinoza tells us that, when we understand that something is necessary, our mind is less affected by the power of the emotions. He gives as an example the fact that infants do not know how to walk, talk or reason, but nobody pities them because that is in the order of necessity of things. "But if most people were born adults, and only a few were born babies, then everybody would feel sorry for babies, because they would then look on infancy itself not as a natural and necessary thing, but as a fault or flaw in Nature."[46] In Spinoza's view, the events of our lives happen with the same necessity as the stages of an infant's life. The difference is that we tend to understand and accept the latter, because we understand the causes, but we resist the former, pitying ourselves and staying in the grip of our emotions, simply because we do not understand the causes shaping them.

For Spinoza, rather than fate determining that everything happens as it *should*, there is only the web of causality ensuring that everything happens as it *must*. Because everything is connected to everything else (and thus every state of affairs is the effect of a previous state of affairs—its cause), the series—or more accurately, the web—of causes is determined as it goes along. In the case of humans, this means that everything we have done in the past is part of the causal web and determines what we do in the future. Thus, we are not just following fate, we are partners in creating it. Either way, however, Spinoza and the Stoics are in agreement on the fundamental point that happiness and freedom can only come when we accept the necessity of nature and live according to it.

The Road Not Followed

In the last chapter, we saw how Descartes' mind-body dualism and mechanism helped shape our modern ideas of the body and the self, largely in a negative fashion by denigrating the body and elevating the mind. As a result, many philosophers and other thinkers, especially feminist thinkers, tend to reject much of the framework of modernity and the seventeenth-century thinkers that shaped it. Spinoza is another matter. We can look to Spinoza from the perspective of what might have been, and, reading him thus, we can call on him rather than reject him. In other words, we can take much from his philosophy of mind and body and recuperate it to support a contemporary view of body that is free of the many dualisms of modernity—not the least of which is the view that mind/reason are masculine (and thus good) and body/emotion are feminine (and thus less than good). Lloyd speaks of the fascination exerted on her when she discovered Spinoza's philosophy: "it was largely because Spinoza spoke in an alternative voice, engaging with, and offering alternatives to ways of thinking that I now see in retrospect as being the residue of Cartesianism in contemporary philosophy."[47] This recognition allowed her to see Spinoza's philosophy as an opportunity to restore the past rather than reject it, something that is beginning to be recognized through changing attitudes to the history of philosophy by critics of modernity:

> This was a moment of the philosophical tradition where the polarization between reason and other aspects—imagination, affect—was not expressed through the male/female distinction. This meant that if one wanted to break down an alignment or dichotomy between reason and its opposites, and thus between "male" and "female," here was a moment of the philosophical tradition that one could turn to, to see how Spinoza did it, how he avoided the dichotomy. There might be potential there for more constructive ways of thinking both the male/female distinction and the reason/affect/imagination distinction.[48]

Thus, we can look to Spinoza as a corrective to many of the dichotomies of modernity, including mind-body; male-female; reason-emotion; thought-imagination; self-nature; individual-collective; etc. A body that does not stand in isolation from the mind or soul, and a self that is immersed in nature rather than detached from it—these are just two of Spinoza's starting points that can be examined for their relevance to contemporary attitudes to mind, body and nature. The relevance of these points to notions of the body in contemporary biomedicine will become apparent in the latter part of this book. Most importantly, we can look to Spinoza as a moment in the history of modern philosophy where the body does not have to be rejected in the mind's quest for knowledge. In Spinoza, the body is a source of knowledge. As we saw in this chapter, for Spinoza knowledge begins with the body, with that direct awareness of the body that occurs at the level of the imagination. Our knowledge becomes more precise, our ideas more adequate, but the level of the imagination is not surpassed or discounted. The body counts in the quest for knowledge.

Notes

1.   From the record of excommunication of 1656, cited in Genevieve Lloyd, *Routledge Philosophy Guidebook to Spinoza and the Ethics* (New York: Routledge, 1996), 1. See also Roger Scruton, *Spinoza: A Very Short Introduction* (New York: Routledge, 1999), 10. A cubit was a unit of measurement based on the length from the middle of a man's body to the tips of his fingers—approximately three feet. Excommunication was not a rare event at that time, and Spinoza could have sought reconciliation, as others who had been excommunicated did. But he did not, and he "calmly removed himself from any further form of Jewish life." Rebecca Goldstein, *Betraying Spinoza: The Renegade Jew Who Gave Us Modernity* (Toronto: Random House, 2006), 5. For an account of the many interpretations of the reasons for and the actual process of the excommunication of Spinoza (the former ranging from his denial of the immortality of the soul to his troubles with the authorities over taxes and problems in the Jewish community), see Richard Popkin, *Spinoza* (Oxford: Oneworld Publications, 2004), Ch. 3.

2.   There are debates in the literature as to whether or not Spinoza wrote in a dual language that could only be understood by the initiated. What is certain is that his ideas were a threat to the established religions of the time and that Spinoza did not publish the *Ethics* in his lifetime.

3.   This is a derogatory term that means "swine."

4.   Scruton, 7. It wasn't just the religious authorities who railed against him. Pierre Bayle, a French philosopher and contemporary of Spinoza, described his philosophy "as having implications that surpassed the fantastic ravings of the maddest heads that were ever locked up." Cited in Genevieve Lloyd, *Part of Nature: Self-Knowledge in Spinoza's Ethics* (Ithaca and London: Cornell University

Press, 1994), 5. On the other hand, DeBrabander finds the idea that Spinoza was threatening to tradition rather misguided and points out that "Spinoza harks back to pre-modern sensibilities, and in fact offers a stirring critique of the direction modernity would take." Firmin DeBrabander, *Spinoza and the Stoics* (New York and London: Continuum International Publishing Group, 2007), 6.

5. Goldstein, 5.
6. Richard Schacht, *Classical Modern Philosophers* (New York and London: Routledge, 1984), 67.
7. Stuart Hampshire, *Spinoza and Spinozism* (Oxford: Clarendon Press, 2005), 68.
8. Moira Gatens, *Feminist Interpretations of Benedict Spinoza* (University Park, PA: Pennsylvania State University Press, 2009), 2.
9. Baruch Spinoza, *Ethics*, trans. Samuel Shirley (Indianapolis and Cambridge: Hackett Publishing Company, 1992), I, Pr. 14. All quotations from the *Ethics* in this chapter are from Shirley's translation. Abbreviations are as follows: Pr. = proposition; Cor. = corollary; Sch. = scholium (or explanatory note); Post. = postulate; Def. = definition; Ax. = axiom.
10. Spinoza refers to the "infinite attributes" of God or Nature, and there are academic debates as to how many this might actually be. The important thing is that, as humans, we perceive only two.
11. *Ethics*, II, Pr. 1 and Pr. 2.
12. Hampshire, 41, 42. *Deus sive Natura* translates as 'God or Nature,' by which Spinoza means that you can call the one Substance God or you can call it Nature.
13. Letter 32, "To the most honourable and learned Henry Oldenburg from Benedict Spinoza," 20 November 1665, in Shirley, 280. Sir Henry Oldenburg was one of the founders of the Royal Society of England, who became a lifelong friend and correspondent of Spinoza.
14. Letter to Oldenburg in Shirley, 281.
15. *Ethics*, IV, Pr. 20.
16. Jonathan Bennett, *A Study of Spinoza's "Ethics"* (Cambridge: Cambridge University Press, 1984), 11.
17. Hampshire, 32.
18. Lloyd, 19.
19. *Ethics*, II, Pr. 7.
20. Hampshire, 52.
21. *Ethics*, II, Pr. 7, Sch.
22. Hampshire, xxii.
23. As pointed out in the chapter on Stoicism, if the most important problem for a dualist is to explain the interaction of mind and matter, the most difficult question for the monist is to account for gradations of being, especially degrees of mind or soul, along a continuum.

24.   *Ethics*, II, Pr. 11, Cor.
25.   *Ethics*, II, Pr. 11, Sch.
26.   This is another reason for considering Spinoza's philosophy heretical: "If all things are modes of the one substance, the atrocities that human beings inflict on one another cease to be the responsibility of individuals and become the self-mutilations of an all-encompassing God" (Lloyd, *Nature*, 5).
27.   *Ethics*, II, Pr. 11.
28.   Hans Jonas, "Spinoza and the Theory of Organism," in *Philosophical Essays* (Englewood Cliffs, NJ: Prentice-Hall, 1974), 210.
29.   *Ethics*, II, Pr. 13, Sch.
30.   *Ethics*, II, Pr. 13, Sch.
31.   Hampshire, xxiv.
32.   Lloyd, *Nature*, 12.
33.   *Ethics*, III, Pr. 6, Pr. 7.
34.   Jonas, 213.
35.   Jonas, 206.
36.   Jonas, 211.
37.   Jonas, 211.
38.   It is interesting to note that there is no chapter on Spinoza in Taylor's book, *Sources of the Self*.
39.   Lloyd, *Nature*, 39.
40.   *Ethics*, II, Pr. 14, Dem.
41.   DeBrabander, 19.
42.   DeBrabander, 41.
43.   *Ethics*, IV, Pr. 17.
44.   Hampshire, 110. "Salvation" is Spinoza's term for achieving happiness, freedom and thus virtue. It is an earthly salvation, not the heavenly salvation of Christian theology.
45.   DeBrabander, 36.
46.   *Ethics*, V, Pr. 6, Sch.
47.   Susan James, "The Power of Spinoza: Feminist Conjunctions (Susan James Interviews Genevieve Lloyd and Moira Gatens)," *Hypatia*, 15: 2 (2000), 41. For other discussions of the relevance of Spinoza to the feminist critique of modernity, see Gatens, *Feminist Interpretations of Benedict Spinoza*.
48.   James, "The Power of Spinoza," 44.

PART II

The Limits of Mechanism: Contemporary Problems and Solutions

In philosophical terms, the seventeenth century represented a turning point, which many consider the beginnings of modernity. Not all philosophers agree with this; some hold that modernity started much earlier, for example, with the Renaissance and the beginnings of humanism, while others see it starting a century later with the Enlightenment and the Age of Reason. From the point of view that is being set forth in this book—the body and its relation to nature and the cosmos—it was the seventeenth century that provided the mechanistic framework that has governed science and philosophy up to the present, and thus represents the beginning of modernity. While many believe that the mechanistic paradigm is shifting, I maintain that, to the extent that this might be taking place, such a shift remains on the fringes of mainstream science and philosophy. There might be many marvellous discoveries in biology, genetics, physics and even medicine, but the reigning paradigm at the level of the day-to-day world is still a mechanistic one based on a dualistic metaphysics of mind and body.[1] Most importantly, for most people and their doctors, the body is still a machine. As we have seen, this approach to the human body, both scientific and philosophical, has its roots in the sixteenth century with the breakdown of the idea of the macrocosm-microcosm resulting from the discoveries of Copernicus and Galileo (the heliocentric view of the universe), and with the subsequent breakdown, directly related to the first, of the connection between the human soul and world soul. The year 1543, with the publications of both Copernicus (on the movements of the planets) and Vesalius (on the fabric of the human body), has already been mentioned as pivotal. But it was Descartes who, in the seventeenth century, provided the metaphysical foundations—based on dualism and mechanism—that have supported Western scientific endeavours, including the disciplines linked to biology and psychology, for the last four hundred years. Mind and body are distinct realms of study, requiring different kinds of explanations.

The application of mechanistic science to the study and explanation of the human body has had an enormous influence on how ordinary people perceive their bodies, as well as on the development of technologies affecting the body. The separation of the subject that knows the body from the body that is known results in an objectification of the body, which is a presupposition of many of the wonders of medical technology as it is applied to the body today, as well as of many practices based on the notion that a person somehow 'owns' or 'uses' his or her body for ends relating to the development of the 'self.'

In this second part of the book, I will examine the legacy of the objectified body, the body-machine, through the lens of several contemporary problems and practices. In Chapter 7, I will address the impact of dualism and mechanism on modern medical practice, in particular organ transplantation and reproductive technologies, and will maintain that these practices are based on notions of the body as an object of knowledge—including medical knowledge. The body in modern medicine is "viewed not primarily as purposive and ensouled; nor as the scene of moral dramas; nor as a place wherein cosmological and social forces gather; but simply as an intricate machine," with the role of medicine being to draw upon "a reservoir of scientific knowledge concerning how the machine works, and [employ] the technologies of repair."[2]

I will also address the impact of dualism and mechanism on current research in robotics and the expressed goal of some of its practitioners of downloading human consciousness into a machine (from the body-machine to the robot-machine). This research and the practices resulting from it bring the Platonic idea of the body as an obstacle to knowledge right into the twenty-first century. The only reason for pursuing the research in the first place is the assumption that our physical bodies simply slow us down and get in the way of the attainment of true knowledge.[3] The fact that much of the literature in this realm refers to a 'post-biological' future or the 'obsolete body' is a clear indication of dualism taken to an extreme, and the idea of 'reverse engineering the brain' in order to download consciousness into a machine represents mechanism taken to the edge of absurdity. These researchers and authors assume that whatever consciousness is (and they do not know), it is something separate from the body and something that would operate much more efficiently without the encumbrance (Plato would say prison) of the body. The body, here, is without question an obstacle to knowledge.

A third prong of Chapter 7 will touch on the modern phenomenon of extreme body modification. Here the body is treated in some cases as an object of an individual self's desires and fantasies, in others as a means of showing that the body is not an integral part of the self, and in still others as a means of turning the body into an art object. In all of these cases, the body becomes a thing that is used (and/or abused) as an instrument that can, ultimately, be done away with. The true self does not need the machine.

In Chapters 8 and 9, I will look at contemporary practices, which can be seen as attempts to recover the holism of the past, and lead us away from the vanishing body so apparent in the trends discussed in Chapter 7. In these chapters, I will be tracing the thread of the body as a source of knowledge (of the world and of the self), which we have seen so clearly in the Stoics and in Spinoza. While these are considered by many people to be on the fringe and not scientifically respectable, I will demonstrate that they represent a return to many of the metaphysical notions of the past—now often updated and supported by much scientific research. I will look first, in Chapter 8, at the explosion in the Western world of the Eastern science of yoga, and, in Chapter 9, at so-called *alternative* medicine, in particular homeopathy. In both cases, holistic notions of consciousness and energy form the basis for a new way of looking at the body. I will demonstrate that these practices represent a return to certain notions of what I have been calling 'cosmic connectors' in their recognition of the connection of mind, body, spirit and cosmos. They fit more easily with Hippocrates and Plato than with Dennett and Dawkins, although many serious writers on these topics do claim scientific legitimacy based on technological breakthroughs in recent decades—the ability to measure acupuncture meridians being one clear example. On the question of macrocosm-microcosm, for example, Yuasa points out that, while modern science has rejected this view of human beings and the world, "the meditation method and the Eastern theory of the body seem to provide us with a starting point to re-evaluate this old view from a contemporary perspective."[4]

It is a fundamental premise of this narrative that the modern materialist and mechanistic view of the body is the logical extension of Descartes' mind-matter dualism. This is not to suggest that Descartes is responsible for how the body of modernity is perceived, nor is it an attempt to lay the blame for our society's objectification and commercialization of the body on his earnest shoulders. Nor do I presume that his particular two-substance theory is explicitly accepted by contemporary thinkers, or even in the popular imagination today. Quite the opposite: many thinkers explicitly eschew Cartesian dualism, and in our secular society few people seriously refer to soul—although they would be hard-pressed to define the mind, if asked to do so. However, even avowed materialists often adhere to some form of mind-body dualism, often unacknowledged, sometimes expressed more as brain-body dualism. The soul has been dispensed with, but no adequate concept of self or mind or consciousness has replaced it in reductionist theories of body. The dualistic framework has survived, although its expression is varied and often hidden, as will become apparent in Chapter 7. If Descartes could visit us in the twenty-first century, he would likely be shocked by what has become of his 'body-machine.'

Notes

1.   To give one example, Yuasa Yasuo points to the fact that acupuncture has been excluded from Western medicine as unscientific: "Although it is recognized in virtue of its actual clinical effects, it has been regarded as unsuited for the academic world. But a moment's reflection reveals that this view is unreasonable. If acupuncture indeed demonstrates actual clinical effects, should not the position of empirical science be to investigate the mechanism of how these effects are obtained?" Yuasa Yasuo, *The Body, Self-Cultivation, and Ki-Energy* (Albany: SUNY Press, 1993), 99. The same question can be addressed to the scientific community regarding yoga, homeopathy, osteopathy and many other alternative therapies that the medical community dismisses as unscientific as a matter of course. This, as we will see, is because of a number of fundamental principles of the mechanistic paradigm that conflict with the principles of holistic therapies, but cannot be given up by mechanistic science and medicine.

2.   Drew Leder, ed., *The Body in Medical Thought and Practice* (Dortrecht and Boston: Kluwer Academic Publishers, 1992), 3.

3.   It should be noted that what is referred to as knowledge in this field is often limited to 'information,' which is not the same thing, although mechanistic and materialist philosophies can easily equate the two.

4.   Yuasa, 109.

CHAPTER VII

THE LEGACY OF MECHANISM: THE FRAGMENTING AND DISAPPEARING BODY

One thing that becomes clear as we follow the philosophers' thinking on the human body through the history of philosophy is that, in the final analysis, we can arrive at no consensus about what the body really is. In philosophical terms, this means that we are actually quite ignorant regarding the ontological status of the human body. At the same time, the sciences that are most particularly linked to the body (biology, physiology and medicine, for example) have all accepted as a presupposition the idea of the body as an object of nature, subject to the same physical laws as any other object of nature. Explanations of soul or mind are excluded from these sciences, as they have been excluded from natural science since the seventeenth century. In spite of the many philosophical arguments that have been made against Cartesian dualism since Descartes' time, his mind-body dualism remains the basis of the sciences of the body today. This fact will be one of the principal points of argument in the chapters that follow, where the dualistic legacy will be demonstrated and an appeal made to a recuperation of some form of philosophical monism of the sort seen in the philosophy of the Stoics and Spinoza.

The Body and Modern Medicine[1]

Chapter 5 demonstrated that, in relation to the body, dualism is only one prong of Descartes' dual legacy, the other being mechanism. It can be said that the first prong is metaphysical (dealing with what the body is) and the second epistemological (dealing with what can be known about the body and how it can be known). As pointed out in Chapter 5, Descartes' lifelong goal was to establish a method that would work for all areas of inquiry, based on the fundamental mechanistic laws of nature that he had articulated. As he wrote in his *Principles of Philosophy*, near the end of his life:

> For I freely acknowledge that I recognize no matter in corporeal things apart from that which the geometers call quantity, and take as the object of their demonstrations, i.e., that to which every kind of division, shape and motion is applicable. Moreover, my consideration of such matter involves absolutely nothing apart from these divisions, shapes and motions.... And since all natural phenomena can be explained in this way ... I do not think that any other principles are either admissible or desirable in physics.[2]

This meeting of Descartes' metaphysics and epistemology is succinctly expressed by Hans Jonas: "To know a thing means to know how it is or can be made and therefore means being able to repeat or vary or anticipate the process of making."[3] This is the true legacy of Cartesian dualism and mechanism, which is particularly evident in biomedical technology today, where a human body can be divided into increasingly smaller parts and *put back together in different ways*. That this represents a slippage from the epistemological plane to the metaphysical is not immediately obvious, and Jonas points out the logical error involved when he states: "from the fact of machines working by natural principles entirely it does not follow that they work by the entire natural principles, or, that nature has no other modes of operation than those which man can utilize in his constructions."[4] In other words, knowing *how* the body *works* (and presuming that one gets this right) does not entail knowing *what* the body *is*. That the workings of the body follow certain laws of physics and chemistry does not entail that the body *is only* physical and chemical. If this distinction between knowing *how* and knowing *what* is accepted, then it can be suggested that modern biomedicine is operating from assumptions that are seriously open to question.

But the error does not stop there. We have seen how mind-body dualism leads to the separation of the knowing subject and the known world of science. Everything in the world becomes an object for the knowing subject or self, including its own body. Notions of purpose, ends, feelings, knowledge—and any other elements connected with consciousness—fall on the side of the subject, or the self, which has become the locus of all attribution of value in the human person.[5] This self-subject is not considered part of the domain of biology; rather, it falls into the realm of psychology.

This epistemological division both reflects and reinforces the metaphysical one. The biologist's object of study is the body; the psychologist's, the mind.[6] This leaves the biologist free to examine and know the human body without considering the person as such, something that is evident when one takes a look at how medicine is taught. In his analysis of the medical school curriculum in France, Didier Moriau demonstrates the unmistakable influence of Descartes' mechanism, an influence that persists to this day.[7] For example, in biology, the first image of the body is as a multitude of cells ruled by chemical and biophysical laws; in anatomy, the dominant image is of a body made of detachable parts: bones, muscles, joints, tubes, systems (digestive, cardiovascular, pulmonary, etc.); in physiology, the body appears as a well-oiled tool, with pumps, filtration system, ventilation system, and so on.

This teaching reinforces the notion of the body as a machine: the heart pumps; the kidneys filter; the lungs ventilate; the digestive tube feeds, cleans and eliminates; the brain (the highest function, physically and morally) manages and controls. The student then learns that the pieces of the machine can break, deteriorate, wear out; that they can be repaired and, if necessary, replaced. Moriau refers to this medicalized body as a cold biological mechanism, devoid of thought, feeling or social context; it is not an individual but a type. The doctor thus learns to see himself as a mechanic, the fixer of broken parts, the one who must do everything in his power to keep the machine in good working order, and to stave off death.

This cold, biological mechanism is also devoid of value. It is, following Descartes' method, broken down and analyzed by purely quantitative criteria, following the laws of physics. As we saw in Chapter 5, the purpose of Descartes' *Treatise on Man* was to describe the body in terms of the size, speed and direction of particles. Being amenable only to quantitative analysis, particles do not have qualities. Whatever is qualitative in the human being (and thus imbued with value) falls on the side of mind or self. The body, as material and objective, is not the seat of the self, nor is it what is unique or sacrosanct about an individual. Mechanistic science, including modern scientific medicine, demands objectivity and moral neutrality from the objects it studies. "First Nature had been 'neutralized' with respect to value, then man himself."[8]

It is interesting to note, however, that the machine metaphor has been transformed by modern technology. Descartes often compared the functioning of the body to the functioning of a clock (with God as the clockmaker) that worked according to the laws of nature but was not amenable to human interference beyond repairing a malfunction. But, as Susan Bordo points out, over time, "a technology that was first aimed at the replacement of malfunctioning parts has generated an industry and an ideology fuelled by fantasies of rearranging, transforming, and correcting, an ideology of limitless improvement and change, defying the historicity, the mortality, and, indeed, the very materiality of the body."[9] We will look at a number of examples of this ideology of limitless improvement and change.

The Fragmenting Body: Organ Transplantation

This vision of the body as objective, neutral and value-free is a condition of possibility for the practice of organ transplantation. It provides the metaphysical support for the establishment and expansion of the practice while at the same time circumscribing and limiting the ethical debates surrounding it. Following the metaphysics of mechanism, an organ is objective, material and above all mindless or soulless. In other words, in the discourse of organ transplantation, it is simply anathema to suggest that my kidney is somehow *me*![10]

In the following pages, I will examine two aspects of organ transplantation that demonstrate my thesis that the dualistic paradigm still rules and that modern medicine is rooted in the concept of a soulless (or mindless) and value-neutral body. The two aspects I will deal with (while recognizing that there are others) are brain death and the rejection phenomenon.

Brain Death
It is crucial to the success of an organ transplant that the organ be fresh and thus 'alive.' On the other hand, in order for the procedure to be legal, this live organ must come from a dead body. This need has been met over the years through the concept of brain death, institutionalized in the United States in 1968[11] and gradually accepted in most developed countries around the world (Japan being a notable exception until 1997). Peter Singer has referred to brain death as "a convenient fiction,"[12] because it allows us to believe that a person is dead and to harvest the organs while the person is being 'kept alive' on a ventilator—thus avoiding accusations of killing the person by extracting the

organs. Assuming that a person is dead because the brain has ceased functioning is a clear demonstration of the non-identification of body and person—and of the fact that the value of the person resides only in the mind.[13] This is not an argument in favour of keeping comatose patients alive indefinitely on ventilators. However, what is in serious need of consideration is the ontological status of the so-called dead person. Some bioethicists have grappled with this question, and different terms have been proposed in the literature to try to define this particular state between life and death—for example 'neo-morts,' 'living cadavers' and 'simulated life.'

Interestingly, the redefinition of death almost forty years ago took place in North America and Europe with little or no public comment. It was quite otherwise in Japan, where mind-body dualism is not part of the metaphysical framework. According to the anthropologist Margaret Lock, the issue of brain death

> caused considerable social angst, even though Japan, for the most part a secular society, is driven by the principles of rational order and scientific progress associated with modernization. What is more, many people in Japan apparently do not understand death as a straightforward event affecting only the physical body.... Dying is widely understood as a process, and cannot therefore be isolated as a moment. What is more, *the cognitive status of the patient is of secondary importance for most people.*[14]

Lock points out further that in Japan the dying person is more than an individual self—even one of mind and body—since a person is part of a web of relations, and because "death in Japan represents more than the extinction of individual bodies: it is above all a familial and social occasion. *Even when medically determined, death becomes final only when the family accepts it as such* ... many people repudiate the idea of tampering with newly dead bodies."[15]

Brain death is a Western invention, supported by a conception of the body as mechanistic, objective and value-neutral. Even thinkers who reject Cartesian dualism will not object to the notion of brain death, since, for many of them, mind is an illusion and can ultimately be reduced to brain processes. If those processes have ceased functioning, the mind—and thus the person—is dead.[16]

The Rejection Phenomenon

With the exception of kidney transplants and partial liver transplants from living donors, most transplanted organs are harvested from dead or brain-dead bodies. There are ethical debates—usually arising out of religious and cultural practices— relating to the integrity of the dead body that I do not intend to address here. What is of interest, here, is not so much the use of the dead body but the status of the organ itself. In order to accept and promote the transplantation practice, it has to be assumed that the living organ is not a person or part of a person. A kidney is a kidney—objective and morally neutral, although it is 'alive.' It is more than a kidney one would buy from the butcher to prepare for dinner—but just what that 'more' consists of is not a subject of debate in the literature of biomedical ethics. In fact, in many bioethics textbooks, the question of the ethics of organ transplants is subsumed under a chapter heading like "Allocation of Scarce Resources," an appellation that would appear to beg the question.

At the same time, while the transplantation of a live kidney from one body to another is not problematic for the medical profession or even for bioethicists, it is problematic from the point of view of the recipient. The recipient body rejects the organ, and it is only because of the invention of very powerful immunosuppressive drugs that organ transplantation is possible on the scale that it is today. Without them, the transplant would fail. These drugs must, however, be taken by the recipient for the rest of his or her life, which means that the host body never adapts to the foreign organ.

The rejection phenomenon appears to be a blind spot for the transplantation community, as well as for bioethicists. It has been described as "the innate and unrelenting intolerance of individuals to grafts of other people's tissues and organs,"[17] and as "a strong biological expression of our individual uniqueness and separateness."[18] But what does this mean in relation to a purely material body? Is our personality, our self, our personal identity expressed biologically? This is a question that is not addressed in the literature, where most writers take for granted that questions of personal identity relate to psychology and not biology.

At the same time, many organ recipients appear to experience a changed sense of self, and, as explained by Renée Fox, "the responses of donors, recipients and their families to the experience of organ transplantation suggest that, on preconscious and unconscious levels, they feel that something akin to the transfer of psychic and social as well as biological qualities of self to the other has taken place."[19]

The literature on organ transplants is replete with anecdotal evidence of changed behaviour, changed tastes and transformed attitudes (suggesting that they are more than "preconscious" or "unconscious"), but the general reaction to these stories is that all of the perceived effects are psychological. This is consistent with the belief that what is transferred is an objective and neutral physical organ, and thus these perceived changes can *only* be psychological. Lock interviewed organ recipients who, after their transplants, developed cravings for foods they had never wanted before—mustard, cheese or chocolate, for example, all of which are seemingly strong physiological reactions—but on interviewing a psychiatrist who deals with organ recipients was told, "Remember, what these patients are thinking is *all* in the imagination, no matter where the organ came from."[20] This attitude is fairly common, but there are a few researchers who are willing to explore, from a scientific perspective, the anecdotal evidence that has been gathered. One of these is the psychoneu-roimmunologist Paul Pearsall, who asks: "Are the remarkable stories by some heart transplant recipients regarding changes in their food preferences, dreams, fantasies, and personality manifestations related on some level to the cellular memories of their donor?"[21] Pearsall believes that they are, but his position is considered radical and, for the moment, the rejection phenomenon remains one of the most difficult and puzzling aspects of the transplantation field. Pearsall is cautious about his own research results, but builds on the work of other scientists, in particular Dr. Candace Pert, whose research led her to a theory about neuropeptides, "tiny chains of amino acids that are keys to our emotional experiences that were first identified in the brain and, her work now proves, are also 'bits of brain' floating all over the body."[22] Pearsall hopes that mainstream science will look more seriously at what is happening with the transfer of an organ (especially a heart), which would include questions about why the recipient body rejects a foreign organ so strongly; for the moment, however, mainstream research appears to aim not at understanding the response but rather at suppressing it.

Why does one body reject an organ from another? If the rejection reaction is "purely somatic, physiological, chemical," as one writer suggests,[23] why does the recipient's body not eventually adapt to and accept the organ? This would appear to be an unanswered question. Is it possible that what is somatic, physiological and chemical is also imbued with mind stuff as Pert's neuropeptides theory might suggest? As pointed out earlier, the fact that bodily functions can be explained in terms of physical and chemical laws does not entail that the body is *only* physical and chemical. Writing about the rejection reaction, one transplant surgeon states that in the beginning "the clinical success of organ transplantation far exceeded justifiable expectations considering its weak scientific underpinnings," and adds that, even after three decades of research, "rejection processes remain multifaceted and unpredictable."[24] This statement alone suggests that more research is needed on the question of the status of a transplanted 'live' organ. However, seriously asking why the body's response to a foreign organ is so total and enduring could put at risk the entire transplantation enterprise. It would also put into question the long-standing assumption that physical explanations are not to be confused with mental or psychological explanations.[25]

I would emphasize that I am not concerned, here, about the rightness or wrongness of the technology of organ transplantation, nor am I making ethical judgments about how it is used or who uses it.[26] My concern in this chapter is highlighting the conditions of possibility for the development of such a technology in the first place, of which a dualistic and mechanistic conception of the human body is the most fundamental. Some might argue that it is possible that with a holistic view of the body we might still have the technology, and perhaps they would be right. However, if this were the case, the practice and the discourse surrounding it might be quite different. We would be forced to accept that a human organ is not neutral matter containing no trace of the person from whose body it was taken. People receiving organs would not be told their concerns about the possibility of receiving aspects of another's personality along with the organ are simply psychological, nor would people who actually experience personality changes be told they are imagining it all. Many people might be less willing to donate organs, but, on the other hand, others might be more willing.[27] Ethical questions regarding the buying and selling of organs or the donation of organs from living persons might be analyzed differently. The strict secrecy surrounding donor and recipient, which makes it difficult or impossible for the two to connect, might be re-examined. Fundamentally, however, with a holistic view of body, a different medical paradigm would have grown up over the centuries, and whether organ transplantation could have found a place in it is an unanswerable question. As already discussed, Japan has a more holistic view of the body and a significant resistance to the notion of brain death, but organ transplantation is still practised there. Modern medicine is global.

Organ transplantation is just one example of how unacknowledged metaphysical presuppositions about the body determine a concrete medical practice and the ethical discourse that surrounds it. Another example is reproductive technology.

The Fragmenting Body: Reproductive Technologies

Several years ago, a story appeared in the newspapers about a case of a sperm-donor child tracing and contacting her biological father.[28] The father was both surprised and worried—surprised because he apparently had not made any connection between his two-hundred-odd 'donations'[29] of sperm many years ago and any living, breathing being; worried, because he knew that ninety-eight of his donations had actually resulted in successful pregnancies. He suddenly realized that, in addition to the lovely young seventeen-year-old who arrived on his doorstep, there were, spread across the continent, ninety-seven of her siblings (all of whom, the young lady said, she was determined to find). It was a heart-warming story—the young woman seeing herself in her biological father and understanding at last why she was so different from everyone in her family; the older man recognizing himself in his biological daughter and immediately feeling both loving and protective toward her. Mother and daughter changed cities to be closer to him and his family, and he declared himself willing to support the child financially, offering to pay for her university studies. However, at the time of the story, he was pleading with the sperm bank not to release his name to any of the ninety-seven 'siblings'!

Is this a story of biology or psychology? In the discourse of reproductive technology, there is only biology; reproductive medicine deals with biomaterials (sperm, ova, embryos). These are the raw materials for making children. They can be combined in various ways so that the resulting children may be biologically related (in whole or in part—sometimes not at all) to the parents who will raise them. Like the biological father in the above story, male university students have been selling their sperm for decades. Young (preferably smart and beautiful) women are solicited (via the Internet and university newspapers) to sell their eggs at prices that are very tempting to the economically vulnerable. Commercial surrogacy flourishes in the United States (although it is now illegal in Canada), and many North Americans are now going to India and other less developed nations to have their reproductive materials implanted in women who bear their children for them. The 'donors' of gametes do not appear to see themselves as reproducing; they are simply providing the raw materials for infertile couples to make children—an altruistic act perhaps, but also financially rewarding. It is essential that anonymity be preserved in most of these processes (surrogacy being an obvious exception) in order to suppress any consideration of paternal or maternal ties to—or responsibility for—the resulting offspring. The gametes are 'neutralized,' divested of any recognition of parentage or kinship, so that the infertile couple can believe they are having their own biological child.

Like the blind spot of organ rejection, this is the blind spot of reproductive technologies: couples who desperately want their own biological child (and thus reject adoption) go to great lengths (and expense) to produce a child who is, in fact, *not* wholly—or in some cases not even partly—their biological child, one who will eventually undertake a search for his or her biological parent or parents.[30] The discourse of *in vitro* fertilization and donor insemination, however, creates and maintains the belief that the gametes coming from third parties are neutral materials of reproduction.

As with the discussion of organ transplantation above, I am not here concerned with the morality of the practice of reproductive technologies, and wish to focus on the practice from a metaphysical perspective. Speaking of the penetration of physics into all provinces of knowledge, including the biological, Jonas states, "If it is shown how things are made up of their elements, it is also shown, on principle, how they can be *made up out of* such elements. Making, as distinct from generating, is essentially putting together pre-existing materials or rearranging pre-existing parts."[31] This is the legacy of mechanism; like all other objects of nature, which have been reduced to resources for human use and consumption, the body itself has been reduced to an object that can be divided into parts that can be used as needed. As with organ transplantation, the body parts of one person become resources for the needs of another.[32]

Having facilitated the separation of the sexual act from reproduction, science and technology now facilitate the separation of reproduction from the sexual act. Gametes have been brought outside the body; they are now detachable from the person and have become 'pre-existing materials' allowing the repetition of the process of reproduction outside the human body. Peter Singer points out that *in vitro* fertilization (IVF), for example, is revolutionary not because of the technology itself, which is really quite a simple process, but "because it brings the embryo out of the human body. Once the embryo is in the open, human beings can observe it, manipulate it, and make life-or-death decisions about it. These possibilities make IVF, and its future applications, a subject of the utmost moral importance."[33] But they also make the whole area of reproductive technology a subject of the utmost *metaphysical* importance. A strong argument can be made to the effect that the moral questions around these practices and possibilities cannot be properly assessed unless metaphysical questions about the body are raised and addressed. These relate fundamentally to the materialist and mechanist assumptions that are implicit in all our medical technologies.

The Fragmenting Body: Tissues and Genes

The development of biotechnology in recent decades has expanded the number of body parts that can be used as products for commercialization, raising even more metaphysical questions about the status of the human body. For decades, blood has been collected for transfusion and saving lives; it is now collected for developing cell lines for research and for the commercial development of pharmaceuticals.[34] Tissues that used to be considered waste (for example, from biopsies or surgeries) can be transformed into genetic material for therapeutic use. The development of markets in these tissues has transformed human tissue into a valuable commodity that doctors and hospitals can now sell to pharmaceutical companies. "Human tissue has become so valuable that it is sometimes a target for corporate espionage and theft."[35] People with rare diseases are finding themselves in a position of having samples of their blood, sperm or other tissues collected, not for their own treatment, but for research purposes (and, ultimately, financial gain for the researchers). An American who had his spleen removed because of hairy cell leukaemia later discovered that his doctor had been selling his blood samples to a pharmaceutical company and that he had become a patent number. "My doctors are claiming that my humanity, my genetic essence, is their invention and their property. They view me as a mine from which to extract biological material. I was harvested."[36] He sued the doctors for malpractice and property theft, but the court decided that he did not own his tissue and that the doctors and the pharmaceutical company were not in the wrong in collecting and using his samples (even for their own profit).

This decision was understandably disturbing for the person who felt that his humanity and his essence had been turned into someone else's property. However, if we examine it in the light of our discussion of the self in Chapter 5, we can return to a fundamental question about ourselves and our bodies: Is the body something we *own* or is it what we *are*? Following the separation of the Cartesian self from its bodily expression, one can argue that the court decision merely followed the logic of dualism and mechanism; the body is an object, and, as an object, it can be owned. The question for the court, in effect, was not about whether or not the body tissue in question was an object (this was already assumed), but rather to whom the particular object belonged. The court decided it properly belonged to the researchers who re-worked it (and added value to it). The complainant might have provided the raw materials (unwittingly perhaps), but the final product belonged to its 'inventors' and became subject to the laws relating to property, patents and inventions.[37]

There is a disturbing thread running through the three issues discussed here; in the logic of mechanism, the body is the sum of its parts, and, with the help of modern technology, it becomes the sum of ever smaller and smaller parts. Who owns these parts—which, with the help of modern technology, have a use-value that goes beyond their usefulness to the 'owner' himself or herself? I have two kidneys and yet I really only need one to survive; does this mean I have an obligation to give one of mine to save the life of another? This is not a frivolous question, as the discourse of organ transplantation moves increasingly toward encouraging live donation (as if parts of our bodies are extras that we have an obligation to share, as the rich must share their extra wealth through taxes[38]). A young fertile woman has infinitely more ova than she can possibly use herself. Does she have an obligation to provide some of hers to help someone who cannot conceive? If my genetic material can be used to help researchers develop a cure for a rare disease, do I have an obligation to provide that material even if I perceive it, as did the complainant above, as my humanity and my essence? Modern medical technology has raised these and many other ethical questions. However, as with organ transplantation, there are serious metaphysical questions regarding the ontological status of the human body that are often masked by the ethical questions, making the ethical questions themselves difficult to answer. As long as we remain in the Cartesian dualistic and mechanistic paradigm, the body and its parts will continue to be perceived as valuable resources whose use must be maximized for the progress of humanity (as well as for the benefit of particular individuals). One can ask where the individual self fits into these scenarios, a question that goes beyond the scope of this book, but one that, in light of our analysis in Chapter 6, elicits another question: What would Spinoza think?

The Obsolete Body

The separation of self and body, which has been one of the hallmarks of modernity, has been a condition of possibility for the medical procedures discussed above, all of which fundamentally rely for their legitimacy on the belief that that the body and its parts do not constitute a person. In Platonic and Cartesian terms, the container, or parts of the container, can be put to use while the person remains intact.[39] There is another branch of science that is actively working to dispose of the container altogether, and to preserve the 'person' in another, more efficient, one. In the dreams of the gurus of the 'posthuman' future, the 'person' is not a body, but only a collection of brain patterns or neuronal circuitry. The body, for these thinkers, is an encumbrance. Writing about the limitations of carbon-based neurons, Ray Kurzweil writes:

> While human neurons are wondrous creations in a way, we wouldn't design computing circuits the same way. Our electronic circuits are already more than 10 million times faster than a neuron's electrochemical processes. Most of the complexity of a human neuron is devoted to maintaining its life support functions, not its information processing capabilities. Ultimately, we will need to port our mental processes to a more suitable computational substrate. Then our minds won't have to be so small, being constrained as they are today to a mere hundred trillion neural connections each operating at a ponderous 200 digitally controlled analog calculations per second.[40]

If this sounds like a quote from a science fiction novel, it is not. Kurzweil is only one of a number of scientists, academics and inventors who are working on what is referred to as the 'transhuman' or 'posthuman' future of our species. These terms tend to be used interchangeably, but they do not have the same roots or precisely the same goals. Transhumanism has its roots in the 1970s, in particular with the psychedelic movement of Timothy Leary, and is geared toward enhancing both the physical and mental powers of humans through technology and psychoactive substances. Posthumanism has its roots in cybernetics and is expressed, in particular, in the work of Raymond Kurzweil, Marvin Minsky and Hans Moravec, among others. The vision of the posthumanists is, to a large extent, encapsulated in the above quote from Kurzweil; our biological brains and bodies are simply too slow and cumbersome. They must be—and in fact will be—replaced by super-powerful computer-machines so that humanity can move through the next stage of evolution. In Kurzweil's words, "the freeing of our thinking from the severe limitations of its biological form may be regarded as an essential spiritual quest."[41]

Kurzweil is uncertain about the exact form the body of the future will take; it might be built up through nanotechnology, or it might be some kind of virtual body, but it is unlikely to be wholly (or even partly) biological. The drastic change will come about gradually, however:

> ...body and brain will evolve together, will become enhanced together, will migrate together toward new modalities and materials.... We will enhance our brains gradually through direct connection with machine intelligence until such time as the essence of our thinking has fully migrated to the far more capable and reliable new machinery.[42]

Nanotechnology will give us the ability to overcome the severe limitations of our current protein-based bodies. Kurzweil believes that we will soon be able to "replicate the physical and chemical functionality of any human cell. In the process, we will be in a position to extend greatly the durability, strength, temperature range and other qualities and capabilities of our cellular building blocks."[43]

According to Moravec, those who criticize the idea that our minds can be ported into another kind of substrate are stuck in what he refers to as the "body-identity position." By this he means that they assume "that a person is defined by the stuff of which a human body is made. Only by maintaining continuity of body stuff can we preserve an individual person."[44] Moravec offers an alternative position for consideration, which he calls the "pattern-identity position." This implies that the essence of a person is a matter of the pattern and processes going on in his or her head: "If the process is preserved, I am preserved. *The rest is mere jelly.*"[45] His main thesis is that the pattern and process can, in fact, be preserved. And if they can be preserved, they can be downloaded into a medium other than a biological body. Kurzweil holds the same view, telling us that it will soon be possible

> ...to scan someone's brain to map the locations, interconnections, and contents of all the somas, axons, dendrites, presynaptic vesicles, neurotransmitter concentrations, and other neural components and levels.

Its entire organization can then be re-created on a neural computer of sufficient capacity including the contents of its memory.[46]

This neural computer, however, will not be a body as we know it.

Those who do not find Kurzweil's predictions outlandish tend at least to find them overly optimistic, but he is adamant that they are wrong; they do not take into consideration the rate of exponential change that is involved in every aspect of computer technology development.[47] On this he is on strong ground based on his past predictions, which even his critics admit have been extremely accurate.[48] His major prediction at the present time is that, by the second half of this century,

> ...there will be no clear distinction between human and machine intelligence. On the one hand, we will have biological brains vastly expanded through distributed nanobot-based implants. On the other hand, we will have fully nonbiological brains that are copies of human brains, albeit also vastly extended.[49]

Ultimately the nonbiological intelligence will reign simply because of its exponential growth rate, while "for all practical purposes biological intelligence is at a standstill."[50]

Whether or not Kurzweil's predictions are accurate is not at issue here. What is at issue for a discussion of the human body is the set of assumptions made by Kurzweil, Moravec and others about what terms such as mind, intelligence, body, brain and even information actually mean. There is, first of all, a fundamental assumption that the mind can be separated from its body, an assumption that represents a clear commitment to dualism. Writing about science fiction writers, Mary Midgley points out,

> they go on as if one person's inner life could be lifted out at any time and slotted neatly into the outer life of someone else, much as a battery goes into a torch. But our inner lives aren't actually standard articles designed to fit just any outer one in this way. The cobbler's mind needs the cobbler's body.[51]

Here, Midgley harks back to a well-known example proposed by John Locke in the seventeenth century about a prince switching minds with a cobbler (and about whether or not either would be the 'same person'), but the example is equally applicable to the futuristic scenario of porting minds (brain patterns) into a different substrate.[52] For Midgley, the cobbler needs the cobbler's body in order to be the same person. For the futurists, neither the cobbler nor the prince needs his own body, which will have been rendered obsolete. While Moravec, Kurzweil and others are considered futurists, the metaphysics upon which they base their futuristic scenarios is quite ancient. As we saw in Chapter 1, Plato posited a realm of Forms to which the soul would return to find perfect knowledge in between its lives in mortal (confining and limiting) bodies;[53] Christianity has its Resurrection, after which souls will reunite with their bodies and achieve perfection in immortality. For our futurists, immortality will be earthly, not heavenly, as minds can be continually updated in the manner of updating software on our computers today. As Kurzweil explains, "if we are diligent in maintaining our mind file, keeping current backups, and porting to current formats and mediums, then a form of immortality can be attained, at least for software-based humans."[54] Further, according to Frank Tipler, since much of our future corporeal existence will actually be virtual, "every immortal human being can pick out his most enjoyable world and realize special corporeal utopias," including, it appears, unlimited sex with beautiful women.[55] These futuristic fantasies are a reminder of early Christian questions about whether Adam and Eve had sex, or whether there will be sex after the Resurrection.

Expressions such as 'mind file' and 'software-based humans' are replete with assumptions about the human mind, which is reducible in these scenarios to patterns that can be duplicated by electronic circuitry, as if our inner life were identical to a software program. This is a major error, according to John Searle, based on the assumption that human activity is mostly computation. From this point of view, "if we can create machines that can compute better than humans, we have equalled and surpassed humans in all that is distinctively human. But in fact humans do rather little that is literally computing."[56] This is not to deny that humans do compute, or that much of human behaviour can be explained by brain activity; but recognizing this does not allow us to conclude that our mind is nothing but brain activity. It is worth once again reflecting on the point made earlier in this chapter regarding the supposition of the mechanists that nature has no other modes of operation than those that scientists can explain by physical and chemical processes. As already pointed out, knowing how the body works does not entail knowing what the body is. The same point can be made here about the mind; knowing how the mind *works* (or more precisely, how the brain works) does not entail knowing what the mind *is*. This represents, once again, a slippage from epistemological claims to metaphysical ones, but in this case the concrete practical results of such assumptions (presuming that the futurists actually succeed in porting brain patterns into different substrates) could be more than worrying. Just *what* would be ported into the new substrate? What would be left behind? What type of posthuman creature would be created? What would be the inner life of the new creation?[57]

This brings up a related assumption about what information is. The futurists assume that it is something distinct from the body that holds it. This is an assumption not limited to the world of cybernetics. N. Katherine Hayles points out that it underlies the discourse of molecular biology (which sees the body as instantiating its genetic code), but she also maintains that "a defining characteristic of the present cultural moment is the belief that information can circulate unchanged among different material substrates."[58] It is a small step from the belief that information is disembodied to the belief that the human body is incidental to human nature or the human mind: "embodiment continues to be discussed as if it were a supplement to be purged from the dominant term of information, an accident of evolution we are now in a position to correct."[59]

The futurists believe that, since the mind can be ported out of its body, then the body is ultimately redundant. This is based on an assumption that the body does not count in the mental life of the person—an assumption that is reflected in Moravec's distinction between the pattern-identity position and the body-identity position referred to earlier. Those who think the person needs the same body to be the same person are making a serious mistake, according to Moravec. But, examined from the perspective of Spinoza's monism and his theory of the *conatus* discussed in Chapter 6, it can be argued that it is Moravec who is making a serious mistake. Remember that for Spinoza there is no separate or separable self. The self is the striving for existence whereby the individual (mind and body) is in constant interaction with—and adaptation to—its environment, of which it is, ultimately, a part.[60] No individual is a whole unto itself.[61] Further, looked at from the point of view of Spinoza's three levels of knowledge, the information-processing aspects of knowledge, including scientific and mathematical knowledge, represent only the second level of knowledge. How would the highest level, intuition, whereby an individual grasps a greater understanding of the whole and his or her place in it, be represented in Moravec's pattern-identity position?[62] As Searle has pointed out, the assumption of human knowledge for these thinkers is computational knowledge—very sophisticated computational knowledge, but computational nonetheless.[63]

There are many aspects of the vision of Kurzweil et al. that can be, and have been, criticized; chapters could be written on any one of the quotes from their work referred to in this chapter. My intention, however, is to focus on those aspects of their work that presume a dualistic and mechanistic vision of the body, a presumption that reduces human consciousness and self to the brain and its information-processing capabilities (and that now presumes that, by isolating and enhancing these capabilities, the human species will be enhanced in the process). Their goal is not surprising, given what Anne Foerst refers to as "the sense of disembodiment that has shaped people in the Western world for centuries."[64] This sense of disembodiment is reinforced with our current use of computers.[65] But "we cannot blame computers for this, as they are constructed under the assumption that our brain works like a computer and that our body is not important for intelligent processing in the brain."[66]

In spite of our secular science and our secular society, the Christian vision of an immortal soul guaranteeing human superiority over everything in nature has not faded; it has simply been transformed. It is now the human intellect that sets us apart from nature—rising above it and living independently of it. We still see ourselves in Cartesian terms as pure intellects, "detached observers, set above the rest of the physical world to observe and control it."[67] Because of this detachment from the world, we tend to see ourselves as detached from the process of evolution, as well. It has become, at least in the minds of many scientists, something that humans can control. The next step in evolution, for many of our futurists, will be to create intelligent machine-children who, in Moravec's words, "will mature into entities as complex as ourselves, and eventually into something transcending everything we know—in whom we can take pride when they refer to themselves as our descendants."[68] Our descendants perhaps—but without our bodies.

The Body as Consumer Object: Modifying the Body, Modifying the Self

The first part of this chapter focused on the body as an object of scientific and medical knowledge, and on the uses to which the objectified and divided body can be put for the good of others (saving lives through organ transplants;

relieving infertility through transfer of gametes; furthering medical research—and corporate profits—through the patenting of genetic material). The second part examined a contemporary vision of the body as an obstacle to knowledge—a biological limitation on the capacity of the human mind to fulfil its true knowledge potential and to become immortal through spiritual machines. My position throughout the chapter has been that none of the scenarios presented so far could exist without an implicit assumption that the mind and self are distinct from the body. They all play a role in bringing to its logical conclusion the dualistic and mechanistic view of the body that has supported Western science since the seventeenth century.

In this section, I want to look at scenarios that stem from similar assumptions about the self and the body, but play themselves out in different ways. These cases also implicitly assume a body-as-property point of view ("It's my body and I can do what I want with it"). In effect, the body becomes a consumer object—"the finest consumer object," in the words of Jean Baudrillard, who states, "In a capitalist society, the general status of private property applies also to the body, to the way we operate socially with it and the mental representation we have of it."[69] Here the question is not so obviously one of the obsolete body; rather, the body becomes something of a fashion accessory that one can acquire and put on in order to enhance the inner self, or to conform to what one perceives as one's *real* self. As we will see, however, taken to its limit, the fashion accessory itself can ultimately be seen as transformable to the point of redundancy.

There is a continuum of body enhancement projects and techniques, ranging from cosmetic surgery to tattooing to dramatic transformations of the body, that consciously and purposefully use the body as an art object. I will deal with a number of these while making the point that, while they represent different degrees of body manipulation, they are all made possible because of widespread acceptance of the body as an object and as property. They reflect the modern notion of the self, whereby one's self—that separated self, discussed in Chapter 5—is, in a sense, one's life, which is then seen as something that one must develop or shape. As Arthur Frank explains, the self becomes raw material that people think they are expected "to do something with." The body then becomes an instrument in this pursuit of self-making, which, taken to extremes, can become one's life project.[70]

The idea of the body as an instrument is not new. For Plato, harmony between body and soul is very important to the overall health of both, although, as we have seen in Chapter 1, he tends to denigrate the body and attribute absolute importance to the soul and to reason, an attitude that has influenced Western thought through the centuries. And we have seen clearly in Descartes that the mind is the seat of the self, which, when combined with a view of the body as an instrument or tool, becomes the user of the tool. In a framework where the mind or soul has an ultimate, and presumed higher, purpose (for Plato, reaching the pure knowledge of the Forms; for Christians, including Descartes, salvation and immortality), the body becomes an instrument for the achievement of that goal or purpose. It becomes in effect an instrument of virtue—moderation in all physical pursuits leading to harmony of body and soul. With the Stoics and Spinoza, one would add harmony with nature to the mix; living in accordance with nature (the Stoics) or one's environment (Spinoza) becomes the goal.

In a mechanistic universe with a mechanistic body as the instrument of a self that looks only to its own self-determined goals and purposes, each person's body becomes a tool for individual self-expression and self-formation. Modification of the body then becomes a means to the end of meeting external norms (e.g., cosmetic surgery) or simply an end in itself (e.g., full-body tattoos; the body as art object). We can make our bodies into anything we want in order to create or transform an identity or a self. For Joe Rosen, a plastic surgeon who dreams of giving humans wings, human flesh "is infinitely malleable.... The body is a conduit for the soul, at least historically speaking. When you change what you look like, you change who you are."[71] The self becomes as malleable as the flesh.

The notion of human flesh as infinitely malleable is, in part and in some quarters, a reaction against mechanism, which is identified with fixity and permanence. Contemporary theorists of the body, in particular feminist theorists, focus on the "socially constructed body—the malleable surface of an internally stable corporeality," often building on the work of the French philosopher Michel Foucault.[72] But even the "internally stable corporeality" is questioned by the discourse of biology, more and more focused not on the organism but on mapping information flows of the genome,[73] a reduction and diminishment of the body comparable to that of Kurzweil and Moravec discussed earlier in the chapter.

In this context, the body becomes a project that a person can fashion to fit his or her desires. And in fashioning the body, people believe they are fashioning (or re-fashioning) the self. In his study of the ever more popular practice of tattooing, Paul Sweetman quotes one heavily tattooed interviewee as stating, it makes you feel individual ... you know like, everyone's born with roughly the same bodies, but you've created yours in your own image [in line with] what your imagination wants your body to look like. It's like someone's given you something, and then you've made it your own, so you're not like everyone else any more.[74]

Some of Sweetman's interviewees spoke of feeling "more complete" or being "a better, more rounded, and fuller person" because of their tattoos.[75]

Extreme Body Modification

Those with tattoos are referred to as either 'lightly tattooed' or 'heavily tattooed.' There are some in the latter category who have tattooed their entire bodies. Along with tattoos, many people have piercings; they can also be described as lightly or heavily pierced. At the far end of this spectrum, we find what is known as "extreme body modification," which, while not in any way mainstream, is becoming more popular, as well as more competitive, as people try to outdo each other in their quest to be original. An example of this is the case of an American, Steve Deerwood, who made it into the *Guinness Book of World Records* in 2006 by having 2,507 surgical needles (each 1.5 inches long) inserted into his body.[76] Mr. Deerwood's piercings were temporary and done to raise funds for victims of domestic abuse. Somewhat more permanent is the tongue modification of Allen Falkner, a thirty-six-year-old Texan who split his tongue down the middle so that when he sticks it out it resembles a snake's tongue. According to a CBS news report, "Falkner did his work himself, experimenting with various methods and instruments that included scalpels and string. Already sporting multiple tattoos and piercings, he said he further modified his body for aesthetic reasons, and in part just to see if he could."[77] The idea of making dramatic changes to the body simply to see if one can is a testament to the body's lack of value (its having been rendered 'value-neutral,' to use Jonas' terminology) as it progresses down the road to obsolescence. The foregoing constitute just two examples; there are many others, as a casual tour through body modification websites will attest, and it is difficult to classify any of the modifications as having been done for aesthetic reasons. It would seem many body modifiers are like Falkner; they do it because they can.

Stelarc

One might want to say that Deerwood and Falkner are very much on the fringe and should not be taken seriously (although the copycat factor of the Internet gives one pause here). They are, however, simply at the far end of a spectrum of tattooing and piercing practices that are used purposefully and consciously by more and more ordinary (especially young) people to turn the body into a project to reflect the self, to make some political or social statement, or just for the sake of it. Others, who because of their fame and recognition in the art world must be taken seriously, take the body-as-project to even greater extremes. The Australian performance artist known as Stelarc, who has performed all over the world, is one example. He refers to the body as a sculptural medium and as evolutionary architecture, rather than as reflecting personality or gender or psyche. Many of his experiments and performances involve a melding of robotic technology with his own body, with a view to showing how our biological body (which he refers to as 'biological architecture') can extend its capacities through technology. In the 1970s and 1980s, his performances involved suspensions of his body in space, first using ropes and harnesses and later using hooks attached through his skin, making the skin become part of the support structure. He sees these suspension performances as "a bridge between primal and technological yearnings" and as "an image of escaping both the planetary pull and by implication, our genetic containment as well."[78] Besides escaping his genetic containment, his objective is to challenge our concepts of "individuality, identity, agency and autonomy," and to ask questions such as the following: "Can we consider a body that can function with neither memory nor desire?"[79] A body without memory or desire would not be a person, and one might ask why anyone should want to consider the question. However, Stelarc does not see the body as a person but as a structure, an object for redesigning. He points out that we have blurred the body with technologies that allow us to sustain the comatose, preserve a corpse cryogenically, transfer blood from one person to another, and so on. As a result, we are living in the age of "the cadaver, the comatose and the chimera."[80] Like Kurzweil and Moravec, Stelarc considers the body obsolete, and he is putting his own body on the line to demonstrate this.[81]

Orlan

Another example is Orlan, the French performance artist,[82] who uses her body as an art object, and in so doing, "pushes to new extremes both the material use of her body as a project and the self as inextricably tied to how that project is realized."[83] Among her more sensational projects is a series of surgeries in the 1990s, which she turned into performances, with herself and the surgeons in costume, the operating room as a theatre, and herself as commentator on her own operations. (Using local instead of general anaesthetic allowed her to observe and comment; one picture shows her lying on her side on the operating table, holding a microphone, while the surgeons, scalpels in hand, remove skin from her buttocks).[84] While these 'performances' are somewhat gory, they have a purpose, here described by the art critic and historian Barbara Rose:

> With self-transformation in mind, and proceeding with a cold, Cartesian logic buttressed by her considerable knowledge of esthetics and art history, Orlan began to deconstruct mythological images of women. Recalling that the ancient Greek artist Zeuxis made a practice of choosing the best parts from different models and combining them to produce the ideal woman, Orlan selected features from famous Renaissance and post-Renaissance representations of idealized feminine beauty ... the nose of a famous, unattributed School of Fontainebleau sculpture of Diana, the mouth of Boucher's Europa, the forehead of Leonardo's Mona Lisa, the chin of Botticelli's Venus and the eyes of Gerome's Pysche as guides to her transformation.[85]

Some see Orlan's project as simply an extreme end of the continuum of plastic surgery, and many feminists criticize her work as buying into male fantasies of the female form. But Orlan sees her plastic surgeries as a path toward self-determination. She purports to be showing women that, in fact, they can regain control over their bodies. "Orlan has to be the creator, not just the creation; the one who decides and not the passive object of another's decisions."[86] She also claims to demonstrate the futility of the male fantasy of the ideal woman. Her objective is not to make herself beautiful, something that becomes clear when one looks at the results of her surgeries. Whether Orlan's work is pro-feminist or anti-feminist (in fact, she dismisses the question by saying she is both) is a secondary issue and not the main reason for including her carnal art in this chapter. Her work represents an extreme example of the rejection of the body as a biological reality; for her it is a social construction, one that modern technology makes increasingly redundant. Referring to Orlan's project of deconstruction of the body, Kathy Davis writes,

Orlan's project takes the postmodern deconstruction of the material body a step further. In her view, modern technologies have made any notion of a natural body obsolete. Test-tube babies, genetic manipulation and cosmetic surgery enable us to intervene in nature and develop our capacities in accordance with our needs and desires. In the future, bodies will become increasingly insignificant—nothing more than a 'costume,' a 'vehicle,' something to be changed in our search 'to become who we are.'[87]

The words 'become who we are' reflect the idea of modification of the body as a project of self-creation, but they are misplaced here, since Orlan is constantly changing what she sees herself as becoming. There is no permanence, either, to the body or the self in her project. She sees her work as exploring the question of identity. But what meaning can the word have in her world of constantly shifting body performances? For example, "since 1998, Orlan has been creating a digital photographic series titled 'Self-Hybridizations,' where her face merges with past facial representations (masks, sculptures, paintings) of non-western civilizations. So far, three have been completed: Pre-Columbian, American-Indian and African."[88] Self-hybridization and identity would seem to be contradictory objectives.

Giving Us Wings

Rosen, the plastic surgeon referred to earlier who wants to give us wings, also sees the fixity and permanence of the biological body as a constraint. He does not understand why we are so 'conventional' with respect to our bodies, or why plastic surgeons are not allowed to help people explore their possibilities. For him, plastic surgery is not only the intersection of art and science, it is also the "intersection of the surgeon's imagination with human flesh."[89] This, in effect, takes the issue a step further than Orlan, who, while using plastic surgeons as tools toward her self-transformation, guides their work according to her own imagination. Rosen would like to use the flesh of others as the medium for the creations of *his* imagination—one of them being human wings. As Lauren Slater describes it, Rosen has "blueprints, sketches of the scalpel scissoring into skin, stretching flaps of torso fat to fashion gliders piped with rib bone. When the arm stretches, the gliders unfold, and human floats on currents of air." He is serious enough about this to give "lectures to medical students on the meaning of wings from an engineering perspective, a surgeon's perspective, and a patient's perspective."[90] He truly believes that the idea of human wings is not a bad one, and is one that will be realized in the not very distant future.

Looking at these different phenomena of extreme body modification, I want to ask: Why? But the response of Rosen, Orlan and the others will simply be: Why not? There is, for them, no notion of the person as body and soul, or of body and soul connected to nature or the environment, as in Spinoza or the Stoics. They see any normative notions of the human body as a constraint. There is only an ever-malleable body (that can be modified into oblivion) and a self that does not seem to be much more than an autonomous human will directing bodily transformations according to its desires. These cases represent the enactment of an idea—the idea of the body as object, as property, as *my* property: "It's *my* body and I'll do what I want with it."

There is, however, an argument Rosen makes that, at least on the surface, poses a challenge to Spinoza's view of the mind as the idea of the body: If Rosen gives the body wings, what happens to the mind? Does it include the idea of wings? And, if so, is that a bad thing? Is it not just a way of transforming the self? Rosen's position, here, is clear: "Our bodies change our brains, and our brains are infinitely moldable [*sic*]. If I were to give you wings, you would develop, literally, a winged brain. If I were to give you an echolocation device, you would develop in part a bat-brain."[91] Why we would want a winged brain or a bat-brain is a question we might be tempted to ask. The answer would likely be simply because we *can*. And in a world devoid of *should* or *must*, 'because we can' is an answer that philosophers have difficulty countering.

So, what would Spinoza say? If the mind and body are the same thing expressed under two attributes, then the mind is as changed as the body by the insertion of 2,500 surgical needles, multiple plastic surgeries (whether for art or for burn therapy) or the implantation of wings. Slater wonders if Rosen's wing technology would "toggle us down the evolutionary ladder,"[92] which is an interesting question. From a Spinozistic point of view, however, one can ask whether such body modifications would strengthen or weaken the *conatus*, which, we must remember, simply *is* the self, persisting in its being, maintaining the ratio of motion and rest in relation to its environment. Spinoza's self is never a whole; it is a part of its environment as well as of its history—and it is determined by both. Rosen's scenario—as Orlan's—presupposes a body detached both from the mind and from the world around it. It also presupposes a Cartesian belief in free will, a position that Spinoza denies.[93] Like the worm in the blood that does not see the web of causation that determines it, nor the role it plays in the organism of which it is a part, Rosen and the others do not see the causes that determine mind and body, or understand that the individual (body and mind), while appearing to be a whole, is really a part of a larger series of parts and wholes.

The postmodern thinkers arguing against fixity in relation to the self are fighting both the mechanistic view of the body and the Cartesian view of the rational, thinking self. I would point them in the direction of Spinoza and the Stoics, and suggest a project that would recuperate a holistic vision of mind, body and nature, one that recognizes all aspects of the person in his or her situation in the world. Orlan may be right in saying that modern technology is rendering the natural body obsolete, but that is because technologies are being developed and used in a mechanistic way on bodies that are seen as machines—a vision that, I would suggest, is anything but natural. Our vision of the natural body disappeared with the Renaissance; Orlan is the *reductio ad absurdum* of the mechanistic vision. Instead of deconstructing the body-machine, we need to recuperate the natural body in its wholeness with the world around it. This would allow possibilities of transformation of self that do not rely on its deconstruction and disappearance, but on its flourishing and fulfilment. Spinoza's individual is anything but fixed; at the same time, it cannot just decide to change itself into something it is not. As the worm cannot decide to give itself horns, we cannot decide to give ourselves wings. For Spinoza, freedom is not the freedom to transform the body from the outside, but to understand the body from the inside *and* its relation to the outside, in all the complexity of its organic development and the web of cause and effect. It is not a machine alone in the world; it is an organic part of the world around it. Rosen would attach wings to the body-machine. Spinoza's body would not grow wings.

One can argue that it is a long road from organ transplantation and reproductive technologies to Orlan's surgeries and Rosen's wings, and I would not want to suggest simplistically that there is a slippery slope from the former to the latter.[94] My intention, however, has been to demonstrate that the practices discussed in this chapter presume the body to be an object—of science, or art, or simply individual will—that is, in different ways, perceived as separate and apart from the self. One can argue about the purposes involved in these various practices from an ethical point of view, and propose that some are useful and beneficial while others are frivolous or harmful. But from a metaphysical point of view, all of them presuppose a body disconnected from nature, mind or soul. For better or worse, they can all be subsumed under the logic of the body-machine.

In the next chapter, I will examine a vision of the body and of personal transformation that is far from postmodern: the world of the ancient practice of yoga, which transcends the idea of the body-machine in its recognition of the unity and inter-relation of body, mind and spirit, and their relation with the world and the cosmos. We will see the body not as a broken machine that risks becoming obsolete, but as the basis of self-transformation, shaping mind and spirit and, in turn, being shaped by them.

Notes

1. This section has been adapted from my article, "The Body and Technology: A New or an Old Anthropology?" in *Technology and the Changing Face of Humanity*, eds. Richard Feist, Chantal Beauvais and Rajesh Shukla (Ottawa: University of Ottawa Press, 2010), 22–40.

2. *The Principles of Philosophy*, Part Two, #64, in CSM, I, 247.

3. Jonas, *Phenomenon*, 204.

4. Jonas, 203.

5. I refer the reader to the discussion of the disembodied Cartesian 'self' discussed in Chapter 5.

6. While psychology occasionally looks in the direction of biology in its explanations, biology does not return the favour. Medicine, however, nods in the direction of psychology as it puzzles over the placebo effect, for example.

7. Didier Moriau, "Le corps médicalisé," in *Quel Corps?* ed. Michel Beaulieu (Paris: Éditions de la Passion, 1986), 128ff.

8. Hans Jonas, *Philosophical Essays* (Englewood Cliffs, NJ: Prentice-Hall, 1994), 19.

9. Susan Bordo, *Unbearable Weight: Feminism, Western Culture, and the Body* (Berkeley: University of Califormia Press, 1993), 245.

10. The notion that my kidney is me may strike one as absurd; and it *is* absurd within the context of a mechanistic and materialist account of the body—which is the account that I am questioning here. In a holistic account of the body, one might perceive the situation differently.

11. The new definition came about as the result of a report by an *ad hoc* committee at the Harvard Medical School. The result of the Harvard committee's work was the establishment of what is called the "whole brain" formulation to determine when death has occurred. This formulation means that a person can be declared dead when the functions of the entire brain have ceased. The World Medical

Association adopted the whole-brain definition of death in August 1968, with the Canadian Medical Association following suit in November of the same year. The guidelines have been amended over the years, but the basic definition entailing the irreversible cessation of all functions of the entire brain has remained stable among Western countries.

12.   Peter Singer, *Rethinking Life and Death* (New York: St. Martin's Griffin, 1994), 35.

13.   There is no doubt that if the ventilator is turned off the person will usually die very quickly (although in rare cases this does not happen). But the same can be said of a person whose life is being maintained by dialysis. Yet, in this case, no one would say that the person on dialysis is dead because his or her kidney has ceased to function.

14.   Margaret Lock, *Twice Dead: Organ Transplants and the Reinvention of Death* (Los Angeles: University of California Press, 2002), 4, 8 (emphasis added).

15.   Lock, 8.

16.   Jonas points to Cartesian dualism as a bridge, "which carried the mind of man from the vitalistic monism of early times to the materialistic monism of our own." Jonas, *Phenomenon*, 12. Once the spiritual was hived off from the physical, it only remained to dispense with it altogether. Midgley puts it a little more colourfully when she states, "With the advance of the physical sciences, matter increasingly looked intelligible on its own. Mind and body did indeed start to look more like ship and pilot, and people began to ask whether the pilot was actually needed." Midgley, "Souls, Minds," Pt. 1, 4.

17.   R. E. Billingham, "Basic Genetic and Immunological Considerations," in *Symposium on Organ Transplantation in Man*, vol. 63, or *Proceedings of the National Academy of Sciences, U.S.A.* (Washington, DC: National Academy of Sciences, 1969), 1020. (Quoted in Stuart J. Youngner, Renée C. Fox and Laurence J. O'Connell, *Organ Transplantation: Meanings and Realities* (Madison: University of Wisconsin Press, 1996), 6.

18.   Renée C. Fox, "Afterthoughts: Continuing Reflections on Organ Transplantation," in Youngner et al., 255.

19.   Fox, 256.

20.   Lock, 327.

21.   Paul Pearsall, *The Heart's Code: Tapping the Wisdom and Power of Our Heart Energy* (New York: Broadway Books, 1998). Psychoneuroimmunology is the study of how the brain and immune system interact with the world. Pearsall's book tackles the radical idea of cellular memory and, in the process, recounts stories of heart recipients who experience changes (including changes in dreams and memories) as a result of their transplant. To give only one example: Pearsall was present at a meeting between a doctor named Glenda and a young man who was the recipient

of her husband's heart (the husband having died in a head-on car crash one night several years earlier). Glenda put her hand on the young man's chest, and, as if addressing her husband, said that everything was "copacetic." The young man's mother, who did not know the meaning of the word copacetic, said that this strange word, one she had never heard him use before, was the first thing her son said after the transplant: "He said everything was copacetic." Glenda explained that every time she and her husband made up after an argument they would both say that everything was copacetic. Further, the young man, who had been a vegetarian, now ate meat and junk food; his musical taste changed from heavy metal to fifties rock-and-roll; and he had dreams about bright lights coming at him. Glenda responded "that her husband loved meat, was a junk food addict, had played in a Motown/rock-and-roll band while in medical school, and that she too dreams of the lights of that fearful night" (Pearsall, 76). In preparing his book, Pearsall recorded the stories of heart and other organ transplant recipients, their families and donor families, as well as the clinical experiences of doctors, nurses and researchers in the transplant field. He includes the story of the eight-year-old girl who received the heart of a murdered ten-year-old girl. When her nightmares and the information that came from them about the murder and the murderer were finally taken seriously by her parents, her therapist and the police, the killer was found and convicted of the crime (Pearsall, 7).

22.	Pearsall, 10. Pert has written hundreds of scientific articles, along with a popular book, *Molecules of Emotion* (New York: Touchstone Books, 1999), exploring the relationship between body, mind, spirit and emotions.

23.	Leslie A. Fiedler, "Why Organ Transplant Programs Do Not Succeed," in Youngner et al., 57.

24.	Barry D. Kahan, "Organ Donation and Transplantation—A Surgeon's View," in Youngner et al., 126.

25.	The notion that the transplanted organ is more than neutral physical matter may be anathema to the medical community, but it could be a factor in the overall resistance of the population to the donation of organs. On this point, see Le Breton, *La Chair à vif*, 270. Concerning the reaction of the medical community to his work, Pearsall states: "I have been told that I would do damage to the transplant movement by bringing attention to the idea that the heart is much more than a pump or that someone else's 'soul stuff' could accompany a transplanted organ" (9).

26.	See Carol Collier and Rachel Haliburton, *Bioethics in Canada: A Philosophical Introduction* (Toronto: Canadian Scholars Press, 2011), Ch. 9, for an analysis of the ethical issues relating to organ transplantation.

27.	In fact, some research has shown that a holistic view of the body is not conducive to donation. See Russell Belk, "Me and Thee, Mine and Thine: How Perceptions of the Body Influence Organ Donation and Transplantation," in *Organ Donation & Transplantation*, eds. J. Shanteau and R. J. Harris (Hyattsville, MD: American Psychological Association, 1990), 139–47, for a discussion of body metaphors that encourage and discourage donation of organs. This article was the result of a conference of psychologists that dealt specifically with different views of the body and their impact on organ donation. The participants concluded that organ donation is more probable when people think of their bodies as machines rather than as sacred or as integral to their identities (145). On the other hand, anecdotal evidence indicates that some families are more willing to donate their loved one's organs when they believe the loved one lives on in the recipient's body.

28.   Paul Kendall, "Anonymous no more," *National Post*, October 1, 2004, A14. The sperm provider's name is Robert Gerandot and the name of the young woman is Katie Whitaker. A follow up to this story can be found at www.lifesupporters.com/forms/politics/sperm-donors-offspring (post-dated June 19, 2005, accessed October 18, 2010). In this article, the wife of the sperm 'donor' remarks on the connection between her husband and the young woman conceived with his sperm: "People don't want to comprehend the power of a biological connection. These kids, they're going to find their donors, they're going to look for their half-siblings—it's going to happen because there's a fundamental drive to do it, and these sperm banks need to start counseling families that this is what could come."

29.   The word 'donation' is always used in relation to gametes when very often they are not donated but sold. Officially, since 2003, all commercial transactions relating to reproduction are illegal in Canada.

30.   This can be done, for example, through the Donors Sibling Registry, a website and non-profit organization that allows children born through artificial insemination by anonymous donors to find their parent and/or other siblings born from the same donor sperm. See donorsiblingregistry.com (accessed October 18, 2010).

31.   Jonas, *Phenomenon*, 202 (emphasis added).

32.   Ethical arguments regarding the buying and selling of reproductive materials usually revolve around issues of individual choice and autonomy. Many ethicists argue in favour of a free market in reproductive materials and procedures. John A. Robertson, for example, goes so far as to state that, "in a liberal society, the invisible hand of procreative preference must be allowed to flourish, despite the qualms of those who think it debases our humanity." Thomas Mappes and David Degrazia, *Biomedical Ethics*, 5th ed. (New York: McGraw-Hill, 2001), 547. Others argue that the values of the marketplace are inappropriate in matters relating to the procreation of children.

33.   Peter Singer, "Creating Embryos," in Mappes and Degrazia, 534.

34. For an interesting story of the development of a cell line for research and commercialization, see Rebecca Skloot's recent book, *The Immortal Life of Henrietta Lacks* (New York: Random House, 2010). Blood cells were taken from the body of a poor Black tobacco farmer without her knowledge and have survived since 1951, being used for research all over the world and the development of medical miracles such as the polio vaccine. They have also made a lot of money for the pharmaceutical industry, while the family of the deceased Henrietta has received no benefit and, in an ironic twist, cannot even afford health insurance.

35. Dorothy Nelkin and Lori Andrews, "Homo Economicus: Commercialization of Body Tissue in the Age of Biotechnology," *The Hastings Center Report*, 28: 5 (September–October 1998), 31.

36. Quoted in Nelkin and Andrews, 32. The patient's name is John Moore, and the pharmaceutical company is said to have paid $15 million for the right to develop the 'Mo' cell line.

37. This is a clear example of the meaning of Jonas' quote about the breaking down and building up of elements.

38. This should not be interpreted as an argument against taxes or income distribution in society. The point is made in order to raise the question of the ontological status of body parts. If they are property, a strong argument can be made that they should be considered resources to be distributed—which, as pointed out in this chapter, is how they are considered in the language of transplantation ethics. Many ethicists argue in favour of mandatory 'donation' at death; it is a small step from there to mandatory donation in life—and there have been court cases in the United States about the obligation of a parent or relative to 'donate' an organ or tissue to save the life of another. So far, arguments about this kind of obligation have been resisted. But these are arguments that follow logically from the assumption that body parts are property.

39. Some philosophers will object to my using the container analogy, here, since Descartes explicitly resisted it in his Sixth Meditation when he stated that he is not in his body as a pilot is in his ship. On the other hand, as we have seen, he was unable to reconcile mind-body union within his dualistic and mechanistic metaphysics, so I do not think using the container analogy here is inappropriate.

40. Ray Kurzweil, "The Evolution of Mind in the Twenty-First Century," in *Are We Spiritual Machines: Ray Kurzweil vs. the Critics of Strong A.I.*, ed. Jay W. Richards (Seattle: Discovery Institute, 2002), 29. The title of Kurzweil's article gives a clue to his vision of the future: advanced neural computers (and robots) modeled on the human brain and able to replicate themselves represent the next stage of the evolution of mind, and, in his view, of humanity.

41. Kurzweil, "Evolution," 53.

42.   Ray Kurzweil, *The Age of Spiritual Machines* (New York: Penguin, 1999), 135. Kurzweil makes the point that—at the time of writing his book—we had already come a long way in transforming our bodies. "We have titanium devices to replace our jaws, skulls, and hips. We have artificial skin of various kinds. We have artificial heart valves. We have synthetic vessels to replace arteries and veins, along with expandable stents to provide structural support for weak natural vessels. We have artificial arms, legs, feet, and spinal implants" (135). The list goes on.

43.   Kurzweil, *Spiritual Machines*, 140. There is a problem with nanotechnology, however, and that is that it is extremely costly. So the nanometer-sized machines "need to come in the trillions," and this would only come about by allowing the machines to build themselves (140). It would seem that whatever form the body of the future takes, it will not be unique to any one individual. Machine bodies replicating themselves will presumably be identical.

44.   Hans Moravec, *Mind Children* (Cambridge: Harvard University Press, 1988), 117.

45.   Moravec, 117 (emphasis added).

46.   Kurzweil, "Evolution," 36. The process by which this will be done is referred to, by Kurzweil and others, as "reverse-engineering the brain." This is a highly complex project, similar in scope to mapping the human genome, but Kurzweil is convinced it will be possible within the next two decades. "There are many projects around the world, which are creating nonbiological devices and which recreate in great detail the functionality of human neuron clusters, and the accuracy and scale of these neuron clusters are rapidly increasing" (Kurzweil, 37). Many of these projects are aimed at the development of medical technologies. "Neurological disorders may someday be circumvented by techno-logical innovations that allow wiring of new materials into our bodies to do the jobs of lost or damaged nerve cells. Implanted electronic devices could help victims of dementia to remember, blind people to see, and crippled people to walk" http://www.engineeringchallenges.org/cms/8996/9109.aspx (accessed September 2, 2010). In one project, a group of neuroscientists, biologists, physicists, engineers and computer scientists are working on reverse engineering the brains of fruit flies. The project, which involves shaving "50-nanometer slices off the top of the infinitesimal fruit-fly brain ... is trying to establish the exact connections among the neurons and synapses of the tiny creature's brain" http://spectrum.ieee.org/biomedical/ethics/reverse-engineering-the-brain (accessed September 2, 2010).

47.   Kurzweil's predictions are based on 'Moore's Law,' which can be roughly stated as follows: "Every two years you get twice as much computer power and capacity for the same amount of money." John Searle, "I Married a Computer," in

Richards, 56. It is possible to calculate the number of synaptic events per second in the human brain (based on the total number of neurons and the number of synapses among neurons), and then estimate the improvement factor needed for computers to match the computational capacity of the human brain. According to Baldi, most experts agree that "the performance gap should disappear, and even begin to reverse, sometime between the years 2020 and 2050." Pierre Baldi, *The Shattered Self: The End of Natural Evolution* (Cambridge: MIT Press, 2001), 93. Baldi adds that "sheer computing power is a necessary component of intelligent systems but is not sufficient per se," a point that Kurzweil does not emphasize.

48. While the accuracy of past predictions cannot be used as proof for the accuracy of predictions about the future, Kurzweil's record is impressive. He accurately predicted the downfall of the Soviet Union based on the fact that new technologies would disempower authoritarian governments. He predicted that a computer would beat out the best chess players by 1998, something that actually happened in 1997, when IBM's Deep Blue computer beat Garry Kasparov in a tournament. He forecast the development of the Internet and its expansion to include worldwide networks of databases, libraries, etc., long before the Internet had become a reliable medium. He also predicted the development of pocket-sized computers, as well as wireless access to electronic networks. These are only a few of his many predictions, most of which have come to pass. He is also an inventor of note and the recipient of numerous honorary degrees; in other words, he is taken seriously by a lot of people.

49. Kurzweil, "Evolution," 55.

50. Kurzweil, "Evolution," 55.

51. Midgley, "Souls, Minds," 3.

52. Kurzweil appears to have an answer to Locke's identity question: "Objectively, when we scan someone's brain and reinstantiate [*sic*] their personal mind file into a suitable computing medium, the newly emergent 'person' will appear to other observers to have very much the same personality, history, and memory as the person originally scanned.... The new person will claim to be that same old person and will have a memory of having been that person. The new person will have all of the patterns of knowledge, skill, and personality of the original" (Kurzweil, "Evolution," 40).

53. Hayles refer to the disembodied information of the futurists as "the ultimate Platonic Form. If we can capture the Form of ones and zeros in a nonbiological medium—say, on a computer disk—why do we need the body's superfluous flesh?" N. Katherine Hayles, *How We Became Posthuman: Virtual Bodies in Cybernetics, Literature, and Informatics* (Chicago and London: University of Chicago Press, 1999).

54.   Kurzweil, "Evolution," 52. Kurzweil does add some nuance to his identity and immortality claims when he says that questions of consciousness and identity, which have been debated since Plato, "will not remain polite philosophical debates, but will be confronted as vital and practical issues" (52).

55.   Oliver Krueger, "Gnosis in Cyberspace? Body, Mind and Progress in Posthumanism," Journal of Evolution & Technology, 14: 2 (2005), 84. Krueger quotes from Frank J. Tipler's book, *The Physics of Immortality: Modern Cosmology, God and the Resurrection of the Dead* (New York: Anchor Books, 1995): "it would be possible for each male to be matched not merely with the most beautiful woman in the world, not merely with the most beautiful woman who has ever lived, but to be matched with the most beautiful woman whose existence is logically possible." This is notable not only as an example of, to use Krueger's words, "paradisiacal male fantasies," but because of its similarity to the claims of radical Islamists for whom dying as a martyr in the cause of Islam will allow the deflowering of large numbers of virgins in heaven.

56.   Searle, 69.

57.   In his book *On the Internet*, Hubert Dreyfus analyzes six stages through which a student advances, moving from instruction to practice to apprenticeship. The early stages, ending at Stage 3, Competence, involve principally the transmission of information in such a way that bodily presence in a classroom or with a teacher is not crucially important. However, "at every stage of skill acquisition beyond the first three, involvement and mattering are essential. Like expert systems following rules and procedures, the immortal detached minds envisaged by futurists like Moravec would at best be competent. Only emotional, involved, embodied human beings can become proficient and expert." Hubert Dreyfus, *On the Internet*, 2nd ed. (London and New York: Routledge, 2009), 47. This is before even considering other dimensions of learning such as the ethical, the philosophical, the spiritual or the artistic.

58.   Hayles, 1.

59.   Hayles, 12.

60.   Remember Spinoza's analogy of the worm set out in Chapter 6.

61.   The self-replicating systems of the futurists are, however, closed systems, isolated from their environment. Their response to their environment is determined totally by their internal self-organization. As Hayles puts it, "Their one and only goal is continually to produce and reproduce the organization that defines them as systems." In the latest paradigm of self-organizing and self-making systems, there are no feedback loops, "for the loop no longer functions to connect a system to its environment" (Hayles, 1).

62. I do not believe that Spinoza's idea of mind and body can be captured by either the pattern-identity position or the body-identity position. It can be argued that both of these positions are rooted in dualistic thinking.

63. Searle draws a distinction between syntax and semantics. Syntactical processes are purely formal; they deal solely with the manipulation of symbols. Semantics provides meaning and content to symbols; in the thinking process, semantics is what the thoughts are *about*. Part of Searle's argument against Kurzweil is that computers only do syntax and that you cannot get to semantics from syntax alone. In short, minds work semantically; computers are syntactical. With respect to the chess game between Deep Blue and Kasparov, Searle says that the "real competition was not between Kasparov and the machine, but between Kasparov and a team of engineers and programmers" (Searle, 63).

64. Anne Foerst, *God in the Machine* (New York: Penguin, 2004), 90. With degrees in computer science, philosophy and theology, Foerst is in the unique position of being a 'robotics theologian,' exploring what robots can teach us about our humanity, including our emotions, our thinking and our actions.

65. Foerst describes research by a German researcher where both computer specialists and high school students who spent considerable time in front of computers were asked to draw portraits of how they saw themselves. In both groups, "people saw themselves reduced to hands, eyes, and brain; most of them felt that their bodies had vanished or been fragmented" (Foerst, 86).

66. Foerst, 90.

67. Midgley, "Souls, Minds," Part 2, 5.

68. Moravec, 1. It should be pointed out that when people like Moravec and others begin speculating about the next stage of evolution—or even about the *purpose* of evolution—they are no longer talking about science but are moving into metaphysics, a subject in which few of them are specialists. They are also supposing what Midgley calls the escalator or ladder theory of evolution (which situates humans—and human intelligence—at the top of a long ladder of progressive development). In her view, this is not Darwinism: "Darwin saw no reason to posit any law guaranteeing the continuation of any of the changes he noted, or to pick out any one of them, such as increase in intelligence, as the core of the whole proceeding." Mary Midgley, *Evolution as Religion* (London and New York: Routledge, 1985, 2002), 38.

69. Jean Baudrillard, *The Consumer Society: Myths and Structures*, trans. Chris Turner (Los Angeles: Sage Publications, 1998), 129. The chapter in which the quotation is found is titled "The Finest Consumer Object: The Body."

70. Frank, 20. Frank's article deals with the ethics of using medical technology for enhancement rather than therapeutic purposes (although there is a continuum here, as well)—for example, limb-lengthening for someone who considers himself

not tall enough vs. limb-lengthening for someone diagnosed with achondroplasia (genetic dwarfism). This is another case where metaphysical concerns hide beneath the ethical issues.

71. Lauren Slater, "Dr. Daedalus: A Radical Plastic Surgeon Wants to Give You Wings," *Harper's* (July 2001).

72. Linda Birke, *Feminism and the Biological Body* (New Brunswick, NJ: Rutgers University Press, 1999), 137. Michel Foucault's (1926–1984) work often emphasizes the body "as preeminently a site of political control, increasingly subject to surveillance" (Birke, 33). Thus the body is not a given, but is 'constructed' by social and political relations, and, in the case of female bodies, these relations are fundamentally gendered, the body of biomedicine, for example, being that of a white male.

73. See Birke, 144, 148: "Within biology as a whole, students now must learn about information flows and their mapping; it is genome projects, not organisms, that mark the centre of biological knowledge … there is no theory of the organism as a self-organising, dynamic, transforming entity, in the way that biology is currently taught. Organisms are simply epiphenomena, accidental byproducts of genetic plans."

74. Anonymous interviewee in Paul Sweetman, "Anchoring the (Postmodern) Self? Body Modification, Fashion and Identity," *Body & Society*, 5: 2–3 (1999). http://bod.sagepub.com/content/5/2-3/51, 68 (accessed September 20, 2010).

75. Sweetman, 68.

76. The previous record was 745 needles. http://www.impactlab.net/2006/03/30/extreme-body-modification (accessed September 20, 2010).

77. http://www.cbsnews.com/stories/2006/08/05/health/main (accessed September 21, 2010). The news report also mentions that Falkner has several websites and gets many inquiries from people interested in "modifying themselves." The Internet facilitates the propagation of these practices and feeds the expressed need of some individuals to turn their bodies into projects.

78. Quoted in Nicholas Zurbrugg, "Marinetti, Chopin, Stelarc and the Auratic Intensities of the Postmodern Techno-Body," *Body & Society*, 5: 2–3 (1999): 110, http://bod.sagepub.com/content/5/2-3/93. The suspensions can be seen in the video "The Body is Obsolete," distributed by Contemporary Arts Media, http://www.artfilms.com.au/Detail (accessed September 20, 2010).

79. Zurbrugg, 111.

80. These are Stelarc's words from the video "The Man with Three Ears," VBS TV (http://www.vbs.tv/watch), June 16, 2009.

81. Although Stelarc does not dwell on this, I am assuming it is painful to have eighteen hooks piercing the skin, allowing him to be suspended in mid-air.

82. One can question whether what Orlan does is really art, but the art historian and critic Barbara Rose reluctantly concludes that it is. See Barbara Rose, "Orlan: Is it Art?" *Art in America*, 81: 2 (February 1993), 83–125, http://www.stanford.edu/class/history34q/readings/Orlan/Orlan2.html (accessed September 21, 2010).

83. Frank, 20.

84. Website for English 114 EM at the University of California Santa Barbara, offered by Prof. Elizabeth Heckendorf Cook in 2003, http://www.english.ucsb.edu/faculty/ecook/courses/eng114em/surgeries.htm (accessed September 21, 2010). See also Kathy Davis, "'My Body is My Art': Cosmetic Surgery as Feminist Utopia?" in *The European Journal of Women's Studies* 4 (1997), 26, http://ejw.sagepub.com/content/4/1/23 (accessed September 21, 2010). Davis reports that Orlan's seventh operation-performance was "transmitted live by satellite to galleries around the world (the theme was omnipresence) where specialists were able to watch the operation and ask questions which Orlan then answered 'live' during the performance." She also has preserved "souvenirs" from her operations in "reliquaries" (bits of skin, scalp, fat cells, surgical gauze drenched in blood). "She sells them for as much as 10,000 francs, intending to continue until she has no more flesh to sell."

85. Rose, "Orlan." These transformations were done in a series of choreographed operations—involving music, dance and elaborate sets—performed by state-certified surgeons.

86. Davis, 30.

87.˙ Davis, 29. Davis adds that, when male plastic surgeons "balked at having to make [Orlan] too ugly ('they wanted to keep me cute'), she turned to a female feminist plastic surgeon who was prepared to carry out her wishes" (Davis, 30). It is worth noting that there are ethical issues involved in this whole project concerning both the misuse of scarce medical services and resources and the doctors' obligation to do no harm (Hippocratic Oath).

88. *Wikipedia*, http://en.wikipedia.org/wiki/Orlan (accessed September 22, 2010).

89. Slater, 59, quoting Joe Rosen.

90. Slater, 61. Rosen is not out on the fringe of his profession. He is a well-respected plastic surgeon, as well as an associate professor of surgery at Dartmouth Medical School. He travels all over the world giving presentations and "has had substantial impact not only scalpeling [*sic*] skin but influencing his colleagues' ethics in a myriad of ways" (Slater, 61).

91. Slater, 66, quoting Rosen.

92. Slater, 66. It should also be emphasized that interaction between body and brain is not the same as interaction between body and mind, unless one assumes that mind is identical with brain processes (which, of course, many thinkers do; Spinoza, in my view, did not assume this).

93.   See Chapter 6 on the difference between Descartes and Spinoza on the will and the self.

94.   It is interesting, however, to note the link made by Orlan and Stelarc themselves between their work and the increasing blurring of the body with technology.

CHAPTER VIII

RECOVERING THE BODY: YOGA

Millions of Westerners, and in particular North Americans, are practising yoga. They pick up their yoga mats, head for a local yoga studio, and spend an hour or two performing the physical exercises (postures) of the many different and evolving forms of hatha yoga. They are taking part in a 5,000-year-old spiritual practice that is also an art, a science and a philosophy[1]—although for many of them it is not perceived as much more than a good workout that gets their bodies into shape and enhances their energy levels. "Yoga has been secularized and turned from a rigorous spiritual discipline into an 'instant' fitness system."[2] Some of these practitioners, however, will see beyond the physical benefits and notice a quieting of the mind, or an emerging dissatisfaction with the materialist direction of their lives; they might begin to search for deeper meaning in the postures they perform on their mats. They might become teachers themselves or disciples of one of the many Indian teachers, whose role has been to transplant this ancient practice into new ground, adapting it to the Western body and mind. They might become serious *yogis* and *yoginis*[3] and, if they do, their lives may be transformed.

Whether they realize it or not, they are also learning a new approach to the body, one that sees mind, body and spirit as so inextricably linked that any disturbance in one is a disturbance in the other. They may also begin to experience spirit as something different from mind and as a new dimension for self-exploration. Georg Feuerstein emphasizes that the traditional purpose of yoga "has always been to bring about a profound transformation in the person through the transcendence of the ego."[4] This goal is reflected in all the martial arts of the East, where self-cultivation means, in effect, a total transformation of the self in relation to the world.

The idea that yoga has been secularized in the West presupposes that it is, or was, a religion, but this is not a position that receives unanimous support. Some writers hold that yoga predates the Hindu religion with which it is often identified. Vivian Worthington points out, for example, that Hinduism actually adopted yoga, since yoga originally existed outside the framework of Brahmanism, as the early form of Hinduism was known:

> Although fiercely contested and often persecuted by the Brahmins, [yoga's] main writings, the Upanishads, were later adopted by the Brahminical establishment and tagged on at the end of the Vedas, thus changing the whole complexion of Hinduism....[5]

Other writers (often writing from an academic and religious studies point of view) hold that the *Vedas* came first and the *Upanishads* came later. Given that these ancient texts were oral before they were written, deciding who is correct is not an easy matter. It can safely be noted, however, that even if yoga itself is not a religion, it has influenced, and has been practised within, different religions for centuries, most notably Hinduism, Buddhism, Jainism and even Sufism.[6] Another claim that it is quite safe to make is that, in its millennia of existence, yoga has existed in many forms and undergone many adaptations. In addition, all commentators emphasize the syncretic nature of the Indian mind and culture, its ability to adapt to new ideas and to accept many different versions of the same general philosophy, even where they might be, or might appear to be, contradictory. In this, the Indian belief system is akin to that of the Renaissance naturalists whom we met in Chapter 4. In the final analysis, finding the 'authentic' yoga history and practice is a task best left to the academics, one of whom tells us that, "as long as there is no agreement on the interpretation of the written sources from the Indus civilisation, such claims about the presence of yoga will remain possible interpretations."[7]

Yoga has a distinctly spiritual dimension, but it does not demand any particular set of beliefs, dogmas, or rituals; it can be practised by people of any religion or no religion. A serious practitioner of the discipline, however, cannot ignore the spiritual goal of self-transformation. The word 'yoga' itself means 'yoke' or 'union,' and refers to the union of the lower, everyday self (ego) and the higher or transcendental Self. Arriving at this latter state entails meditative practices that many do tend to perceive as religious. Writing about yoga from the perspective of academic religious studies, Elizabeth De Michelis states that, as it developed "under rapidly secularizing Western conditions, Modern Yoga came to be described more and more as an inward privatized form of religion."[8] Thus, while yoga has been practised mainly in a religious context for centuries, in the West it is now more often practised in a secular context as a path to individual spirituality and self-transformation. It continues, however, to be "a free-thinking experimental and experiential discipline requiring self-effort, compassion and knowledge."[9]

Indian philosophy was studied in Europe in the eighteenth century, and colonial administrators and scholars brought yoga to Britain in a limited fashion when they returned home. But the person who did the most to bring yoga to the West was Swami Vivekananda, who caused a sensation when he attended the Parliament of Religions held in Chicago in 1893.[10] A disciple of Ramakrishna, he believed, like his master, in the unity of all religions;[11] at the same time, it was his conviction (and his experience) that no one should take religion on faith: each person must experience God directly. Nobody can be religious unless and until he or she has had the same experiences as the founders of the great religions, who "all saw their own souls, [and] saw their souls' future and their eternity; and what they saw they preached."[12] Like most authentic yoga teachers, Vivekananda's watchword was to believe nothing until one has experienced it. "Do not believe a thing because you read it in a book. Do not believe a thing because another has said it is so. Find out the truth for yourself. That is realization."[13] That yoga is based on personal experience rather than faith gives it a subjective dimension that can make it a difficult subject for academic study.

Vivekananda did more than simply bring yoga to the West; he also transformed it to fit the place and the times—in particular, the esotericism that was popular in certain parts of nineteenth-century American society, represented by such groups as the Theosophists or the Christian Scientists.[14] Many of his essays, for example, bring in Christian themes and symbols, suggesting a kind of cross-fertilization as Vivekananda both influenced and was influenced in turn by American ideas. The result was a blend of Eastern and Western spirituality that became the basis for modern yoga in the West, but also for a renaissance of yoga in the East.[15]

Many other yogis contributed to the development of yoga in the West during the twentieth century. Two among these were especially influential. Paramahansa Yogananda, author of the very popular and influential *Autobiography of a Yogi*, came to America in the 1920s, eventually establishing an *ashram* in Los Angeles and starting the Self-Realization Fellowship, which now runs five hundred temples, *ashrams* and meditation centres around the world. The other was Swami Sivananda of Rishikesh, who, although he never came to the West himself, trained a number of disciples who contributed much to the development of yoga in the West. One of his many disciples was Swami Sivananda Radha, whose work is discussed later in this chapter. Worthington tells us that Sivananda's *ashram* "was a powerhouse of yoga teaching, and he was himself a very powerful man."[16] There are Sivananda centres and *ashrams* around the world.[17]

Because of the many traditions and lineages represented by these different yogis,[18] yoga in the West has developed branches and sub-branches; even a cursory examination of them is beyond the scope of this chapter. Yoga is included here because it is a tool for self-knowledge through the body, one of the main themes of this book. The body in yoga is neither the body-machine of Descartes, nor the body of modern medicine. It corresponds more to Spinoza's monistic vision of mind and body, where there is nothing in the mind that is not in the body, and vice versa. But it also encompasses a more clearly spiritual dimension than Spinoza—a dimension that cannot be reduced to mind. The important thing to remember is that, in doing the postures of hatha yoga, one is also working on the mind and spirit, since, in yoga, body, mind and spirit are all one.

In this chapter, I will examine several dimensions of yoga and relate them to philosophies of the body that have been discussed earlier in the book. I will be looking at hatha yoga (the most common form of yoga known in the West), along with a particular approach to hatha yoga called the hidden language of hatha yoga, a very effective practice for letting the body speak. I will also include a discussion of the yoga of sound (mantra yoga), which includes a cosmic dimension that can be related back to ancient ideas of cosmic harmony. I will be looking, as well, at the yoga of breath (*pranayama*) and relating it back to the *pneuma* of the Stoics and of pre-Cartesian metaphysics. The links between mind, body, spirit and nature (or cosmos) will be central to each of these discussions. We will see different ways of explaining and expressing what I call the 'cosmic connectors.'

The Metaphysics of Yoga

First, however, it is essential to come to grips with some of the metaphysics of yoga, which is not a simple matter, since there are so many branches of yoga philosophy; while there are significant similarities, there are differences, as well. Most of the focus in this chapter will be on non-dualist or monistic Vedanta, often referred to as Advaita Vedanta,[19] which holds that if there is a God, "not only is He the creator, but He is also the created. He Himself is this universe."[20] There is no supernatural god who is separate from the universe, his creation. Everything in the universe is, in effect, God. We are all God; we are all one: "There is no supernatural, says the yogi, but there are in nature gross manifestations and subtle manifestations. The subtle are the causes, the gross the effects. The gross can be easily perceived by the senses; not so the subtle."[21] The purpose of yoga is to provide the *yogi* or *yogini* with access to the subtle, in order to understand the causes of what manifests in the world.

There are more poetic and metaphorical ways in which this unity is described. Sometimes it is explained as the dance of *Siva* and *Sakti*:[22] *Siva* is the masculine principle of the universe, the Unmanifest, the power behind creation; *Sakti* is the feminine principle of the universe, the whole of creation, the Manifest. Thus, the whole of creation is feminine—sometimes referred to as Divine Mother—which is a very non-Western idea. *Siva* and *Sakti* are one, inseparable, and are sometimes spoken of in terms of energy or consciousness or light:

> The oneness of Siva and Sakti is described like fire and heat, which cannot be separated. From this perspective, Siva and Sakti are not different, and are only the names of philosophical ideas. The male/female principles are not separate entities but are a unit—the same source of Energy manifesting different qualities. Power simply is. It is not male or female. Just as the air is not he or she and the air can have various conditions, so Energy and Power are not separate.[23]

However one wants to think of this power and the manifestation of this power (in creation), the most important point is that it is in each and every person. Everyone has access to this power—his or her higher self—and the practices of yoga (postures, breath, chanting, meditation) can help foster a connection with this higher self (sometimes referred to as *Atman*). While *Siva* and *Sakti* are popularly conceived as a god and goddess, this is only a way of thinking about them to help people understand what they represent. The vast cosmic power is called *Siva*, for example, "to personify it so the human mind can communicate with it and about it."[24] It is difficult to communicate with, or feel love or reverence for, a principle—just as it is difficult to communicate with creation as a whole. So it is called *Sakti*, or Divine Mother, or *Saraswati*,[25] or any number of names and forms, all of which serve to bring out different aspects of reality, which, ultimately, are different aspects of the self that the practitioner wants to reach, communicate with and bring to consciousness.

Following the belief that humans are, ultimately, one with the universal reality or the divine principle, yoga teaches us that the world of everyday experience, as well as our everyday idea of our individual selves, is an illusion. This is often spoken of as *maya*, which refers to the cosmic illusion resulting from the fact that the true reality is veiled from us. We can access it only by transcending the world and the self through *Samadhi* (discussed below).

Although much of yoga philosophy is framed in terms that are foreign to the Western mind, it is possible to practise yoga, even in its broadest and deepest sense, without using any of the personified gods, goddesses, images, myths or metaphors for support.[26] The ultimate reality, for an enlightened person, is none of these things—it is beyond all of them. Those who might be uncomfortable thinking of their higher self as God, or Atman, can simply call it light, or intuition, or cosmic consciousness. After all, few people know what it *really* is.[27]

The Tree of Yoga

The aspect of yoga that most North Americans are familiar with is usually called hatha yoga, which refers principally to the yoga of the postures or *asanas*. *Asana* is only one of the eight limbs of classical yoga set out in the *Yoga Sutras* (or *Aphorisms*) of Patanjali,[28] one of the highest authorities of yoga philosophy. And hatha yoga can also refer to the eight limbs as a whole, adding another level of terminological confusion.[29] It is helpful to list the eight limbs in order to be able to situate the practice of *asana* and to understand how it is linked to the others.

The first limb consists of the *yamas*, ethical guidelines governing one's actions in the world and with other people. The *yamas* are five in number: *ahimsa* (non-harming, non-violence); *satya* (truthfulness); *asteya* (non-stealing); *bramacharya* (control of sensual pleasure); and *aparigraha* (detachment). The second limb is the five *niyamas*, internal guidelines for one's own spiritual development. They are *sauca* (cleanliness or purity); *santosa* (contentment); *tapas* (discipline); *svadhyaya* (self-study); and *isvara-pranidhana* (devotion; worship).

The third limb of yoga is *asana*, the yoga of postures, the objective of which is the "cultivation of profound physical and psychological steadiness and ease in mind, breath, and body."[30] The *asanas* represent the physical aspect of yoga, but, as already mentioned, it is a mistake to think of the *asanas* as *only* physical. Traditionally, the *asanas* were designed to bring the body into the stillness and flexibility necessary for meditation: "The body must be so supple it can bend any way you want it to. Such a body will always be healthy and tension-free. The moment we sit down for meditation in such a body, we'll forget it."[31] But in the process of developing flexibility, one also releases physical and mental toxins that are part of the reason the body is stiff and tense to begin with. So, even if meditation is not one's aim in beginning a hatha yoga practice, it might well be the result of achieving clarity and stillness. More will be said about this later in the chapter.

The fourth limb of yoga is *pranayama*, the yoga of breath, a practice that works to still the mind through stilling the breath. But *prana* is more than breath; it refers to the vital or life force. Thus, regulation of breathing is also regulation of energy in the body.

The fifth limb is called *pratyahara*, often translated as withdrawal of the senses, but referring more precisely to discrimination and the ability to have sense experiences that are not predetermined by past experience and memory. With *pratyahara*, according to Iyengar, intelligence "guides the mind not to depend completely on memory and its impressions,"[32] allowing for more intuitive insight in perception.

The last three limbs (*dharana*, *dhyana* and *Samadhi*) relate to the different levels of concentration and meditation, the first involving focus on a single object (breath, sound, an image); the second, being a deeper meditation where the meditator and the object of meditation (observer and observed) become one; and the third, being a state where "the body, the mind and the soul are united and merge with the Universal Spirit."[33] These last three limbs are the goal of the first five; in other words, one cannot reach the highest levels of meditation until one has achieved stillness of mind, body and spirit, which the practice of the first five limbs makes possible.

Since our concern, here, is knowledge of and through the body, we will focus on the *asanas* and on *pranayama*.[34] While these are usually treated separately in the literature, in hatha yoga they are often intertwined in practice, where arriving at stillness is a fundamental objective. As Michael Stone writes,

> What we mean by 'stillness' is psychological stillness. We tend to the body and its infinite layers and our spreading of breath throughout these layers without being apart from the experience. We use the experience to wake up. We use the body to study the mind and the mind to study the body so that we come to see the inherent interpermeation [*sic*] of mind and body and world.[35]

Hatha Yoga (The *Asanas*)

According to its practitioners, it is impossible to do hatha yoga seriously and not meet the mind, which often confronts the student with the recognition of patterns of thought and behaviour that he or she might otherwise not care to look at. "It's not just the body that becomes more flexible in yoga postures, but the mind as well.... The mind moves in grooves with qualities similar to those of a stiff arm bone in a shoulder socket—tightness, discomfort, and stress."[36] Working with the tightness, discomfort and stress of the shoulders can lead one to ask what kinds of tightness, discomfort and stress are in the mind. It is easy to understand how the *asanas* might help relax tight muscles and thus relieve mental stress; but the mind-body connection in hatha yoga goes deeper than that. Every posture can be a map into the interior of the mind and body, unveiling unconscious patterns of behaviour, forgotten memories, unexpressed emotions. Loosening up that constricted shoulder can actually loosen up a constricted pattern of behaviour or thinking. Stone invites us to think about physical inflexibility as being expressed psychologically, as well:

> When the mind is unable to hold several viewpoints simultaneously, when it is impossible to listen in a conversation, or when we find ourselves clinging to one perspective, we are caught in inflexibility. It is not just the body that becomes more flexible in yoga postures, but the mind as well.[37]

How does this come about? Yoga philosophy provides an explanation of the mind-body-spirit connection that runs counter to our usual mechanistic view of the body. According to yoga philosophy, mind and body as a whole are actually made up of five different sheaths (called *kosas*—which means sheath or subtle body), which are interacting and interpenetrating. When we are practising hatha yoga or *pranayama* or meditation, these sheaths are all working together. "The kosas represent the interconnection of mind, body, emotion, thought and stillness—aspects of human experience that cannot ultimately be separated from one another."[38] The five *kosas* are as follows:

1) *Annamaya kosa:* anatomical sheath (bones, tendons, muscle groups);

2) *Pranamaya kosa:* physiological sheath (circulation, respiratory system, nervous system, lymphatic and immune systems);

3) *Manomaya kosa:* psychological sheath (mind, feelings and the processes that organize experience);

4) *Vijnanamaya kosa:* the frame responsible for intellect and wisdom; and

5) *Anandamaya kosa:* feeling of the body as energy or impersonal flow.[39]

These five sheaths are like a matrix: they work together, and any activity in one has effects in the others. This is a different way of looking at mind and body, which are normally perceived in our culture as, if not completely separate, at least requiring different kinds of explanation. It is interesting to note that the mind forms a different sheath from the intellect (mind and intellect are not identical in yoga philosophy). It is also interesting to note that the 'unconscious,' which we normally associate with mind and look to psychologists to explain, is, in yogic philosophy, considered to be a bodily phenomenon. Further, because mind constitutes just one of the five parts of this matrix, it does not have priority over body: we cannot argue for the priority of consciousness "because mind, breath, body, and stillness are of one piece, and if the kosas are truly interdependent, one aspect cannot operate without interactions with all the others."[40] Memory is lodged in all five sheaths, as well, and this can explain why the movements of the *asanas*, the fluctuations of the breath, and the stillness of meditation can all work to bring to the fore forgotten or suppressed emotions and allow precious insights into what is happening to oneself as a whole being.

Some might argue that the concept of the five sheaths is not based in reality, or that there is no empirical evidence for their existence. But the *yogi* could ask what empirical evidence exists for the separation of mind and body, a view that has dominated Western thought for centuries, or for the mechanical view of the body that is still current in Western medicine. Who is to say the Eastern view of the body is wrong and the Western view is right? We might take a step back and ask which model of mind, body, spirit and breath has greater explanatory value. We can also, from a practical point of view, take a good look at where the mechanistic view of the body in the West has taken us, and our bodies. The philosopher Richard Shusterman writes that our consciousness of our bodies is "flawed in ways that systematically hamper our performance of habitual actions that should be easy to perform effectively but yet prove difficult, awkward, or painful."[41] He also suggests that we need to increase our philosophical understanding of body consciousness through training in disciplines that encourage reflective awareness of the body. Yoga is such a practice.[42] In becoming conscious of the body through the postures of hatha yoga, one can become conscious of its essential oneness with mind and spirit. Thus, yoga corrects a fundamental assumption of much Western philosophy that the self (and knowledge of the self) is a matter of mind, not body. In yoga, awareness of the body increases awareness of the self.

Whether or not one accepts the yogic explanation of the effects of performing *asanas*, meditation and breathing exercises, it is an empirical fact that these activities do have both physical and mental health benefits for those who practice them. Studies have shown that yoga (including meditation techniques and *pranayama*) has therapeutic benefits for a number of chronic health conditions, including hypertension and diabetes. It has been shown to reduce body weight, stress, blood pressure, glucose levels and cholesterol levels.[43] Given the holistic nature of the practice, however, and the fact that psychological and spiritual factors are part of any individual's reaction to the practice, it is very difficult to set up clinical trials that meet the objective criteria of medical science. As we will see below, yoga is a very personal experience, and each person will integrate its effects in different ways.

The Hidden Language of Hatha Yoga

Writers such as Stone describe the awareness that results from performing the yoga *asanas*. They recommend staying with whatever arises in the mind and/or body, working through it, not fighting it. But they often remain at the level of the abstract, and do not explain how or why certain poses might cause certain insights (comfortable or uncomfortable) to arise. Can different poses bring up different issues? Do different parts of the body hold different types of patterns of thought or behaviour?

These questions are addressed through a unique approach to hatha yoga developed by Swami Sivananda Radha, one of the many disciples of Swami Sivananda. While she was at Sivananda's *ashram* in India, he instructed her to investigate the mystical aspects of the poses. As a result, she developed a method for using the poses as an exploration of mind and body to increase awareness of the patterns of thought and behaviour that govern our lives. This method is set out in her book, *Hatha Yoga, The Hidden Language: Symbols, Secrets & Metaphor*. Today, the hidden language approach to hatha yoga is one of the central practices at the Yasodhara Ashram, which Swami Radha founded in the Kootenay region of British Columbia upon her return to Canada.

For example, in a simple but well-known pose, the Tree, one is invited to think about key words that come up in thinking about a tree, or in visualizing a favourite tree. Different words will come up for different people in a class: some will think of roots going deep into the ground, or branches reaching toward the sun; others about balance or sturdiness, or sturdiness balanced with flexibility; still others might think about the fruit of a tree or the need to prune back a tree to aid its growth. Students will be asked to choose a key word that speaks to something within them (which is, ideally, a word that has spontaneously come to them), and take that word into the pose for reflection. The possibilities for metaphorical association with their own lives are endless. Standing in the pose (on one leg, with the foot of the other balanced on the thigh of the standing leg, the arms reaching up to the sky like the branches of a tree), one can ask oneself questions such as: What are my roots and how are they nourished? Am I flexible enough to withstand the storms of my life? Am I growing in an environment that fits my needs? Are there parts of my personality that need pruning? By focusing on a key word and/or a key question in any pose, "one can now begin to look at the postures as symbols and find in them an unsuspected significance."[44] In the stillness of the pose, the intuitive part of the mind starts to work, and, if one stays with any uncomfortable associations that come up (often in images or memories, but also in words or phrases), important insights can be gained. In hidden language classes, students come with notebooks and have time to write reflections on their experiences and insights.

The need to let go of the strong sense of self and the mental constructs that determine one's perceptions of the world has already been referred to in relation to Stone's holistic approach to yoga, which points to the connection between rigidity of thought and rigidity of body. Radha mirrors Stone when she points out that "a person who has a neck and shoulders as unyielding as a piece of steel is probably unyielding in daily life."[45] One of the poses that works on the neck and shoulders, and provides the symbolic inspiration for reflecting on the connection between being physically and psychologically unyielding, is the Plough. This pose, in which the feet are brought over the head as one lies on the ground, is full of symbolism relating to ploughing up old ground, making the earth receptive for new growth, planting new seeds. This pose demands flexibility in the spine, the neck and the shoulders—all areas that an overly strong will can render quite inflexible—and, as these parts of the body open up in the pose, so does the mind become more flexible:

> Even to sow the seeds of understanding, the ground of the mind must be ploughed. The weeds (concepts that have, like crabgrass, grown deep) are hard to remove. The seeds of understanding can only grow in a fertile soil, one that is receptive, and in which the nourishment is of high quality. At the same time, discrimination is needed to distinguish good, healthy thoughts from the weeds of self-importance and fear—weeds that will crowd out new growth.[46]

When a person is relaxed and receptive to the process of hidden language, the logical and rational part of the mind can rest and let the body speak. According to Swami Lalitananda, a disciple of Swami Radha, "in Hidden Language you learn to trust your body and establish a firm foundation in your own intelligence."[47] Following the discussion of the five sheaths, above, and the notion that every one of them contains memories, it is not surprising that opening the shoulders or the hips can release forgotten memories or emotions, for example, or that insights can be gained into certain concepts that, though perhaps useful at one point in a life, might still play too large a role in a person's perception of reality. The words 'hidden language' suggest that at some level we already know these things—the body speaks a language that can be unveiled and listened to. As Lalitananda puts it,

> The human body is the holder of all the secrets, the teller of truths. And when the truths are revealed—good or not so good—they are gifts. Seeing a pattern that creates pain, do I want to keep it or let it go? Can I decide on a new course of action by inviting in a new way of thinking? The value of Hatha Yoga is not just in stretching the muscles, but also in stretching the mind.[48]

The Yoga of Breath: *Pranayama*

We saw earlier that the fourth limb of the yoga tree is *pranayama*, the yoga of breath. The reader might find it strange that there is a branch of yoga devoted to something as common as breathing. However, as one investigates this fourth limb of yoga, it quickly becomes obvious that breathing is not as simple an activity as it appears. In his book, *The Yoga of Breath*, Richard Rosen refers to his *pranayama* students as "beginning breathers," which does seem just a little bit odd. We might ask what his students are doing when they are not in *pranayama* class; are they not breathing? According to Rosen, many of them—like the rest of us—are breathing very badly, often with serious consequences ranging from stress to poor posture, a sagging spine, a sunken rib cage and weak or constricted respiratory muscles. In fact, he tells us, "each of us has a unique breathing behavior or breathing identity. Some of us are very efficient breathers, while others—many others—aren't."[49] Aside from the simple health benefits of proper breathing, there is, in yogic philosophy, a strong relationship between breath and consciousness. As with *asana* practice, the practice of *pranayama* is meant to slow down the fluctuations of the mind. As Stone puts it,

> Asana and pranayama practice have to do with following the flow of the breath and the flow of energy within the body. Once some concentration and ease is established, we notice where energy flows and where it is interrupted. We give immediate attention to the patterns and disruptions of the breath, the nervous system, the heart rate, and the feeling tone in the muscles, fascia, and so on.[50]

The ultimate goal of this for the *yogi* is the attainment of the stillness that is necessary for concentration and meditation and, finally, enlightenment. But even if enlightenment is not one's goal, the regulation of the breath—on its own or in conjunction with *asana*—is a way to self-discovery through the body.

Prana is usually translated into English as 'breath,' but this is a simplification. "Prana is a subtle energy that pervades every corner of the universe. While we can't see and touch it directly, *at least not as beginning breathers*, we can do so indirectly, through one of its most obvious physical manifestations and significant vehicles, our breath."[51] It can be compared to the Chinese *chi*, the Japanese *ki* or the Stoic *pneuma*. The latter, we will recall from Chapter 2, was seen not only as breath but as the vital principle of all living things and the world's active—or seminal—principle, accounting for the immanence or self-directedness of the world's activity as an intelligent whole. In a similar vein, Vivekananda explains *prana* as that out of which everything that we call energy or force is evolved: "It is prana that is manifesting as motion; it is prana that is manifesting as gravitation, as magnetism. It is prana that is manifesting as the actions of the body, as the nerve currents, as thought-force."[52] *Prana* plays a similar role to what I refer to in this book as the 'cosmic connectors'—what links mind, body, soul and cosmos.

In the *Yoga Sutras* of Patanjali, several aphorisms are devoted to the control of *prana*, or the practice of *pranayama*. Patanjali tells us that the "modifications of the life-breath are either external, internal, or stationary. They are to be regulated by space, time and number and are either long or short."[53] The 'life-breath' is *prana*, which, as pointed out above, is not simply breath but cosmic energy or force; however, as Vivekananda tells us, "we begin by controlling the breath as the easiest way of getting control of the prana."[54]

There are many different exercises relating to this simple aphorism of Patanjali's, but I will mention only two. The first, as outlined by Rosen, looks at four qualities of the everyday breath: time, texture, space and rest. With respect to time, at first one simply observes the speed of the breathing and the time of the inhalation and the exhalation. There is no attempt to slow down the breath, although this may happen once one begins to observe it. Texture and space relate to observing how the torso fills up with breath, whether the breath goes to one side more than the other, whether one is a 'front' breather or a 'back' breather. Rosen asks his students to "notice when the breath is disturbed, when it speeds up, when it becomes rough or shallow, or when it stops altogether."[55] He encourages them to do this exercise while standing in line at a grocery store or sitting in traffic, for example, so that they can learn much about their feelings of the moment and their reactions to what is going on around them. The fourth part of the exercise, rest, entails simply observing that the breath tends to rest at the end of an inhale and an exhale; observing this will tend to lengthen the rest period, which many people find very relaxing.

A second practice is alternate nostril breathing with retention. This consists in blocking one nostril and breathing in slowly; blocking both nostrils and retaining the breath; then unblocking the second nostril and breathing out slowly; then blocking both nostrils and holding the breath. The purpose of retention is not to stop the breath as an end in itself, but to stop the fluctuations of the mind that block discovery of the true self. As Rosen explains, "for the yogi what we understand as breathing is a means to an end, a tool that both increases and conserves the aspirant's vital energy and intensifies and channels its transformative powers."[56] *Pranayama*, as we have seen, is another step on the ladder of enlightenment for the aspirant; it can also have health benefits for anyone who practices it.

The Yoga of Sound: Mantra

Another aspect of yoga, which is not a limb in itself but is linked to the limb of concentration, is mantra or chanting—the yoga of sound. The importance of mantra is based on the central idea that the world is vibration, and that the repetition of certain key sounds is a way of linking into that vibration.

The best-known mantra is the universal sound "OM," around which many religious practices of the East revolve. It is considered a primal sound, one of several seed syllables. As Joachim-Ernst Berendt explains, the "sages of India and Tibet as well as the monks of Sri Lanka feel that if there is a sound audible to us mortals that comes close to the primal sound that is the world, then it is the sound of the sacred word OM."[57] OM is here referred as to the primal sound that *is* the world: the "seed from which the mantras sprout is the same as the one from which Lord Brahma [who is God] grew."[58] This conforms to the title of Berendt's book, *The World Is Sound: Nada Brahma*. 'Nada' is the Sanskrit word for 'sound,' and *Brahma* is one of the names and forms of the divine, which means 'the universe' or 'the cosmos.' In other words, in yogic philosophy, the cosmos *is* sound or vibration. This is not as novel an idea as it might seem; modern science has been teaching us that the entire universe, from the planets to the atomic structure of chemicals, functions according to recognizable rhythmic and harmonic patterns that are remarkably similar. "It has been said since ancient times that the nature of reality is much closer to music than to a machine, and this is confirmed by many discoveries in modern science."[59] We saw that Plato described the harmony of the heavens in terms of the musical scale, as did Pythagoras before him and Johannes Kepler much later in the seventeenth century.

Cosmic Sound

That the world is vibration is now accepted as scientific fact. But it is more than that: it is harmonic vibration. As Berendt writes:

> From the standpoint of physics, there are billions of different possible vibrations. But the cosmos—the universe—chooses from these billions of possibilities with overwhelming preference for those few thousand vibrations that make harmonic sense.[60]

This can be observed from the smallest things in the universe to the largest—from atoms to planets. Experiments have been done for many years, now, on the musical preferences of plants and how they will shy away (or even shrivel up) with certain music while they move toward other music and thrive when it is played. But photo-acoustic spectroscopy has allowed researchers actually to hear, for example, the sound that a rose makes as it bursts into bloom—an organ-like sound that resembles a Bach toccata! Hans Kayser, a twentieth-century scientist and specialist in Pythagorean harmony, translated the sound of certain rock crystals into musical notation that can be played on a keyboard. The sounds are individual—garnet, for example, being quite different from topaz—but the result is often what Kayser called "utterly magnificent sequences of notes."[61]

While modern interpreters have not seriously considered ancient depictions of the harmony of the spheres as a description of reality, Berendt reports that, in the mid-twentieth century, two Yale University scholars demonstrated that it might be so. They programmed the angular velocities of the planets into a synthesizer and then made a recording of the results—which corresponded to the musical ideas attributed to the planets by astronomers such as Kepler. Berendt makes specific reference to one "moving" piece called "Duo in the minor mode danced by Earth and Venus," in which Venus "dances around" E sharp while Earth "dallies" between two G sharps.[62] Moving to the infinitely microcosmic level, atoms have been shown to exhibit harmonic proportions; for example, the carbon atom produces the tone scale C-D-E-F-G-A, a Gregorian chant scale.[63] The harmonic relations of the universe—from atoms to the periodic table of chemical elements to DNA to plants, animals and planets—are becoming serious subjects for study, and some of the ideas of the ancients are being brought back to life.[64] With all of the harmonic vibrations that are around us, one can easily see that hooking into them in order to blend harmonically with the universe is not necessarily just a "New Age" notion.

Chanting Mantra

For a *yogi*, chanting a mantra differs from the Western notion of prayer, the latter being supplications that evoke thoughts and concepts. Reciting or chanting a mantra is not linguistic in the sense of encompassing ideas or cognitive meaning; it expresses feelings rather than ideas; it is more about tuning oneself to the vibrations of the world than about asking for favours or help (although it is said that being 'tuned' or in harmony may help to bring about the things that one needs or wants). As Radha explains it:

> The chanting or recitation of Mantras activates and accelerates the creative spiritual force, promoting harmony in all parts of the human being. The devotee is gradually converted into a living center of spiritual vibration which is attuned to some other center of vibration vastly more powerful. This energy can be appropriated and directed for the benefit of the one who uses it and for that of others.[65]

However, unlike prayer, mantra is not *necessarily* a spiritual or holy activity: "Mantra is a power which lends itself impartially to any use."[66] It is generally believed that mantra can be used to kill or injure, as well as to reach spiritual and meditative heights.[67] It is an energy or power that is, in itself, neutral.

In the Christian New Testament, the Gospel of John opens with the words, "In the beginning was the Word, and the Word was with God, and the Word was God."[68] Similar words are found in the *Vedas*: "In the beginning was Brahman; with whom was Vak or the Word; and the word is Brahman."[69] In Christianity, Jesus is seen as the Word incarnate, the Word made flesh. In Hinduism, the Word is incarnated in every being—all beings and things. As John Woodroffe explains,

> The Word as Vak became flesh, not on one particular date in one particular place and in one particular historic person. It appeared and now appears in the flesh and other forms of matter of all limited beings.... Vak manifests Herself in every man and is knowable and known as She is in Herself....[70]

In yogic terms, the Word (*Vak*) is sound, cosmic sound; this cosmic sound is part of each and every one of us, and, according to yoga practitioners, we can learn to resonate with it and live in harmony with it. Mantra is a practice designed to develop and cultivate this harmony. Chanting mantra aloud "calms the senses which are fully engaged outside enjoying external objects, and leads the mind to its true nature, consciousness-in-itself."[71]

Mantras are linked to *rishis*, or ancient seers, to whom the mantras are said to have been divinely revealed, and from whom they were passed down through the centuries from guru to disciple.[72] The transmission of mantras and their "repetition billions of times by countless devotees over the centuries has brought about a vast reservoir of power which augments the inherent spiritual potency of the Mantras."[73] Each mantra has a *raga* or particular melody attached to it, which is considered an integral part of the mantra. Ideally, the key of the melody should not be changed, since the rate of vibration is intimately tied to the effectiveness of the mantra. The same rigour is attached to the pronunciation of the words.[74] Ultimately, however, the effectiveness of mantra may simply depend on the spiritual attitude of the chanter: "The *sabda* or sound of the mantra is not a physical sound (though it may be accompanied by such a one) but a spiritual one. It cannot be heard by the ears but only by the heart, and it cannot be uttered by the mouth but only by the mind."[75]

Mantras are also linked to a name or form of the divine (e.g., Krishna, Siva, Tara). This is the *Devata*, or presiding deity, the source from which the power of the mantra is presumed to derive. This can serve the purpose of allowing the chanter to feel a personal connection with the divine. But another way of seeing this is to think of the *Devata* as "one facet of a diamond representing Cosmic Intelligence. A diamond with many facets will reflect many rays of Light at the same time, but one particular ray will especially appeal to the individual as he or she begins travelling the spiritual road."[76] As was pointed out earlier, it is difficult to feel love for, or connection with, a principle; similarly, it is difficult to chant to the cosmic intelligence itself. It is believed that a personal relationship with Krishna, for example, can serve the aspirant until he or she has reached a point of being able to relate to the divine energy itself—as in the eighth limb of yoga, *Samadhi*.

Most Westerners (as well many people of the East) believe that chanting mantra is simply muttering gibberish. At the same time, Indian religion and philosophy are replete with lengthy treatises on sound, on the levels of sound that precede the actual utterance of human sound, and on the relationship of these primal sounds with cosmic energy and the origins of the universe. One can ask why the Indian sages would spend so much time investigating human and cosmic vibrations if they found nothing meaningful in the exercise. Or why they would chant mantra for centuries, even millennia, if they did not find in it some power or effect.[77] Woodroffe suggests that Westerners do not necessarily have to accept the Indian practices relating to mantra, "but they should at least first understand what they condemn as worthless."[78] Perhaps the sages of the East knew (and know) something that we don't (or have forgotten). We can, however, suspend disbelief for a moment and ask: Assuming that mantra does work in some fashion (since people persist in doing it), *how* might it work? For Berendt and other writers on the subject, the explanation is very simple:

> Mantras consist of vibrations. Our nerves, our ganglia, and our cells also vibrate. The law of resonance teaches us: Anything that vibrates reacts to vibrations, even (as recent discoveries have shown) to the most minute vibrations, and to those that only a few years ago could not be measured— brainwaves, for instance—and hence logically also to vibrations that have yet to become measurable.[79]

We all know that sound is vibration—that our vocal cords vibrate and that sound is produced from that vibration. But the vibration is not only in the vocal cords; vibration moves through our entire body, right down to our cells. If we understand that, then we can also understand "that sound is 'heard' not only through our ears but through every cell in our body."[80] There is a well-known phenomenon called 'entrainment,' whereby the vibrations of one object can cause the vibration of another object that has a similar frequency. The two objects vibrate in resonance. Thus can sound resonate both through the body and outside of the body. The *yogis* believe that even our thoughts are vibrations, which is why yoga places so much emphasis on the proper use of language (both spoken and unspoken). In yoga philosophy, the vibrations of our words can have a great impact, which is why the vibrations of mantra are considered to be so special: they are sounds that have been cultivated and repeated to have maximum resonance in the universe of sound and vibration. We may not understand exactly *how* it works, but the *yogis* claim to know *that* it works.

How does ultrasound work? Do the millions of pregnant women who rely on it for a picture of the health of the fetus they are carrying really know how or why it works? It has become a standard medical practice that they find useful, and therefore they use it. One medical doctor who uses sound in healing points out that "the same properties of sound that enable it to penetrate the body and produce legible images of hearts, bladders, and fetuses offer hints about how vibratory waves of sound might also be used as tools of healing."[81] If the vibrations of the heart can be measured, why not the vibrations of the voice itself? Sound is vibration, and it has many names and forms. Mantra is a way of connecting vibrations.[82]

Yoga and Philosophy

The above explanations of yoga are, for the most part, based on the testimonies and experiences of yoga practitioners and, in some cases, ancient texts; in addition, the descriptions of hatha yoga, the hidden language of hatha yoga, and mantra, in particular, have been coloured by my own experience in this domain, mainly at the Yasodhara Ashram in BC, and with the teachings of Swami Radha. This is a philosophy book and most of the previous chapters have followed the thinking of philosophers, past and present. How do the philosophy and practice of yoga measure up within a philosophical framework?

Yuasa Yasuo points to a very important difference between Eastern and Western philosophy, one that can be a barrier to acceptance of Eastern ideas in the West. Philosophical knowledge in the East is not abstract or merely intellectual; it is experiential and even assumes some practical knowledge on the part of the reader that will aid in his or her understanding:

> The books on self-cultivation methods in Buddhism and Daoism [as well as Yoga] are not designed to give intellectual proofs or ratiocinations. Rather, they are guidebooks for attaining practical experience. The books dealing with theoretical doctrines are written by pre-supposing practical experience.... In the case of Eastern philosophy, it is important to acquire practical experience rather than an intellectual proof.[83]

Western philosophy was not always so biased in favour of intellectual proofs and ratiocinations, and prior to the seventeenth century many thinkers wrote about concrete experience, as shown in the discussion of Montaigne in Chapter 4. During the Renaissance, there was room for both abstract thought and concrete experience; and philosophers such as Montaigne had "respect for the rational possibilities of human experience."[84] The historical shift from practical philosophy to purely theoretical philosophy that had its beginnings with Descartes' *Discourse on Method* has not brought the world closer to understanding human experience. One very strong reason for this is the fact that theoretical philosophy is divorced from the body and its activities. Because of its abstract and general nature, it is devoid of context. But embodiment is, by its very nature, steeped in context. And the practices of yoga are embodied practices, carried out by individual people in concrete situations. So, the results of these efforts at individual self-transformation will elude scientific and philosophical explanations as long as scientists and philosophers cling to their current methods. "Yoga requires empathy to be commented on satisfactorily. Scholastic aloofness from the subject, much prized in many fields, is not a proper attitude for its study."[85]

Yoga's goal of self-cultivation or self-transformation is, in itself, problematic for modern Western philosophy, since these terms are neither objective nor quantifiable and would be considered value-laden. Questions about what is good or what constitutes a good or fulfilled life, for example, are avoided in modern philosophy, because, ultimately, they require assumptions about the purpose of life that would be seen as teleological. The top branch of the yoga tree, *Samadhi*, the union of the Self with the Universal Spirit (or God) is teleological, and the roots and trunk, represented by the *yamas* and *niyamas*, form an ethical system that is value-laden at its core. Aristotle might be comfortable with the tree of yoga, but modern philosophers would shy away from it or confine it to philosophy of religion or comparative philosophy, where it could be studied objectively without regard to its experiential nature.

On the other hand, we can ask if philosophy would not be better served if it re-examined its avoidance of questions of self-cultivation and self-fulfilment. We can also ask how much that avoidance is related to the general neglect of the body in philosophical discourse, as well as an overemphasis on reasoning and the mind. Shusterman recommends that "we put aside philosophical prejudice against the body and instead simply recall philosophy's central aims of knowledge, self-knowledge, right action, happiness, and justice...."[86] If we look at these aims from the point of view of yoga, we will see that the attention to body awareness is useful in the pursuit of them all.

We have seen that, in the Stoics and Spinoza, both knowledge and self-knowledge ultimately come from the body. The practices of yoga fit readily with these holistic visions of human nature and human knowledge. In the metaphysics of Spinoza and the Stoics we can see the possibility of a meeting of Eastern and Western philosophies and, perhaps, a road to greater acceptance of the former by the latter. It was pointed out in Chapter 6 that Spinoza's philosophy offers a corrective to the many dichotomies of modernity. Yoga offers a similar corrective, working as it does to link mind and body, head and heart, individual and cosmos, self and community. As such, it can be seen as providing a link back to Spinoza—and the Stoics.

Concerning the aim of right action, Shusterman points out that right action requires not only self-knowledge but effective will. However, "[b]ecause action is only achieved through the body, our power of volition—the ability to act as we will to act—depends on somatic efficacy."[87] In other words, we cannot exercise our power of volition unless we have an efficiently functioning body. But many people's bodies do not function efficiently, and they are unable to perform even simple tasks—often, Shusterman suggests, being quite unaware of their lack. The Greeks would understand the value of somatic efficacy, since they valued good health as a virtue and, as we saw with Plato, advised that intellectual activity be balanced with physical activity so as to achieve the goal of a sound mind in a sound body. In the final analysis, this is the basis of the self-cultivation and self-transformation that the yoga practitioner seeks, and this is not a goal that is foreign to Western philosophy in its ancient and more holistic forms.

At the same time, Eastern philosophy has one basic assumption that is not shared by modern Western philosophy: mind and body cannot be described in material and mechanistic terms. Concepts such as *ki*, *chi* or *prana* are essential to Eastern explanations of the body because they help to bridge the world of mind and body; they are psycho-physiological concepts that Yuasa and others believe can dissolve the conceptual and methodological difficulties of the mind-body split. The Western thinker, however, is going to ask for proof of their existence, something that is very difficult to provide, at least at this point.[88] This will likely remain a point of divergence for some time to come. But if Western thinkers stop and examine what is being said and written about the disappearing body in various disciplines, they may come to see the extremes to which the mechanistic view of the body has taken us and the need for a new paradigm of body and nature. The body wisdom of yoga can lead the way.

Notes

1. Evidence of yoga practice has been found in archaeological excavations. Depictions of men in the lotus position or in meditation have been estimated to date back to the third millennium BCE. See Vivian Worthington, *A History of Yoga* (London: Routledge & Kegan Paul, 1982), 9.

2. Georg Feuerstein, *The Deeper Dimensions of Yoga* (Boston and London: Shambhala Publications, 2003), 11.

3. A *yogi* is a male practitioner, and a *yogini* a female practitioner, of yoga.

4.   Feuerstein, 3. Some writers on yoga attempt to avoid the term 'ego' because of
     Westerners' understanding of Freud's use of the term. Stone, for example, uses
     the term "I-maker," meaning a "mechanism in the mind that creates a story
     of self," and that is, in yogic theory, an impediment to happiness. In fact, it
     is the cause of suffering—what Stone refers to as an extension of Freud's idea
     of narcissism. "It's not so much that we have fallen for our image of ourselves;
     rather we are constantly overlaying each moment with a story of self, preventing
     a direct experience of reality, creating a case of mistaken identity!" It is this sense
     of self that the practice of yoga works to transcend. See Michael Stone, *The Inner
     Tradition of Yoga* (Boston and London: Shambhala Publications, 2008), 68.

5.   Worthington, 5.

6.   See Worthington, 136ff. for a discussion of the connection between yoga and
     Sufism, which, he tells us, represents the first movement of yoga westward in
     the seventh and eighth centuries CE. See also Craig Davis, "The Yogic Exercises
     of the 17th Century Sufis," in *Theory and Practice of Yoga: Essays in Honour of
     Gerald James Larson*, ed. Knut A. Jacobsen (Dehli: Motilal Banarsidass, 2008).
     Davis analyzes an essay by a seventeenth-century Sufi scholar and prince that
     describes yogic practices that the prince traced back to the prophet Muhammad.

7.   Jacobsen, 7.

8.   Elizabeth De Michelis, *A History of Modern Yoga: Patanjali and Western Esotericism*
     (London and New York: Continuum, 2004), 183.

9.   Worthington, 145. Worthington also points out that Western systems of thought,
     such as Scientific Humanism and Marxism, which are agnostic or even atheistic,
     became popular in India in the twentieth century. "Yoga is practised just as
     assiduously as by followers of the theistic Vedanta." The question of whether
     there is a God is "irrelevant to the mainstream of yoga practice" (70–71).

10. One woman who attended the event said later that, when Vivekananda "got up
     and said 'Sisters and Brothers of America,' seven thousand people rose to their
     feet as a tribute to something, they knew not what; and when it was over, and
     I saw scores of women walking over the benches to get near him, I said to myself,
     'Well, my lad, if you can resist that onslaught, you are indeed a god.'" Quoted
     in Swami Vivekananda, *Vedanta: Voice of Freedom* (St. Louis: Vedanta Society of
     St. Louis, 1990), 32.

11. Ramakrishna (1836–1886) was a yogic holy man who, though illiterate, not only
     studied yoga (and reportedly spent much of his life in a trance), but seriously
     studied both Islam and Christianity in his efforts to understand the unity of all
     religions. His work was carried on after his death by the Ramakrishna Mission,
     which now has centres all over the world.

12. Swami Vivekananda, *Raja-Yoga* (New York: Ramakrishna-Vivekananda Center,
     1956, 1982), 9.

13.   Vivekananda, *Vedanta*, 25. Carl Jung referred to religion in the East as "cognitive religion" or "religious cognition," and believed that the fact that Eastern religions were not based on faith explained why there was no conflict between religion and science in the East. See Yuasa, 98.

14.   What is referred to as Western esotericism has its roots in antiquity but flourished in the Renaissance, especially with the work of Ficino (see Chapter 4). These esoteric currents (which emphasize, among other characteristics, a living universe and a cosmic hierarchy) also flourished in nineteenth-century America and, according to De Michelis, "contributed to the formation of Neo-Vedantic esotericism, and thus of Modern Yoga" (20). See pages 21ff. for her detailed discussion of the characteristics of Western esotericism. See also Wade Dazey, "Yoga in America: Some Reflections from the Heartland," in Jacobsen, 423, who states that yoga "has resonated with psychological and philosophical tendencies already present in American culture from as early as 1800 and manifested in such religious movements as the Second Great Awakening, Transcendentalism, Mormonism, Christian Science, and Vedanta. Yoga has from the time of its introduction appealed to Americans on many levels: philosophical, spiritual, psychological, and physical."

15.   De Michelis states that the publication of Vivekananda's *Raja-Yoga*, setting out what she refers to as his secularized and rationalistic science of yoga, "immediately started something of a 'yoga renaissance' both in India and in the West." Although not much research has been done on what she calls Modern Yoga, in her view, most discussions "agree that Vivekananda had a pervasive influence on its development" (182).

16.   Worthington, 141.

17.   Most of the Sivananda centres and *ashrams* were established by Sivananda's disciple, Swami Devananda. One of the most important *ashrams* is situated in Val Morin, Québec. Swami Radha established only one *ashram*, the Yasodhara *ashram* in Kootenay Bay, British Columbia, although there are Radha centres in a number of Canadian cities.

18.   Yoga practices are passed down from guru to disciple through what are called lineages. The existence of a lineage in any particular type of yoga is somewhat of a guarantee of the authenticity of the teachings and the practices—that they have been transmitted from teacher to teacher and maintain the original power and intent of the founding guru.

19.   There are different schools of yoga philosophy, some based on a dualist metaphysics and others on a non-dualist or monist metaphysics. Even the non-dualist schools are not necessarily in agreement on their specific interpretation of metaphysical unity. The metaphysical position outlined here, Advaita Vedanta, holds that there is only one Reality (*Brahman*), that there is no

separation between humans and the Divine; everything is interconnected. Vedanta is often opposed to another school, Samkhya, which holds a dualistic metaphysics.

20. Vivekananda, *Vedanta*, 65. This is very reminiscent of Spinoza's one substance, which is God or Nature.

21. Vivekananda, *Raja-Yoga*, 4.

22. Pronounced *Shiva* and *Shakti*.

23. Swami Sivananda Radha, *Light &Vibration: Consciousness, Mysticism & the Culmination of Yoga* (Kootenay Bay, BC and Spokane, WA: Timeless Books, 2007), 35.

24. Radha, *Light & Vibration*, 34.

25. Saraswati is the goddess of knowledge, speech, music and the arts. She is also considered to be the consort of Brahma.

26. Stone's book, for example, is a very detailed discourse on yoga, which strongly emphasizes the moral and spiritual dimension, and contains hardly a reference to gods or goddesses and only one reference to *Siva* and *Sakti* as male energy and female energy respectively.

27. The ambiguity of the language of self-realization in contemporary yoga practice leaves it open to criticism from academic commentators and others who tend to see it as a New Age or counterculture phenomenon. The ambiguity of terms such as 'self' and 'God' leaves the relationship between 'self' and 'God' ambiguous, as well. "And if such relation is *not* defined, or defined in contradictory ways within the same text … the readers will be free to interpret it according to their inclinations…" (De Michelis, 224). However, given the experiential nature of yoga, practitioners are bound to interpret their relation to the divine (whatever it is called and whether they think of it as divine or not) according to their own experience. Many advanced *yogis* (as well as religious mystics) have, of course, had mystical experiences and do know (from their own experience) what these terms mean. For them, the terms are not ambiguous, or, more to the point, they lose their normally understood meaning.

28. It is not certain when Patanjali lived, or even whether he was actually the author of all of the two hundred aphorisms, or whether there were different authors all using the same name. He is thought to have lived around 150 CE, but this is debated.

29. De Michelis avoids the terminological confusion by referring to the practice of *asanas* as Modern Postural Yoga, or MPY. This is not, however, a common reference in the yoga literature and also neglects the fact that hatha yoga as it is practised today often includes aspects of the other eight limbs, such as *pranayama*, concentration or meditation, and also mantra. Yet another level of terminological confusion is evident when the term hatha yoga is used to name just one particular

approach to the *asanas*—or postural yoga, the most traditional or classic. Newer approaches include, just to name a few, Ashtanga yoga (in which the poses are performed in a more energetic fashion, linking one pose to another, always in the same order); Bikram yoga (which is like Ashtanga yoga, but is performed in a very hot room with participants working up a sweat); and Vinyasa or Flow yoga, also emphasizing linked poses, with an emphasis on moving in and out of poses on the breath). All types of yoga will usually include a certain amount of breath work and often some chanting. All of these use the basic hatha yoga postures in different ways.

30. Stone, 45.

31. Sri Swami Satchidananda, *Integral Yoga: The Yoga Sutras of Patanjali* (Yogaville, VA: Integral Yoga Publications, [1985], 2007), 48.

32. B. K. S. Iyengar, *Yoga Vrksa: The Tree of Yoga* (Oxford: Fine Line Books, 1988), 64.

33. Iyengar, 8.

34. Iyengar describes the eight limbs of yoga by using an analogy of the tree: the roots are the *yamas*; the trunk represents the *niyamas*. The *asanas*, or postures, form the branches of the tree. The leaves of the tree are *pranayama*, the bark is *pratyahara*, the sap—which reaches from leaf to root—is *dhyana*, and the essence or fruit of the tree is *Samadhi*, or bliss. Thus, it can be seen that the practice of *asanas* is a small part of classical yoga; it is, however, a prerequisite to concentration, meditation and, ultimately, bliss (Iyengar, 7–8).

35. Stone, 92.

36. Stone, 104.

37. Stone, 104.

38. Stone, 97.

39. Stone, 97.

40. Stone, 111.

41. Shusterman, xii.

42. Shusterman's own experience is with the Feldendrais Method, "a form of somatic education for improved self-awareness and self-use," rather than hatha yoga, but he also acknowledges his debt to yoga and several other disciplines (e.g., t'ai chi) "that promote heightened somatic consciousness and body-mind attunement." Disciplines of the East such as yoga also recognize "somatic training as an essential means toward philosophical enlightenment and virtue" (Shusterman, 7, 17).

43. Kyeongra Yang, "A Review of Yoga Programs for Four Leading Risk Factors of Chronic Diseases," *eCAM*, 4: 4 (2007). (Note: 'CAM' is an acronym for Complementary and Alternative Medicine).

44.   Swami Sivananda Radha, *Hatha Yoga: The Hidden Language* (Spokane, WA and Kootenay Bay, BC: Timeless Books, 2007), 25.

45.   Radha, *Hidden Language*, 32.

46.   Radha, *Hidden Language*, 100.

47.   Swami Lalitananda, *The Inner Life of Asanas* (Spokane, WA and Kootenay Bay, BC: Timeless Books: 2007), 12.

48.   Lalitananda, 14.

49.   Richard Rosen, *The Yoga of Breath: A Step-by-Step Guide to Pranayama* (Boston and London: Shambhala Publications, 2002), 22.

50.   Stone, 116.

51.   Rosen, 18 (emphasis added).

52.   Vivekananda, *Raja-Yoga*, 35. Compare this to the following statement from Irwin, quoted in Chapter 2, regarding *pneuma*: "The *pneuma* explains the cohesion of the particles in a rock, and, at a more complex level, the growth of a plant, the behaviour of an animal, and the rational action of a human being; soul and reason are simply particular manifestations of *pneuma*."

53.   Satchidananda, 50.

54.   Vivekananda, *Raja-Yoga*, 180.

55.   Rosen, 133.

56.   Rosen, 266.

57.   Joachim-Ernst Berendt, *The World Is Sound: Nada Brahma: Music and the Landscape of Consciousness* (Rochester, VT: Destiny Books, 1983), 28.

58.   Berendt, 27.

59.   Berendt, 11. This quote is from the foreword by Fritjof Capra.

60.   Berendt, 90.

61.   Quoted in Berendt, 86.

62.   Berendt, 66. He comments further that "Mars slides up and down across several notes. Jupiter has a majestic tone reminiscent of a church organ, and Saturn produces a low, mysterious droning."

63.   Berendt, 69. In addition, "depending on the saturation state of the atom, all three Gregorian hexachords exist in carbon."

64.   See in particular reports of the work of Barbara Hero, who invented a Lambdoma Keyboard based on what is known as the Lambdoma Matrix of Pythagoras, a keyboard that translates Pythagoras' ratios into musical notes. Hero uses the keyboard as a therapeutic tool, but she refers to others who are using it, for example, to communicate with dolphins or to help the lettuce grow and the compost pile to mature faster. See http://www.lambdoma.com/.

65.   Swami Sivananda Radha, *Mantras: Words of Power* (Spokane, WA and Kootenay Bay, BC: Timeless Books, 1994), 2.

66.   Arthur Avalon (Sir John Woodroffe), *The Serpent Power: The Secrets of Tantric and Shaktic Yoga* (New York: Dover Publications, 1974), 83.

67.   Alper reports on the disclaimer included at the beginning of an Indian publication, the translation of a sixteenth-century treatise on mantra, which stated, in part: "If any person on the basis of the Yantras [mantras] as provided in this book commits any nefarious act which causes loss, etc., to anybody, then for his actions the authors/editors/translators, printer and publisher will not be responsible in any way whatsoever." Harvey P. Alper, ed., *Understanding Mantras* (Albany: SUNY Press, 1989), 1.

68.   New American Bible.

69.   See Sir John Woodroffe, *Garland of Letters: Studies in the Mantra-Sastra* (Madras: Ganesh & Co., 2004), 4.

70.   Woodroffe, *Garland*, 5. Remember that the world is feminine in Hindu (and yogic) philosophy.

71.   Sthaneshwar Timalsina, "Meditating Mantras: Meaning and Visualization in Tantric Literature," in Jacobsen, 216.

72.   "In the original Sanskrit tradition, the mantras have been handed down for nearly five thousand years orally, without the slightest change of annotation in a single vowel. Thus the effectiveness of the mantras as sound vibrations is maintained." Pandit Usharbudh Arya, *Mantra & Meditation* (Honesdale, PA: Himalayan International Institute of Yoga Science & Philosophy of the U.S.A., 1981), 126. (A sceptic might ask how we know that not a vowel has been changed after 5,000 years!) Woodroffe reports that, in mantra initiation (the transference of a mantra—and its power—from guru to disciple), it can happen that the disciple "swoons under the impulse of it...." Woodroffe, *Serpent Power*, 84.

73.   Radha, *Mantras*, 2.

74.   Both of these criteria for mantra recitation or singing would appear to be exaggerated, since, as Alper points out in relation to pronunciation, "The Vedic ideal notwithstanding, there is no single absolutely correct way to pronounce Sanskrit, as regional variations in pronunciation, not to mention the migration of mantras from India to Central Asia and East Asia, abundantly prove" (443). This is even before taking into consideration the lack of knowledge of Sanskrit by most English speakers who are reciting or chanting mantra. Further, the same mantra might be chanted to a different melody, depending on the *ashram* visited and the lineage practising it.

75.   Alper, 443. Alper is here quoting Lama Anagarika Govinda from his book *Foundations of Tibetan Mysticism, According to the Esoteric Teachings of the Great Mantra* (London: Rider and Co., 1959), 27.

76.   Radha, *Mantras*, 4.

77.   Berendt points out that the Tibetans, who are a very practical people and have survived for centuries in a harsh climate, would hardly recite mantras to the extent they do, "had they not tested and experienced again and again the power of such syllables and sounds in themselves" (41).

78.   Woodroffe, *Garland*, ix.

79.   Berendt, 40.

80.   Mitchell L. Gaynor, *The Healing Power of Sound: Recovery from Life-Threatening Illness Using Sound, Voice, and Music* (Boston and London: Shambhala Books, 2002), 17.

81.   Gaynor, 51.

82.   The use of sound in healing will be discussed in more detail in the following chapter on holistic medicine. Gaynor points out that high-tech medicine has a "blinkered concept of the human body-mind," which prevents it from seriously exploring the healing power of sound. This blinkered concept of the mind and body will also be discussed at length in the following chapter.

83.   Yuasa, 98.

84.   Toulmin, 27.

85.   Worthington, 4. At the same time, it can be said that insistence on experience in yoga causes some practitioners and commentators to look on academic analyses of their practice with disdain. See De Michelis, 7, concerning the need to redress the imbalance on both sides.

86.   Shusterman, 19.

87.   Shusterman, 20.

88.   Yuasa shows how acupuncture meridians—the passages along which *ki* travels—can be shown to exist, not in substance but in function (experiments have shown a galvanic skin response at acupuncture points, but no nerve or other connections between the points), something he describes as being "like hearing a voice without seeing the person producing it" (116). Kirlian photography shows that stimulation of certain points results in luminescence showing up at others, but does not demonstrate the actual existence of the channel itself. It would seem that the technology for proving the existence of meridians is getting closer, but is not there yet. For those who have been successfully treated with acupuncture, however, proof of the existence of the meridians is not necessary.

CHAPTER IX

RECOVERING THE BODY: ALTERNATIVE MEDICINE

So far in this narrative, we have been following the metaphysical threads of holism and dualism and examining how they relate to Western concepts of the body; in the last chapter we looked at competing Eastern and Western paradigms through our discussion of yoga. We have seen that the dominant contemporary Western view of the body is rooted in dualism and mechanism, and, since the scientific revolution, treats the body as an object of knowledge (particularly medical knowledge). The Eastern approach to the body is much older and, in spite of competition from Western, technology-based medicine, is enjoying a renaissance in the East and a transposition to the West. It is perhaps appropriate to ask what Western medicine might learn if it looked back at some of the holistic conceptions of the body that were discarded *in toto* in the seventeenth century.

In the West, so much priority has, over the centuries, been given to the rational mind that we have even arrived at a point where it makes perfect sense in some circles to refer to the body as obsolete and to envision the 'human' of the future as a post-biological combination of mind and machine. Mind, consciousness, self—whatever we call the supposedly non-material part of ourselves—is perceived as being so different from the body in this scenario that it can be detached from it and downloaded into a machine. A less fantastic example, as we have seen, is brain death; there is little resistance in the general public to the idea that a person whose brain has ceased to function is dead and can be harvested for organs—even if he or she is being 'kept alive' on a ventilator.

The chapter on yoga has shown that these ways of conceptualizing the body are foreign to Eastern philosophy,[1] where holistic views of the body predominate and where the body is clearly seen not only as a source of knowledge about the self but also as a means to self-cultivation. This chapter will carry these ideas further, into the domain of medicine. Some of the discussion in this chapter will touch on Eastern approaches to medicine, but it will also be shown that many of the so-called New Age and 'alternative' views of health and healing are rooted in our very own Western tradition. Homeopathy, for example, is based on ideas of Hippocrates, and originated in the West.

While Western science and medicine have given us much biological and physiological information about the body, there remains one simple fact that Western philosophy and science have yet to deal with adequately: nobody knows exactly what the mind is. If this is the case, then the logical conclusion is that nobody knows exactly what the body is. We make assumptions about the mind and body, and we freely use terminology such as 'outer world' and 'inner world' to explain facts relating to a body that interacts with its environment (in objective and observable ways) and a mind that cogitates and reflects on itself (in subjective and non-observable ways). Given that the objective and observable predominates in the Western scientific attitude, "modern theory has altogether excluded the problem of mind from the investigation of body. Taking the body as an objective (material) substance, it has relegated the problem of consciousness to philosophy."[2] To think in terms of 'inner' and 'outer' may be useful as metaphor, but it can lead to strange conclusions if taken as scientific fact. Yuasa Yasuo reminds us, for example, that "it is contrary to common sense to regard one's own body as matter existing outside of oneself" and thus "there is a discrepancy between common sense and scientific knowledge which leaves psychological problems and physiological (and physical) problems totally unrelated ... [which] suggests that the logic of science is divorced from our human life, and proceeds independent of us," a comment that can be extended to the logic of medicine.[3]

This presents us with a methodological difficulty. Health and illness cannot be confined to what we classify as physiological, and yet the methods that we are most dependent upon tend to deal only with physiology, or the material and mechanical aspects of our bodies and our health. The so-called inner and subjective aspects of health and illness are given short shrift, if not discounted entirely, in a medical system governed more and more by technology and objective testing. From an Eastern point of view, however, there is a mediating factor that allows both inner and outer to be taken into consideration in medical diagnosis and healing, and this mediating factor is *ki*,[4] since *ki* affects both mind and body. As a factor in meditation, it can be seen as psychological (although even there it has physiological effects, as well); in yoga (*pranayama* and *asana*) it is both psychological and physiological; and in acupuncture therapy, its effect is physiological. *Ki* circulates internally, but it is also connected to the external world through certain acupuncture points on the skin surface, which allow an exchange of energy with the outer world. For example, the activation of *ki* through meditation can serve to control emotional disturbances; but this can also be accomplished through the insertion of acupuncture needles into the skin. In other words, *ki* is a mediator between the psychological and physiological aspects of the emotions.[5]

Ki plays the role of a 'cosmic connector,' as it mediates internal and external, human and nature, soul and body. As such, it can be seen as a form of *vitalism*, a concept that modern science rejects, but one that is present in most forms of alternative medicine, whether Traditional Chinese Medicine (or TCM— of which acupuncture forms a part), homeopathy, Ayurvedic medicine,[6] or the many forms of energy medicine that have become popular. These systems all perceive the human body as "animated and sustained by a special type of force, energy, or essence which may in turn be connected with a universal cosmic source or reservoir."[7] Whatever this force, energy or essence is cannot, in fact, be explained by science at the present time (although there is much experimentation on the frontiers of science that points to possible answers). The result of this is that, no matter how convincing the empirical evidence of healing with these therapies might be, if the reasons for the success cannot be explained, science will reject the therapy. This fact is clearly admitted by two physicians who are, at the same time, open to homeopathy and working on ways to try to explain it scientifically. In their view, the "scientific validity of a therapeutic method does not depend so much on its success rate as on the fact that the clinical result should be consistent with a pathophysiological, biochemical, and pharmacological theory or rationale."[8] In other words, for a therapeutic system to be considered scientifically valid, it must fit the paradigm of modern medicine, which is based solely on physiological and biochemical premises. The notion of a mental, spiritual or psychological dimension *inherent* in the physiological cannot be accepted. Mechanism is based on purely materialistic principles, and has been since the seventeenth century. Thus, while there are many open-minded participants in the medical system (both as practitioners and teachers) who are promoting *integrative* medicine where allopathic and alternative approaches can come together,[9] their efforts will be incomplete, as long as the biomedical paradigm remains unchanged.

While many argue that alternative medicine is not scientific, others question whether scientific medicine itself is really scientific enough. René Dubos, for example, believes that "the scientific medicine of our time is *not* scientific enough because it neglects, and at times completely ignores, the multifarious environmental and emotional factors that affect the human organism in health and in disease, and to which the organism can consciously respond in an adaptive, creative way."[10] The limits of our medical model can also be seen in the following account of the healer in Native American medicine:

> In the Native American traditions, the notion of healing takes on broader dimensions. Healing occurs on various levels that interact with one another: bodily, emotional, social, and spiritual. The last two levels are especially important. Illness is brought on not only by physical ailments, but also by the quality of one's interrelationships with family, friends, co-workers, and so on. Furthermore, illness is produced by an individual's state of spirituality, not in a church-going sense but in terms of one's relationship with one's own self, or spirit. An imbalance among these various levels acts as a catalyst for the development of symptoms of illness.[11]

The perspective reflected in Native American medicine is shared by most alternative systems. In fact, this perspective forms a core that is missing from conventional or allopathic medicine; all alternative systems "regard the body as inherently healthy in its natural state and endowed with an ecological capacity for self-regulation and balance. All conceive of the physical body as interconnected with other key aspects of persons such as mind, will, spirit, psyche, or emotions, all of which affect and are affected by health and illness."[12] In addition, health, in these systems, is defined not as the absence of disease, but as harmony or balance, both internal and external. In short, they all describe the human body in holistic terms and recognize its fundamental connection with mind, soul, spirit and cosmos. They all reject the concept of the body-machine and its materialistic premises.

Any medical system is based on certain assumptions (explicit or not) about the human body, mind and spirit (and how and if they are related).

These assumptions determine how that medical system judges health and illness, and how and if a diseased body should be treated. We tend to think of our concept of the body—as well as our notions of health and disease—as simple facts of nature, but they are not. As Bonnie O'Connor points out, such conceptions "always reflect broader cultural worldviews, values, and concerns as well as—indeed as part of—their observations of natural facts. This is as true of biomedicine as it is of any other system of health belief, knowledge, and practice."[13] As we have seen, Western medicine is based on assumptions relating to the separation of body and mind (spirit being usually left out of the equation). It is not a brute fact of nature that the body is a machine, or, as it is popular to say today, that the brain is a computer! Nor is it a brute fact of nature that the body is a garden (a metaphor often used in relation to Eastern medicine). These are ways of perceiving the body that tell us more about the perceiver than the perceived, although they can have far-reaching effects on the latter, as a moment's reflection on the words 'machine' and 'garden' will reveal.

In fact, it is not only the science of medicine that reflects cultural worldviews and values. Although not readily admitted by the general public, or even many scientists, science itself is not simply an accumulation of brute facts, nor is it a progression of knowledge moving ever closer to the world *as it is*. It can be said that the philosophical questions regarding the world *as it appears to us* and the world *as it is* that occupied the ancient philosophers (as discussed in Chapter 1) are still with us as philosophers (and scientists) argue about whether scientific theory truly corresponds to reality or whether it is a theoretical construction that explains the world in different ways at different times. Grant Gillett tells us that it "comes as a surprise to many medical scientists that shifts in scientific theory are a pervasive feature of scientific thought," and he quotes a well-known philosopher of science who states that, from the point of view of the search for eternal truth, "scientists (even physical scientists) are a fickle lot. This history of science is a tale of multifarious shiftings of allegiance from theory to theory."[14] This is clearly applicable to medicine, as well. Gillet points out that, when he was in medical school, an answer that was 'wrong' then (regarding the theory of gastric ulcer formation) would be considered 'right' now. What is instructive for him in this realization is that, while this shift came about within the biomedical paradigm, the challenge at the moment is "to explore ways in which non-positivist approaches, such as holistic health care with its focus on the individual rather than statistical generalities, can hope for similar authentication within the methods that define clinical science."[15]

At the present time, we are faced with two competing paradigms in relation to allopathic and alternative medical systems—each with a fundamentally different view of the human body and its relation to mind, soul and cosmos, and each with fundamentally different methods for determining the meaning of illness and the modalities of healing. Some of the assumptions and the limits of biomedicine have been discussed in Chapter 7. In what follows, I will set out three examples of the alternative paradigm, along with the assumptions about the body on which they are based: Traditional Chinese Medicine, homeopathy and healing with sound. While there are considerable differences among these systems, they all share similar assumptions about the human body and its relation to the world, assumptions opposed to those of conventional biomedicine.[16]

Traditional Chinese Medicine

What is referred to as Traditional Chinese Medicine (TCM) has been in existence for several thousand years. Interestingly, although China easily accepted Western medicine in the twentieth century, TCM was not discarded or replaced, principally because of the large population and the impossibility of bringing expensive modern technological medicine to everyone. In fact, China has kept the ancient system and even carried out comparative studies in order to show its efficacy. As a result, TCM is still flourishing in China, where it can be studied at university, including at the MA and PhD levels. It is being taught more and more in the West, as well, and thousands of students are studying it in the United States and Canada.[17] It is a holistic medical system, emphasizing the need to balance the physical, emotional and spiritual aspects of life and the body in order to maintain health and prevent illness. It uses natural and non-invasive techniques and therapies, including acupuncture, herbal medicine and massage. "The human body is conceptualized as a microcosm, linked with, reflecting, and manifesting the same processes as those acting in the physical and social environment and in the cosmos," the latter being understood as a web of interrelated things and events.[18]

The framework of TCM is based on the theory of *yin* and *yang*, described by Ted Kaptchuk as a "dialectical logic that explains relationships, patterns, and change."[19] These terms can be used to describe the characteristics of everything in the cosmos—including the human body. *Yin* and *yang* do not represent opposites, as is often supposed. Nothing is completely *yin* or completely *yang*. Everything is both one and the other (although more of one than the other, depending on the circumstances), and can be transformed from one into the other "as the shady side of the hill in the morning hours becomes the sunny side in late day, and vice-versa."[20] As Kaptchuk explains,

> These complementary opposites are neither forces nor material entities. Nor are they mythical concepts that transcend rationality. Rather they are convenient labels used to describe how things function in relation to each other in the universe. They are used to explain the continuous process of natural change. But Yin and Yang are not only a set of correspondences; they also represent a way of thinking. In this system of thought, all things are seen as parts of a whole. No entity can ever be isolated from its relationship to other entities; no thing can exist in and of itself. There are no absolutes. Yin and Yang must, necessarily, contain within themselves the possibility of opposition and change.[21]

In relation to the dynamics of the body, while *yin* and *yang* are always transforming into each other, a balance is necessary in order for a person to remain healthy. "A deficiency of one aspect implies an excess of the other. Extreme disharmony means that the deficiency of one aspect cannot continue to support the excess of another."[22] Because disharmony shows itself in the pulse, a very subtle and complex system of pulse diagnosis allows the TCM therapist to assess the balance of *yin* and *yang* in the body and determine the proper treatment for rebalancing.[23]

We have already discussed *ki* in the previous chapter in relation to Eastern philosophy and medicine, particularly in Japan. The counterpart of *ki* in China is *qi* (or *chi*). Like *ki*, it is both physiological and psychological; it is often referred to as a type of vital energy that is in everything in the universe. According to Kaptchuk, "Chinese thought does not distinguish between matter and energy, but we can perhaps think of Qi as matter on the verge of becoming energy, or energy at the point of materializing."[24] Further, it is not completely comparable to *ki*, since there are two other elements that share some of the characteristics of the Japanese *ki*: *shen*, which is comparable to the Western idea of spirit or consciousness, and is unique to humans; and *jing*, which is the source of all organic life and "gives rise to processes of organic change such as generativity, growth, development, and decay."[25] These three, along with blood and other body fluids, are the fundamental substances that nourish and sustain the body.

Rooted in the Eastern tradition, TCM sees the body not as a collection of parts but as a holistic system where each part affects every other part. Thus, its diagnoses do not focus on particular parts of the body, but on processes relating to the body fluids, organs and patterns of energy flows.[26] Yuasa explains that this can be understood in terms of the holographic model, which holds that each part contains information about the whole. "In short," he tells us, "the theory of the body held by Eastern medicine attempts to grasp the whole of the bodily functions from a holographic viewpoint, which is in principle different from the theory of the body held by modern medicine where the whole is constructed by gathering the sum of its parts."[27]

Of the elements mentioned above, the most important is *qi*, the vital energy that flows through the meridians. The meridians, as O'Connor tells us,

> are understood to be actual physical channels of conductivity. The fact that they have no corresponding anatomical structures and cannot be located on dissection is a non-issue in the Chinese framework, focused as it is on function and relationality, rather than structure, as the crucial aspects of anatomy and physiology. The system of meridians interconnects and unifies all parts of the body, providing the pathways through which the harmonious balance of health is maintained or regained.[28]

Although the meridians cannot be located upon dissection, some of the energy travelling through them has been captured (at certain acupuncture points) by Kirlian photography, as pointed out in the previous chapter.

Depending on the diagnosis and the imbalance detected, the insertion of acupuncture needles at certain specified points will help to correct the flow of *qi*. There are twelve major meridians and 350 points distributed along them. The meridians are divided into *yin* and *yang* groups and are generally named after solid organs or viscera—for example, the 'kidney meridian' or the 'lung meridian.' "Although some of these names correspond to the names of viscera given by Western medicine, these organs may be thought of as a functional unit working in connection with the twelve major meridians."[29] This point is extremely important, reflecting the integrative and holographic model of the body noted above. It is not the kidneys as such that are the object of diagnosis and treatment; it is the flow of *qi* through the kidney meridian and the resulting impact of any disturbance in that meridian on other meridians (and thus other organ systems). In effect, in this theory of the body, "all the physiological functions of the viscera are resolved into functions of the meridians on the surface of the body. They are arranged as an integrative system ... [or] 'viscera-meridian system'—a circulatory system of *ki*-energy."[30]

Here we come up against a major difference between the two systems. Based on its conceptualization of the body, Western medicine must find ways of investigating the state of the organs *within* the body, while Eastern medicine focuses on the *surface* of the body, where most of the meridians are found and where the acupuncture points are located. There is less focus on the body's interior (something Yuasa admits can be seen as a shortcoming) in what is really a "medicine of the somatic surface."[31] Eastern medicine sees the skin as a boundary between the interior world and the external world, the location of relation that allows an exchange of energy between the two. Yuasa underlines this important distinction between East and West:

> Modern medicine has first separated the body from the external world, taking it as a closed, self-contained system, and then by dissecting its structure into various organs has attempted to understand their respective functions. In contrast, Eastern medicine has from the outset understood the body as an open system connected to the external world. In so doing it has conceived that, although undetectable by sensory perception, there is an exchange of life-energy of some sort between the body and the external world, that is, there is an absorption and release of *ki* between them. Here we see a view of the human being as a microcosm corresponding to the universe as a macrocosm, and of the human body as a vessel for the flow of *ki* in the universe.[32]

This view of the body is reminiscent of that of the Stoics and their *pneuma*, as well as that of Ficino and his medical spirits, since both of these systems rely on an explanatory framework of macrocosm-microcosm and an exchange of life-energy between the two. Reading Yuasa in light of the Stoics and Ficino underscores the possibility that important aspects of the body and its relation to the external world have been lost to Western medicine, and that something might be gained by looking back at our own Western holistic concepts.

Homeopathy

Looking back at ancient holistic conceptions of the body is exactly what Samuel Hahnemann did in Germany in the late eighteenth century. Hahnemann was a physician, but he was also a linguist (he spoke about ten languages) and a competent chemist. He practised medicine for a short time, but gave it up, convinced that the medicine of his day was causing more harm than good. He became a translator of scientific and medical texts, and then a writer of his own treatises on medicine, including his work on homeopathy. In one of these, "Essay on a New Principle for Ascertaining the Curative Power of Drugs (with a Few Glances at Those Hitherto Employed)," he describes the three ways that medicine can relieve illness. The first and most elevated is to remove or destroy the fundamental cause of disease. But since no one had succeeded in uncovering the knowledge of the fundamental causes of disease, this method had not worked. The second method is to seek to remove the symptoms through medicines that produce the opposite condition (for example, an alkaline medicine to combat an acidic stomach). This is the method on which medicine generally relies, and, according to Hahnemann, it works only in acute situations; its effect can only be considered temporary. "In chronic diseases it only gives relief at first; subsequently stronger doses of such remedies become necessary, which cannot remove the primary disease, and thus they do more harm the longer they are employed."[33] In his text he called upon his colleagues to abandon this practice of treating by contraries and instead move to a third method (one that he was then developing), which seeks to cure a disease by administering a drug "which is able to produce another very similar artificial disease."[34] In other words, to reject the principle of *contraria contrariis curantur* in favour of the principle of *similia similibus curantur*, or 'like cures like,' a principle that can be traced back to Hippocrates in the fifth century BCE.

According to Hahnemann in the above-mentioned treatise, "every powerful medicinal substance produces in the human body a kind of peculiar disease; the more powerful the medicine, the more peculiar and marked and violent the disease."[35] He believed that, by testing medicines on healthy subjects and judiciously noting the reactions, he could then apply that medicine to cases of illness where the symptoms matched the reactions to the drug in healthy subjects. Thus was homeopathy born (the word itself comes from the Greek *homoios pathos* and means 'similar suffering'), along with two of its fundamental premises: the principle of 'like cures like,' and the principle of 'provings,' which refers to testing every medicine to discover the symptoms it can cause in healthy individuals.[36] Drug provings, as well as re-provings, continue to be carried out by contemporary homeopathic doctors and students today as the *materia medica* is continually refined and updated. "In fact, for a particular remedy to be introduced and used in the homeopathic pharmacopoeia it is not enough for it to be capable of causing symptoms in a healthy subject; it must show proven ability to cure patients presenting the symptoms detected during the provings."[37]

Hippocrates first articulated the principle that 'like cures like'; Aristotle reiterated the principle a century later. Hahnemann was aware of these ancient philosophers and their beliefs, and even quoted Hippocrates. So, Hahnemann was not the creator of the principle, but he was "the first to discover and formulate the very exact laws of cure which gave birth to homeopathic medicine as a total and precise system."[38] While it might appear that there was a vacuum between Aristotle and Hahnemann, this is not true. During those centuries, Elizabeth Danciger sees "a pattern, a tapestry, linking various traditions and pointing to a line of thought and practice."[39] Within this tapestry were elements of thought that might have been familiar to Hahnemann from his translations and also from his vast knowledge of chemistry and the history of medicine.

A major figure in the tapestry is the controversial Renaissance physician Paracelsus (usually associated with the suspect science of alchemy), who, from his treatment of the diseases of miners in the sixteenth century, came to the conclusion that they should be treated "with remedies made from the exact metals which had caused the specific illnesses."[40] This historical picture is too detailed to pursue here, but what is interesting and relevant to the subject of this book is the fact that at least part of the tapestry is coloured with the threads of a debate in medicine between the vitalists and the mechanists of the seventeenth century, as the Cartesian notion of the body-machine came into greater and greater prominence.[41] This reflects the debate in natural philosophy generally, which, as we have seen, motivated the mechanism of Descartes. The body-machine model eventually became the only model for modern biomedicine, and the animistic and vitalist options came to be considered suspect and even dangerous to scientific thought. The seventeenth-century debate continues today in the field of medicine and the body.

The principle of 'like cures like' is not the most controversial element of homeopathy. In fact, it might be the least controversial, since it is one that is recognized, at least in part, in the practice of vaccination.[42] There are several other aspects of homeopathy that are not only controversial but invite the outright scorn and rejection by the orthodox medical profession. These are: 1) the vital force; 2) the interpretation of symptoms; and 3) the minimum dose.

The Vital Force

Fundamental to the vision of the body underlying homeopathy is the notion of a life force, a *vital force*, which Hahnemann called the *spirit-like dynamis*—a force by which the body reacts to external stimuli, including pathogens. Most modern commentators emphasize that Hahnemann's terminology was not meant to be taken as a mystical approach to medicine: "life force is no more than a metaphor to indicate a dynamic self-regulatory capability which all living creatures are undeniably endowed with in order to give them a better chance of survival."[43] As pointed out earlier, Hahnemann did not believe that it was possible to discover the fundamental cause of all disease, and he approached the vital force in the same manner—as a philosophical question that goes beyond the ability of the doctor to answer. Hahnemann was not trying to describe the essence of living things, only his conviction of the body's inherent ability to heal itself. Thus, it is impossible to say whether or not the vital force as he conceived it is comparable to the *ki* of Eastern medicine. At the very least, however, it is a kind of energy by which the body maintains internal harmony, as well as harmony with its environment. When that harmony is disturbed, whether due to internal or external factors, it is the vital force that reacts. In Hahnemann's view, "every disease (not entirely surgical) consists only in a special, morbid, dynamic alteration of our vital energy."[44] To that extent it is similar to *ki* and to the vitalist assumption shared by all types of alternative medicine, namely that the human body is animated by an energy or force essential to life and to health, and that disruption of the force leads to illness. Whether Hahnemann thought this energy was cosmic energy is unclear, but he did see it as both spiritual and dynamic, insisting that it "rules with unbounded sway, and retains all the parts of the organism in admirable, harmonious, vital operation, as regards both sensations and functions."[45]

The Interpretation of Symptoms

In homeopathy, the vital force or power is directly linked to the symptoms of a disease situation: "Disease symptoms represent the form taken by this power when reacting to a morbific stimulus in the internal or external environment."[46] In other words, any symptom, no matter how intense or disagreeable, is a manifestation of the body's reactive power; the body is doing the work of rebalancing itself. This is why Hahnemann was so adamant about not treating a symptom with a contrary remedy; such a method stops the body's own mechanism for cure. "Since the body's reactive force endeavors to cope with a given stress by producing *a particular set of symptoms*, the physician's duty is to promote the development of this very set of symptoms."[47] Because allopathic medicine cannot accept the principle of the vital force, its practitioners will not understand the homeopathic principle that administering medication to counteract or suppress symptoms is actually harming the body. For example, suppressing natural eruptions of the skin "can give rise to serious systemic disorders. Skin eruptions are the manifestation of nature's effort to throw off some internal toxin or waste matter. The suppression of eczema by local applications has been known to produce colitis, asthma, and bronchitis."[48] The more any symptoms are suppressed, the deeper a disease moves into the body. Continuous suppression of the body's curative force weakens the body; eventually a person becomes less and less healthy. On the other hand, according to the principles of homeopathy, working with the symptoms by administering a medicine in line with the principle of 'like cures like' strengthens the body's own inherent force and heals the patient.

Symptoms vary from patient to patient even when they have the same disease, such as influenza. Allopathic medicine looks to the common symptoms among patients ignoring the particular and idiosyncratic symptoms of individual sufferers. This is because it views disease as the active element and the patient's body as a passive recipient of an external pathogen. It also relies on tests that are designed to test the presence of objectively studied disease patterns. The symptoms described by the patient are considered secondary information, perhaps taken into consideration after the examination of test results, perhaps not. Homeopathy takes an opposite view in regarding the patient's symptoms, as expressed by the patient and in their totality—as the primary source of information in assessing the disease condition. This is, again, because the homeopath views the symptoms as a manifestation of the vital force in action. Even with the same influenza strain, for example, patients will react differently and will manifest different symptoms (and many people, exposed to the disease germ, will never fall victim to it and will have no symptoms). Thus, for the homeopath, it is not the symptoms common to all sufferers of the disease that are of interest; it is the particular and unique symptoms of each individual that are the key to finding the right medicine for each. In Hahnemann's view, the common symptoms observable in all sufferers of a disease were simply "empirical trifles."[49] They did not reveal how any individual patient's body was reacting to the disease in its own unique way, and they could not aid the physician in finding the unique remedy that would allow an individual patient's vital force to do its work. Paolo Bellavite and Andrea Signorini describe how a homeopathic practitioner faced with the symptom of fever will analyze the situation in order to choose a remedy:

> ...fever with heat sensations, reddening of the skin, perspiration, a very high pulse rate, a throbbing headache, mydriasis, and photophobia indicates that the patient needs *Belladonna* (deadly nightshade). Fever of sudden onset after a cold, with anxiety even to the point of fearing death, reddening of the skin (without perspiration), and a strong, hard pulse, but also with miosis, intense thirst and an aversion to blankets, indicates *Aconitum* (monkshood) as the remedy of choice.[50]

There is no remedy for fever as such, only different remedies for different kinds of fevers.

Thus, it can be seen that uncovering all the subtle symptoms can be a considerable task for the homeopathic physician, who must also pay attention to the way in which any symptom works in a patient:

> Is the particular symptom aggravated or relieved by heat, cold, motion, rest, noise, quiet, wetness, dryness, and changes in the weather? In the homeopathic view all these symptoms are important in giving the detailed knowledge of the patient's state, which the physician must have if he is to effect a cure. These changes in the symptoms produced by different environmental conditions are often the key to the correct medicine.[51]

It goes without saying that the patient must also be very observant about his or her bodily reactions to a disease situation, and very precise in recounting them to the physician. The physician must know what questions to ask; the patient must also be attentive in answering them.

The Minimum Dose

Many of the substances used in the preparation of homeopathic remedies—and they may be of animal, vegetable or mineral origin—are toxic in their natural state and cannot be administered unless they are highly diluted. This brings up what is probably the most controversial point about homeopathy: the use of substances that are so highly diluted that the critic or sceptic will maintain that the remedy is nothing but a placebo. Homeopaths agree that some extremely high dilutions in fact no longer contain any molecules of the substance, but they do not agree that the remedy is nothing but a placebo. The use of highly diluted substances "constitutes one of the cornerstones of homeopathy, and at the same time is perhaps the main problem which research is called upon to confirm and possibly explain."[52] To make matters even more challenging, according to homeopathy, the more highly diluted the remedy, the stronger it is. Part of the process of diluting the substance is shaking (succussion) and grinding (trituration), which "actually increase the power of the remedy, so that the 'high dilutions' provoke a more powerful response, by the organism, than the 'low dilutions.'"[53] One does have to sympathize with the sceptic here, since, on the face of it, this claim is, at the very least, counterintuitive. Further, the idea that the succussion process itself (which is referred to as *potentization* or *dynamization*) makes the remedy more powerful tends to bring the theory to the edge of the magical in the eyes of the doubter!

Effectiveness of Homeopathy

As pointed out earlier, homeopathy does appear to work. For example, Bellavite and Signorini report that,

> in the 1854 London cholera epidemic the mortality rate was 53.2 percent for patients treated in conventional hospitals as against only 16.4 percent in those treated in the homeopathic hospital. During the yellow fever epidemic which spread throughout the southern states of America in 1878 the statistics show that the mortality rate in patients receiving homeopathic treatment was one-third of that in patients on conventional treatment.[54]

Today, millions of people all over the world are using homeopathy and insist on its effectiveness in treating conditions that allopathic physicians have given up on. Further, clinical trials have shown very positive results for homeopathic treatments in certain kinds of diseases. Using the rigid criteria of trials for allopathic medicine, a 1991 Dutch study examined 107 clinical trials; the majority of these trials showed positive results. For example, of nineteen trials for respiratory infections, thirteen showed positive results; for hay fever, five out of five; for rheumatic disease, four out of six; for trauma and/or pain, eighteen out of twenty; for psychological or mental problems, eight out of ten.[55]

It can be said that, in the past as well the present, the barrier to acceptance is not that homeopathy is ineffective; it is that its effectiveness cannot be *explained* within the scientific paradigm. In the nineteenth century, homeopathy was very popular and was taught in universities and medical schools. In spite of its effectiveness, it was actively suppressed by the medical establishment. Bellavite and Signorini suggest that it "brought ideas which were apparently too advanced for the primitive state in which medicine found itself at the time."[56] The medical establishment reacted to the threat of homeopathy by denying recognition to graduates of medical schools that taught it, and downgrading these schools based exclusively on standard medical criteria. This approach proved effective, as the number of American medical colleges teaching homeopathy dropped from twenty-two in 1900 to two in 1923 and zero by 1950.[57] Since the 1970s and 1980s, homeopathy has been on the rise, but the resistance of the medical establishment is still strong, even though medicine no longer finds itself in the "primitive state" it did in the nineteenth century. This resistance is not about homeopathy's effectiveness, but about the *explanation* of its effectiveness. This, in itself, suggests that, when comparing homeopathic and allopathic medicine, we are dealing with two fundamentally different paradigms—particularly in relation to the human body.

Energy, Sound and Healing

There are many other branches of alternative medicine that share the same fundamental assumptions of mind and body as TCM and homeopathy, and they cannot all be explored here. Many of them can be said to be at the frontier of the spectrum of what Western scientific medicine can accept. A number of therapies often described under the rubric of religious and/or spiritual healing can be said to fall near this frontier: faith healing, the laying on of hands, prayer, and so on. These tend to be accepted to the extent that they are seen as part of religious belief or ritual. From this point of view, any positive effects on a patient can be seen by the medical establishment as being psychological, explainable perhaps by the religious faith of the sick person. This cannot, of course, be the complete explanation, since some studies have shown the healing power of prayer at a distance in cases of patients who do not realize they are being prayed for. But as long as such healing techniques remain in the realm of the religious, they can be seen as supernatural by believers, or explained away by sceptics.

But more and more, techniques loosely referred to as spiritual or energy healing are not practiced as part of any religion, and practitioners may make no appeals to any idea of God or any kind of religious worship. This makes it difficult to dismiss them as based solely on faith or religion, and thus subjective and not scientific. From the point of view of standard medicine, massage is an acceptable practice because it relieves sore muscles and back pain, and appears to reduce stress. But what about the massage therapist who incorporates therapeutic touch or Reiki[58] into his or her techniques, and claims to be working not only (or at all) on muscles, but on energy? While the term 'energy healing' can be seen as vague, it encompasses a wide variety of concepts about healing and energy that scientific medicine, with its mechanistic conception of the body, finds hard to accept. Different therapies explain the movement and transfer of these energies in different ways, but they all make use of non-material causes that, as shown above in relation to homeopathy, cannot be easily explained within the framework of allopathic medicine.

One of these approaches to energy healing that might be considered to be at the frontier end of the spectrum is healing through sound, voice and music. Some forms of music therapy have been accepted in certain hospital settings, especially in palliative care,[59] but other forms of sound therapy more in line with the theory and practice of mantra discussed in the previous chapter are practiced on the fringes of conventional medicine. Many therapists are using sound in a holistic approach to healing the body, the mind and the soul in ways that appear to work wonders but are difficult to explain within the scientific medical paradigm.

There is a story, now quite well known, about Alfred Tomatis, whose work as an eye, ear, nose and throat doctor eventually led him to research the effect of music on health and healing. In the late 1960s, Tomatis was called on to advise the abbot of a Benedictine monastery in southern France, where many of the monks appeared to be in a serious state of ill health. They were exhausted and listless, and were falling ill at an abnormal rate. After studying the situation and speaking to the monks, Tomatis concluded that their problem was related to the sudden cessation of chanting that had resulted from new rules imposed by the Catholic Church regarding the Latin liturgy. The monks had been used to singing Gregorian chant six to eight hours a day. Their abbot, young and modern, forced them to abandon this practice in order to spend time on more useful activities. Suddenly, they were no longer chanting, and Tomatis was convinced this was the key to the abbot's problem. At his recommendation, the monks began chanting again, and within several months their former robust health returned. Clearly, "the chanting provided spiritual and emotional nourishment to the monks, who lived otherwise Spartan, unadorned lives."[60] Dr. Gaynor saw a parallel between this story and the stories of his many cancer patients who lacked any form of spiritual sustenance in their therapy, and he began to develop a type of sound therapy based on the use of Tibetan singing bowls.

Hazrat Khan gives one explanation for the efficacy of sound therapy, whether it be the traditional chanting of the monks or a special therapy designed for cancer patients:

> Man is not only formed of vibrations, but he lives and moves in them: they surround him as the fish is surrounded by water, and he contains them within him as the tank contains water. His different moods, inclinations, affairs, successes and failures, and all the conditions of life depend upon a certain activity of vibrations, whether these be thoughts, emotions or feelings.[61]

Tibetan singing bowls are bowls that, when tapped, send out the vibrations of a core note plus its overtones, stimulating different vibrations in the body of the person absorbing them. Through the process of entrainment (discussed in the section on mantra in Chapter 8), the vibrations of the sound resonate with the vibrations of the person's body, thus helping to restore the disturbed vibrations of the person or patient. Dr. Gaynor recounts his own experience with the bowls:

> I am not the same person I was before I started using the bowls during my meditation practice. Like most people, I was accustomed to seeing the world purely from the limited perspective of my personal awareness. I had to deal with the same stress that all doctors confront. Through my practice with the bowls, I became more in touch with my essence. If I was holding on to a stressful feeling or thought, all I had to do was play one of my bowls, and that feeling or thought would be transformed.[62]

Gaynor began experimenting with the bowls, playing them for patients who were undergoing chemotherapy, "and saw their anxiety dissipate as they submerged themselves in the sounds." He watched them "take extraordinary emotional, physical, and spiritual leaps forward."[63] This was the case even with the most reluctant patients, many of whom thought the idea of the bowls was crazy or New Age, but who went along with it, thinking that they had nothing to lose. Some of these sceptics were the most transformed by their experiences, eventually buying their own bowls and continuing to use them in meditation. Gaynor believes that the use of sound is one of the most powerful healing techniques available. Here is the testimony of one of his cancer patients:

> I really got into it…. The sound enters your mind and soul, so that every part of you is filled with energy. I visualized the cancer disappearing. At the same time, I used visual imagery to rid myself of the stress in my body, to find peace and harmony, and to find a way to love myself. It was like a cleansing that came over me.[64]

What is going on here? What is it about the singing bowls that they can change inner conflict into feelings of calm and harmony that go right to the cellular level? The answer can be found in the quote from Khan above: we live and move in vibrations, and vibrations live and move in us. As we learned in the last chapter, the world *is* vibration (*nada brahma*). We are each a tiny part of the universal, cosmic vibration. Our body vibrates, our mind vibrates and our soul vibrates. And, in our chaotic world, we become like a badly tuned piano: if the piano is out of tune, nothing played on it will sound right. If our bodies are out of tune for too long, disease results.

Hippocrates, for whom health was harmony and disease disharmony, would understand this very well. Why is it so hard for modern medicine to understand? The answer can only be that these kinds of therapies that use energy and sound (both of which are, in the final analysis, vibrations) do not fit the mechanistic paradigm. They take us back to the naturalists of the Renaissance, for whom resonance was an accepted form of causal explanation and the concept of macrocosm-microcosm was a given. The fundamental principles of TCM, homeopathy, spiritual and energy healing all look back to earlier conceptual frameworks that could account for the connection between the human body, soul and nature (or cosmos). The belief that there was life everywhere in nature—and thus different levels of soul or intelligence—was

284 THE LIMITS OF MECHANISM

a fundamental underpinning of this unity. From the ancients to Descartes, these ideas ruled; but they were too tied up with religion, and science had to rid itself of notions considered spiritual or religious. Henceforth, the physical would be the domain of science; the spiritual and metaphysical the domain of religion and, for a while, philosophy.

What is interesting about all these alternative approaches to health and healing is that they are, for the most part, divorced from any formalized religion. They all have a more or less spiritual dimension, but it is more Platonic than Christian, based on the unity and intelligence of the universe, with human beings participating in that unity and intelligence. Whether one thinks of this intelligence as divine or not does not matter in the ultimate process of connection with it. For all these approaches to body, health and illness, we are light, we are vibration; whether or not we are God becomes a matter of personal belief and experience. Whether we call on God, Brahma or cosmic sound or light, we are calling on the same source, a source that has the power to heal and to make us whole. We are not machines.

Notes

1. I am here ignoring the rather ironic fact that much advanced robotics research is taking place in Japan.

2. Yuasa, 107. It could also be added that, for the most part, philosophy has ceded its place to psychology in most of what concerns the mind or the 'inner world' (outside of the area of morals or ethics).

3. Yuasa, 108. Extending this statement to the logic of medicine is perfectly legitimate. Many people who have chronic health problems that biomedicine appears unable to treat (and that their doctors dismiss as psychosomatic) turn to alternative medicine, which is in turn often dismissed by their doctors as unscientific. "Finding compelling and pragmatically useful knowledge in personal experiences which the scientific community dismisses when approached for explanations or assistance, they could logically claim that it is science which is rejecting them, and not the other way around." Bonnie B. O'Connor, "Conceptions of the Body in Complementary and Alternative Medicine," in *Complementary and Alternative Medicine: Challenge and Change*, eds. Merrijoy Kelner and Beverly Wellman (Amsterdam: Harwood Academic Publishers, 2000), 60.

4. As pointed out in Chapter 8, *ki* performs a similar function as *qi* (from Chinese medicine—pronounced, and sometimes spelled, *chi*) and *prana* (Indian medicine), although none of these terms can be reduced to the other, since there are subtle and important differences among them. Like *prana*, which was discussed in Chapter 8, *ki* and *qi* can be compared to the Stoic *pneuma*, long ago discarded in Western science and medicine.

5. One could take as an example the emotion of anger; through meditation, the emotion can be calmed and controlled, but anger is also seen as having a physiological expression in the liver—and this can be controlled through acupuncture affecting the liver meridian. In both cases, *ki* is the activating or mediating factor—and both kinds of therapy are necessary if the anger is to be truly dealt with.

6. Ayurvedic medicine is the traditional medicine of India.

7. O'Connor, 51.

8. Paolo Bellaite and Andrea Signorini, *Homeopathy: A Frontier in Medical Science* (Berkeley: North Atlantic Books, 1995), 3.

9. Allopathic medicine refers to conventional biomedicine. It is a term used mainly by alternative practitioners.

10. René Dubos, "Health and Creative Adaptation," in *Ethical Health Care*, eds. Patricia Illingworth and Wendy E. Parmet (Upper Saddle River, NJ: Pearson Education Inc., 2006), 24.

11. Michael C. Brannigan and Judith A. Boss, *Healthcare Ethics in a Diverse Society* (McGraw-Hill Higher Education, 2000), 110.

12. O'Connor, 50.

13. O'Connor, 50.

14. Grant Gillett, "Clinical medicine and the quest for certainty," *Social Science & Medicine*, 58 (2004): 728. Gillett is quoting from W. H. Newton Smith, *The Rationality of Science* (London: Routledge, 1981).

15. Gillett, 735. In giving this example, Gillett is illustrating his point that academic and institutional medicine "has become theory-bound and paradigm-dominated in a highly positivistic mode of scientific practice.... In innumerable areas, medicine has succeeded by imposing the rigid and positivist model on those ideas that it accepts as true. But it has also ruled out as being deviant ideas that have later proved to be important in understanding a given problem" (734).

16. It is worth noting that many homeopaths also practice Traditional Chinese Medicine—in particular, acupuncture.

17. See, for example, the website of the Toronto School for Traditional Chinese Medicine (www.tstcm.com) or the Alberta College of Acupuncture and Traditional Chinese Medicine (www.acatcm.com), which offers a program affiliated with that of the Beijing University of Chinese Medicine and has

recently announced new MA and PhD programs for 2010–2011 (accessed July 15, 2010).

18.   O'Connor, 43.

19.   Ted J. Kaptchuk, *The Web That Has No Weaver: Understanding Chinese Medicine* (Chicago: Congdon & Weed, 1983), 7.

20.   O'Connor, 43.

21.   Kaptchuk, 8.

22.   Kaptchuk, 12.

23.   The pulse is taken using three fingers on two wrists and palpating at three different levels of pressure. Kaptchuk describes and classifies twenty-eight classical pulse types (for example, a pulse may be thin or big, empty or full, slippery or choppy, etc.). The pulse positions correspond to particular organs (e.g., the first position on the left wrist to the heart, the second position on the right wrist to the spleen) and the type of pulse can indicate the type of disharmony in an organ. See Kaptchuk, 160–74.

24.   Kaptchuk, 35.

25.   O'Connor, 44. In fact, following Yuasa, there are several kinds of *ki*: *shin-ki* and *sei*-ki. *Shin* can be seen as 'spiritual power,' corresponding to the Chinese *shen*, and *sei* as 'power for procreation,' which is part of the role of *jing*. In the final analysis, *qi* and *ki* might be seen as very similar, or at least as having the same explanatory value.

26.   The TCM physician is looking for disharmonies, which show up in pulse diagnosis, but also in facial colour, qualities of the tongue, mood, movement, pain and other elements. "When these bits and pieces of information are put together, they create the image of a disharmony" (Kaptchuk, 138).

27.   Yuasa, 101. Iridology is another form of alternative therapy that is based on similar assumptions. It holds that every aspect of health is indicated in different parts of the iris of the eye. Examination of the iris can show where there are particular problems or pathologies.

28.   O'Connor, 45.

29.   Yuasa, 208 (fn. 2).

30.   Yuasa, 103. As already pointed out, *qi* and *ki* are treated as being equivalent, both referring to the energy circulating through the meridians.

31.   Yuasa, 107.

32.   Yuasa, 107.

33.   Quoted in Elizabeth Danciger, *Homeopathy: From Alchemy to Medicine* (Rochester, VT: Healing Arts Press, 1987), 6.

34.   Quoted in Danciger, 8.

35.   Quoted in Danciger, 7.

36. Hahnemann carried out provings on himself, his colleagues and his students over his lifetime and accumulated the results in a *materia medica* that has continually been updated since his time. During his lifetime he proved the effectiveness of ninety-nine substances. By the end of the nineteenth century, more than six hundred had been added.

37. Bellavite and Signorini, 9.

38. Danciger, 11.

39. Danciger, 12.

40. Danciger, 23. It is interesting to note that Paracelsus' teachings were very controversial and his works were suppressed—just as homeopathy was suppressed later in the nineteenth century.

41. Danciger, 74. Danciger reports that, at the medical school in Montpellier, for example, the animistic vision, along with the principle of the 'vital force,' held sway, while at the Paris medical school, mechanical medicine reigned. It was, as she says, a confused period for physicians.

42. Vaccination actually represents a *variation* on the principle, but there is a subset of homeopathy called 'isopathy,' whereby a disease is treated by the same agent that is capable of causing it. In the case of vaccination, the goal is *prevention* through building immunity to a disease by administering a dose of the agent capable of causing it.

43. Bellavite and Signori, 16.

44. Quoted in Bellavite and Signorini, 15.

45. Quoted in Bellavite and Signorini, 16.

46. Harris L. Coulter, "Homeopathic Medicine," in *Ways of Health*, ed. David S. Sobel (New York and London: Harcourt Brace Jovanovich, 1979), 290.

47. Coulter, 290.

48. Coulter, 290.

49. Quoted in Coulter, 297.

50. Bellavite and Signorini, 10.

51. Coulter, 297. Needless to say, a homeopathic doctor must spend more time with his or her patient than an allopathic doctor.

52. Bellavite and Signorini, 12. According to Avogadro's Law, "dilutions of any substance beyond 10^{24} (24x or 12c in homeopathic terms) presented an increasingly remote chance of containing only a single molecule or atom of the original compound" (23). A dilution of 1c means the proportion of substance to diluting solution is 1 to 99. Homeopathic remedies are diluted far beyond the limit of Avogadro's Law.

53. Coulter, 306.

54. Bellavite and Signorini, 21.

55. See Bellavite and Signorini, 43.

56.   Bellavite and Signorini, 20.

57.   A similar attempt was made in the United States in the twentieth century against chiropractic, when the American Medical Association launched a lawsuit against a chiropractor. In this case, the judge found that the AMA's Committee on Quackery (a not-unbiased appellation) had undertaken a nationwide conspiracy to eliminate a licensed profession, and dismissed the AMA accusations.

58.   Reiki is a form of energy healing that originated in Japan, but is widely practiced in the West and has become 'westernized.' It is a holistic therapy that involves transference of the energy of the palms of the healer in a form of therapeutic touch designed to cure a specific illness, whether it be physical, mental or spiritual.

59.   The work of Therese Schroeder-Sheker is an example of a practice called music thanatology, a form of music therapy for the dying. See www.chaliceofrepose.org.

60.   Gaynor, 14.

61.   Hazrat Inayat Khan, *The Mysticism of Sound and Music* (Boston and London: Shambhala Books, 1996), 120.

62.   Gaynor, 116.

63.   Gaynor, 118.

64.   Gaynor, 160.

CONCLUSION

Hans Jonas refers to the road through dualism as irreversible. In his view, dualism represents "the most momentous phase in the history of thought, whose achievement, however overtaken, can never be undone."[1] Having sundered the world of matter and the world of spirit, we cannot think them back together again. If he is right about this, then what I have been proposing in this book is a pipe dream. The road not followed cannot be travelled now. He goes on to suggest, however, that while we cannot undo the polarity, we can attempt to absorb it "into a higher unity of existence from which the opposites issue as faces of its being or phases of its becoming."[2] I do not know if he had Spinoza in mind as he wrote this, but his statement calls to mind Spinoza's metaphysics of mind and matter as expressions (or faces) of the one substance, rather than as substances in their own right that need to be fitted back together. And if I am right, then perhaps we can still find our way on the road not followed.

The problem, of course, is finding our way to the "higher unity of existence" or the one substance (which, for Spinoza, is God or Nature), and here our mechanistic science of nature (and of body) is the stumbling block along the road. We cannot perceive the higher unity or the one substance. We cannot touch it, objectify it or quantify it. Therefore, from the point of view of mechanistic science, it does not exist. Whatever names the ancients gave to it or its forms (e.g., *pneuma*, world-soul), or whatever names Eastern science or religion attaches to it or its forms (e.g., *qi* or *Siva*), these are simply fanciful terms for the animism that was banished with the scientific revolution. No matter how many infinitesimally small subatomic particles the physicists discover (and they now number in the hundreds), the idea of some fundamental, all-pervading reality is still anathema to Western science. The result of this is that science cannot explain life, or the living human body. It can tell us how living things work, and it can even work to create life and living things in the laboratory. But it cannot tell us what they *are* in philosophical terms. In other words, we have no ontology of life or of the living body. We have only mechanistic explanations that stand in for ontological ones. Dualism and mechanism have given us the body-machine; but they are incapable of giving us back the living body.

I have attempted in this book to demonstrate how we arrived at our Western conception of the body-machine, and to point to alternative approaches that could lead us away from it. As shown in Chapter 7, materialistic mechanism has brought us to the brink of losing the body. We have learned to see our bodies as objects of scientific investigation, then of medical diagnosis and treatment, then as objects to mould to our wishes (to match our conception of a 'self' that is somehow not properly reflected by the body that 'contains' it). Now we are asked to believe that the body, which is an obstacle to achieving the true potential of our minds, should be disposed of and replaced by more efficient, nonbiological machines. We have been drawn into a medical paradigm in which the body is a collection of interchangeable parts, and many of us are not shocked at the idea of buying and selling those parts (organs, gametes, genetic material). In our dualistic and mechanistic world, our bodies are not us.

What we do consider 'us' is the self, which we see as in some vaguely defined way different from our body—but just how and why neither biologists nor psychologists can tell us. I have tried to show in Chapter 5 how this modern, separated self is linked to a dualistic view of mind and body, and how it differs from more holistic views. The effort we invest in, and the importance we attribute to, this constructed self is part of the great divide between the holistic and dualistic visions that I have been exploring in this book. In a holistic view of mind-body-soul-cosmos, the self is not divorced from the world in which it is situated. If we think of Spinoza's *conatus* or the Stoic's *oikeiosis*, we have an idea of a self deeply embedded in the world. In the case of the Stoics, this is a determined self—determined by fate. In Spinoza, it is determined by all of its past actions and all of the events that it has experienced. The need to think of our 'self' as free, divorced from the world around it and even from its past, ready and able to re-form itself at any given moment, is a modern,

Western invention. It is the source of the exaggerated importance that we put on individual autonomy and free will—something both Spinoza and the Stoics would find misguided.

Ironically, the 'self' that we in the West have spent four centuries cultivating is precisely what the philosophy of yoga suggests we must forego if we wish to be happy. Not that we don't need an 'everyday' self with which to deal in the world—but we should not be fooled into thinking that this so-called self is our real Self. If the *yogis* are right, we have been spending time and effort, along with considerable philosophical reasoning and psychological experimentation, building a mirage that has taken us further and further away from the essence of our being. More importantly, from a practical and perhaps less spiritual point of view, this mirage of the self has taken us further and further away from our bodies. As shown in Chapter 8, many of us do not know how to move properly, to breathe properly or to quiet the incessant noise in our heads—all of which contributes to stress and illness. Mechanistic science may have brought miracle cures to heal the body-machine, but, to a large extent, it's the body-machine that is making us sick in the first place.

We have lost our connection with our bodies, with nature and with the cosmos. In the quest to rid scientific explanation of the cosmic connectors that served to keep human beings linked to the natural world, we have, perhaps, thrown out the baby with the bathwater. It is true that in Descartes' time the bathwater of the philosophy of nature was imbued with ideas that were too easily seen as religious, and that theological orthodoxy played a large—and often impeding—role in the progress of scientific discovery. Divesting the physical of its spiritual elements made the physical easier to study and explain, but the reductionism this manoeuvre entailed has left a legacy of incompleteness—at least in relation to the living human body. This incompleteness comes first and foremost from reductionism's incapacity to explain life. Or, as Jonas puts it, from "denying organic reality its principal and most obvious characteristic, namely, that it exhibits in each individual instance a striving of its own for existence and fulfilment, or the fact of life's willing itself."[3] Descartes' reduction of the principle of life (the heat of the heart) to the 'fire without light,' which we saw in Chapter 5, represents a deliberate conceptual shift that was instrumental in that denial of life—in nature and in the body—that has persisted to our day.

The incompleteness of our body explanations is reflected in our Western approach to medicine, with its inability to deal with chronic ailments that do not display measurable symptoms and known pathologies. The result of this is a public that turns increasingly to alternative therapies, many of which come from the Eastern tradition. Yoga, Tai Chi, TCM and other practices and therapies give us a more complete account of the body than we have in the West. These practices have made their way to the West and are very popular here now because they add something to the lives of the people who make use of them for healing and/or for personal development. There is much to be learned from them. There is also much in them, as we have seen in Chapters 8 and 9, that harks back to visions of the body in the history of Western thought and that deserves to be seriously studied by Western science. In the spirit of Paul Feyerabend, quoted in the Introduction, these practices and their key concepts should be taken seriously and investigated by science, not rejected out of hand because they do not fit into the mechanistic paradigm. Rejecting whatever does not fit and refusing to allow challenges to the established framework simply perpetuates this paradigm, with its many unanswered questions.

This is not to say that mechanistic explanations are not useful; they are. But if they are applied to everything in the universe, then the universe, along with everything in it, becomes a machine. As Carolyn Merchant wrote almost thirty years ago, "Mechanistic assumptions about nature push us increasingly in the direction of artificial environments, mechanized control over more and more aspects of human life, and a loss of the quality of life itself."[4] This is the end of the road of dualism and mechanism that has been followed for almost four centuries. The universalization of these mechanistic principles needs to be rethought.

The idea of recuperating notions that were sidetracked by Descartes should be taken seriously—and has been in certain circles. Plato, in the *Timaeus*, describes the world as a living, breathing, intelligent being. The Gaia Hypothesis (which has advanced to the level of a theory), launched in the twentieth century by James Lovelock and Lynn Margulis (both eminent scientists), holds that the Earth is a living, self-regulating system that can be compared to the workings of any individual organism. This is a theory that many take very seriously and, in the past twenty years, scientists have identified many of the mechanisms by which the Earth self-regulates.[5] This is just one example of an ancient theory, discarded as myth, which has re-appeared as science. The holism that is present in Stoic philosophy and in Spinoza is reflected in the modern science of ecology, which recognizes the interconnectedness of all things, along with the assumption that nature is active and alive, and that "[n]o element of an interlocking cycle can be removed without the collapse of the cycle."[6] There is scientific evidence of the existence of acupuncture meridians, which, until quite recently, were considered imaginary.[7] The notion of the macrocosm-microcosm, long ago discarded in the West, has survived in Eastern philosophy, where it has explanatory value in linking the human body to the cosmos in the sense of part to whole. Modern experiments in sound and vibration hark back to Ficino's *Concordia mundi* and Kepler's music of the spheres. As shown in Chapter 4, even astrology, long ridiculed by science, can now be considered seriously as a result of advances in psychology and technology.

It is not unrealistic to suggest that the cosmic connectors that I have pointed to in earlier philosophies of the body (as well as in Eastern practices and therapies) could be re-examined for their explanatory value in understanding the body and its relation to the world. As has been pointed out regularly throughout this book, the question is not whether the conceptual frameworks about the body that we have seen are right or wrong; the question is: What were they meant to explain? The vision of the body that forms the presuppositions of modern science and medicine is not a brute fact of nature. It represents a conceptual framework intentionally constructed by Descartes to explain a body whose workings followed the mechanistic laws of nature (also conceived mechanistically). A century from now, it may appear as quaint as Ficino's astrological instructions to doctors. Nor is Descartes' dualism of material body and spiritual soul a brute fact of nature—nor is the idea that only humans have minds or intelligence, or that humans are a superior species representing the peak of evolution. As Mary Midgley has observed, this is an idea left over from the Christian belief in an immortal soul that is the preserve of humans. If we want to find the connections between all living things or between the body and the cosmos, we have the tools to look for them. But we won't find them if we refuse even to look, assuming in advance that they are not there.

The body-machine is not a fact of nature; it is a man-made creation that has a history—a history that can be rewritten. It began in the seventeenth century and has survived science and medicine for close to four hundred years; but its usefulness has been surpassed by its inability to serve human physical and spiritual needs. It tells only a partial story about what the body can do. It is time to revise the story by allowing a conception of the body's unity with soul and with nature. A holistic account is needed to recover the whole story—to recover the body.

Notes

1. Jonas, *Phenomenon*, 16.
2. Jonas, *Phenomenon*, 17.
3. Jonas, *Phenomenon*, 61.
4. Merchant, 291.
5. Martin Ogle, "Understanding Gaia Theory," http://www.gaiatheory.org/synopsis.htm (accessed 5 November 2010).
6. Merchant, 293.
7. Dr. Hiroshi Motoyama uses a machine called the AMI (Apparatus for Meridian Identification), which monitors the electrical conductivity and capacity at specific acupoints at the tip of fingers and toes. His research has shown a close correlation between the electrical conductivity of meridians and the flow of *ki* (or *chi*) in the meridians. See the California Institute for Human Science website: www.cihs.edu/AMI/.

BIBLIOGRAPHY

Alper, Harvey P., ed. *Understanding Mantras*. Albany: SUNY Press, 1989.

Aristotle. *De Anima*. Translated and edited by Hugh Lawson-Tancred. London and Toronto: Penguin, 1986.

————. *De Anima*. Translated and edited by R. D. Hicks. Cambridge: Cambridge University Press, 1907.

Arya, Usharbudh. *Mantra & Meditation*. Honesdale, PA: Himalayan International Institute of Yoga Science & Philosophy of the U.S.A., 1981.

Augustine. *Confessions*. Translated and edited by Henry Chadwick. Oxford: Oxford University Press, 1992, 2008.

Avalon, Arthur [John Woodroffe]. *The Serpent Power: The Secrets of Tantric and Shaktic Yoga*. New York: Dover Publications, 1974.

Baldi, Pierre. *The Shattered Self: The End of Natural Evolution*. Cambridge: MIT Press, 2001.

Barnes, Jonathan. *Aristotle*. Oxford and New York: Oxford University Press, 1982.

Baudrillard, Jean. *The Consumer Society: Myths and Structures*. Translated by Chris Turner. Los Angeles: Sage Publications, 1998.

Beck, L. J. *The Method of Descartes*. Oxford: Clarendon Press, 1952.

Belk, Russell W. "Me and Thee versus Mine and Thine: How Perceptions of the Body Influence Organ Donation and Transplantation." In *Organ Donation and Transplantation*, edited by James Shanteau and Richard Jackson Harris. Hyattsville, MD: American Psychological Association, 1990.

Bellavite, Paolo, and Andrea Signorini. *Homeopathy: A Frontier in Medical Science*. Berkeley: North Atlantic Books, 1995.

Bennett, Jonathan. *A Study of Spinoza's 'Ethics'*. Cambridge: Cambridge University Press, 1984.

Berendt, Joachim-Ernst. *The World is Sound: Nada Brahma: Music and the Landscape of Consciousness.* Rochester, VT: Destiny Books, 1983.

Biondi, Paolo. *Aristotle: Posterior Analytics II.19.* Québec: Les Presses de l'Université Laval, 2004.

Birke, Linda. *Feminism and the Biological Body.* New Brunswick, NJ: Rutgers University Press, 1999.

Bitbol-Hespériès, Annie. *Le principe de vie chez Descartes.* Paris: Librairie philosophique J. Vrin, 1990.

Bitbol-Hespériès, Annie, and Jean-Pierre Verdet, eds. *Descartes: Le Monde, L'Homme.* Paris: Éditions de Seuil, 1996.

Bordo, Susan. *The Flight to Objectivity: Essays on Cartesianism and Culture.* Albany: SUNY Press, 1987.

_____. *Unbearable Weight: Feminism, Western Culture, and the Body.* Berkeley: University of California Press, 1993.

Brannigan, Michael C., and Judith A. Boss. *Healthcare Ethics in a Diverse Society.* McGraw-Hill Higher Education, 2000.

Brown, Peter. *Augustine of Hippo.* Berkeley: University of California Press: 1967, 2000.

_____. *The Body and Society.* New York: Columbia University Press, 1988.

Burrus, Virginia. "Word and Flesh: The Bodies and Sexuality of Ascetic Women in Christian Antiquity." *Journal of Feminist Studies in Religion,* 10 (1994): 27–51.

Bynum, Caroline Walker. *Holy Feast and Holy Fast.* Berkeley: University of California Press, 1987.

_____. "Fast, Feast, and Flesh: The Religious Significance of Food to Medieval Women." *Representations,* 11 (Summer 1985): 1–25.

Bynum, Terrence Ward. "A New Look at Aristotle's Theory of Perception." In *Aristotle's DeAnima in Focus,* edited by Michael Durant. London and New York: Routledge, 1993.

_____. *The Resurrection of the Body in Western Christianity, 200–1336.* New York: Columbia University Press, 1995.

Cicero. *De Finibus Bonorum et Malorum.* Translated by H. Rackham. Loeb Classical Library, 1914.

Cohen, Michael H. *Healing at the Borderland of Medicine and Religion.* Chapel Hill: University of North Carolina Press, 2006.

Collier, Carol. "The Body and Technology: A New or an Old Anthropology?" In *Technology and the Changing Face of Humanity,* edited by Richard Feist, Chantal Beauvais and Rajesh Shukla. Ottawa: University of Ottawa Press, 2010.

Collier, Carol, and Rachel Haliburton. *Bioethics in Canada: A Philosophical Introduction.* Toronto: Canadian Scholars Press, 2011.

Cornford, F. M. *The Republic of Plato.* New York and Oxford: Oxford University Press, 1951.

————. *Plato's Cosmology: The Timaeus of Plato*. London: Routledge & Kegan Paul, 1956.

Copenhaver, Brian P., and Charles B. Schmitt. *Renaissance Philosophy*. Oxford: Oxford University Press, 1992.

Cottingham, John. "A Brute to the Brutes? Descartes' Treatment of Animals." In *René Descartes, Critical Assessments*, edited by Georges J. D. Moyal. London: Routledge, 1991.

————. *Cartesian Reflections: Essays on Descartes' Philosophy*. Oxford: Oxford University Press, 2008.

Cottingham, John, Robert Stoothoff, and Dugald Murdoch. *The Philosophical Writings of Descartes, Vols. I and II*. Cambridge: Cambridge University Press, 1984.

Cottingham, John, Robert Stoothoff, Dugald Murdoch, and Anthony Kenny. *The Philosophical Writings of Descartes, Vol. III; The Correspondence*. Cambridge: Cambridge University Press, 1991.

Coulter, Harris L. "Homeopathic Medicine." In *Ways of Health: Holistic Approaches to Ancient and Contemporary Medicine*, edited by David S. Sobel. New York and London: Harcourt Brace Jovanovich, 1979.

Crombie, I. M. *Plato: The Midwife's Apprentice*. London: Routledge & Kegan Paul, 1964.

Danciger, Elizabeth. *Homeopathy: From Alchemy to Medicine*. Rochester, VT: Healing Arts Press, 1987.

Davis, Craig. "The Yogic Exercises of the 17th Century Sufis." In *Theory and Practice of Yoga: Essays in Honour of Gerald James Larson*, edited by Knut A. Jacobsen. Delhi: Motilal Banarsidass, 2008.

Davis, Kathy. "'My Body is My Art': Cosmetic Surgery as Feminist Utopia?" *The European Journal of Women's Studies*, 4: 1 (1997): 23–38, http://ejw.sagepub.com/content/4/1/23 (accessed September 21, 2010).

Dazey, Wade. "Yoga in America: Some Reflections from the Heartland." In Jacobsen, *Theory and Practice of Yoga*, 409–33.

DeBrabander, Firmin. *Spinoza and the Stoics*. London and New York: Continuum International Publishing Group, 2007.

De Michelis, Elizabeth. *A History of Modern Yoga: Patanjali and Western Esotericism*. London and New York: Continuum, 2004.

Dijksterhuis, E. J. *The Mechanization of the World Picture*, translated by C. Dikshoorn. Oxford: Oxford University Press, 1961.

Dreyfus, Hubert. *On the Internet*. 2nd ed. London and New York: Routledge, 2009.

Dubos, René. "Health and Creative Adaptation." In *Ethical Health Care*, edited by Patricia Illingworth and Wendy E. Parmet. Upper Saddle River, NJ: Pearson Education Inc., 2006.

Dupré, Louis. *Passage to Modernity*. New Haven and London: Yale University Press, 1993.

Edwards, Paul, ed. *The Encyclopedia of Philosophy, Vol. 1–VIII.* New York: Macmillan and The Free Press, 1967.

Feuerstein, Georg. *The Deeper Dimensions of Yoga.* Boston and London: Shambhala Publications, 2003.

Feyerabend, Paul. *Against Method.* London: Verso, 1979.

Fiedler, Leslie A. "Why Organ Transplant Programs Do Not Succeed." In *Organ Transplantation: Meanings and Realities,* edited by Stuart J. Youngner, Renée C. Fox and Laurence J. O'Connell, 56–65. Madison: University of Wisconsin Press, 1996.

Foerst, Anne. *God in the Machine.* New York: Penguin, 2004.

Foss, Laurence. *The End of Modern Medicine: Biomedical Science Under a Microscope.* Albany: SUNY Press, 2002.

Fox, Renée C. "Afterthoughts: Continuing Reflections on Organ Transplantation." In *Organ Transplantation: Meanings and Realities,* edited by Stuart J. Youngner, Renée C. Fox and Laurence J. O'Connell, 252–67. Madison: University of Wisconsin Press, 1996.

Frank, Arthur. "Emily's Scars: Surgical Shapings, Technoluxe, and Bioethics." In *Hastings Center Report,* 34: 2 (2004): 18–29.

Galen. *Selected Works.* Translated by P. N. Singer. Oxford: Oxford University Press, 1997.

Galileo Galilei, *Dialogo dei due massimi sistemi del mondo,* 1632. In *Dialogues Concerning the Two Chief World Systems—Ptolemaic & Copernican,* translated by Stillman Drake. Berkeley and Los Angeles: University of California Press, 1953.

Garber, Daniel, and Michael Ayers. *The Cambridge History of Seventeenth-Century Philosophy.* Cambridge: Cambridge University Press, 1998.

Garin, Eugenio. *Astrology in the Renaissance.* London: Routledge & Kegan Paul, 1988.

Gatens, Moira. *Feminist Interpretations of Benedict Spinoza.* University Park, PA: Pennsylvania State University Press, 2009.

Gaukroger, Stephen. *Descartes: An Intellectual Biography.* Oxford: Clarendon Press, 1995.

———. *Francis Bacon and the Transformation of Early-Modern Philosophy.* Cambridge: Cambridge University Press, 2001.

———. *Descartes: The World and Other Writings.* Cambridge: Cambridge University Press, 1998.

Gaynor, Mitchell L. *The Healing Power of Sound: Recovery from Life-Threatening Illness Using Sound, Voice, and Music.* Boston and London: Shambhala Books, 2002.

Gillett, Grant. "Clinical medicine and the quest for certainty." *Social Science & Medicine,* 58 (2004): 727–38.

Goddard, Jean-Christophe, and Monique Labrune. *Le Corps.* Paris: Vrin/Intégrale, 1992.

Goldstein, Rebecca. *Betraying Spinoza: The Renegade Jew Who Gave Us Modernity.* Toronto: Random House, 2006.

———. *Incompleteness: The Proof and Paradox of Kurt Gödel*. New York: W. W. Norton & Company, 2005.

Govinda, Anagarika. *Foundations of Tibetan Mysticism, According to the Esoteric Teachings of the Great Mantra*. London: Rider & Co., 1959.

Grosholz, Emily. *Cartesian Method and the Problem of Reduction*. Oxford: Clarendon Press, 1991.

Grube, G. M. *Plato's Thought*. Indianapolis: Hackett Publishing Company, 1980.

Hackforth, R. *Plato's Phaedo*. Cambridge: Cambridge University Press, 1972.

Hallie, Philip P. "Stoicism." In *Encyclopedia of Philosophy, Vol. VIII*. New York: The Macmillan Company and The Free Press, 1967.

Hampshire, Stuart. *Spinoza and Spinozism*. Oxford: Clarendon Press, 2005.

Hankinson, R. J. "Philosophy of Science." In *The Cambridge Companion to Aristotle*, edited by Jonathan Barnes. Cambridge: Cambridge University Press, 1996.

Harris, R. Baine, ed. *Neoplatonism and Indian Thought*. Norfolk, VA: International Society for Neoplatonic Studies, 1982.

Hawthorne, Susan. "Diotima Speaks Through the Body." In *Engendering Origins: Critical Feminist Readings in Plato and Aristotle*, edited by Bat-Ami Bar On. Albany: SUNY Press, 1994.

Hayles, N. Katherine. *How We Became Posthuman: Virtual Bodies in Cybernetics, Literature, and Informatics*. Chicago and London: University of Chicago Press, 1999.

Hillman, David, and Carla Mazzio, eds. *The Body in Parts*. New York and London: Routledge, 1997.

Hooper, Wallace. "Inertial Problems in Galileo's Preinertial Framework." In *The Cambridge Companion to Galileo*, edited by Peter Machamer. Cambridge: Cambridge University Press, 1998.

Irwin, Terence. *Classical Thought*. Oxford: Oxford University Press, 1989.

Iyengar, B. K. S. *Yoga Vrksa: The Tree of Yoga*. Oxford: Fine Line Books, 1988.

Jacobsen, Knut A., ed. *Theory and Practice of Yoga: Essays in Honour of Gerald James Larson*. Dehli: Motilal Banarsidass, 2008.

James, Susan. "The Power of Spinoza: Feminist Conjunctions—Susan James Interviews Genevieve Lloyd and Moira Gatens." *Hypatia*, 15: 2 (2000): 40–58.

Jaquet, Chantal. *Le Corps*. Paris: Presses Universitaires de France, 2001.

Jonas, Hans. *The Phenomenon of Life: Towards a Philosophical Biology*. New York: Harper & Row, 1966.

———. *Philosophical Essays*. Englewood Cliffs, NJ: Prentice-Hall, 1974.

Kahan, Barry D. "Organ Donation and Transplantation—A Surgeon's View." In *Organ Transplantation: Meanings and Realities*, edited by Stuart J. Youngner, Renée C. Fox and Laurence J. O'Connell, 126–41. Madison: University of Wisconsin Press, 1996.

Kaptchuk, Ted J. *The Web That Has No Weaver: Understanding Chinese Medicine.* Chicago: Congdon & Weed, 1983.

Kaske, Carole, and John R. Clark. *Marsilio Ficino: Three Books on Life.* Binghampton: Center for Medieval and Renaissance Studies, SUNY at Binghampton, 1989.

Kendall, Paul. "Anonymous No More." *National Post,* October 1, 2004.

Khan, Hazrat Inayat. *The Mysticism of Sound and Music.* Boston and London: Shambhala Books, 1996.

Klibansky, Raymond, Erwin Panofsky, and Fritz Saxl. *Saturn and Melancholy.* London: Thomas Nelson & Sons, 1964.

Kuriyama, Shigehisa. *The Expressiveness of the Body and the Divergence of Greek and Chinese Medicine.* New York: Zone Publications, 2002.

Kurzweil, Ray. *The Age of Spiritual Machines.* New York: Penguin Group, 1999.

_____. "The Evolution of Mind in the Twenty-First Century." In *Are We Spiritual Machines? Ray Kurzweil vs. the Critics of Strong A.I.,* edited by Jay W. Richards. Seattle: Discovery Institute, 2002.

Lalitananda. *The Inner Life of Asanas.* Spokane, WA and Kootenay Bay, BC: Timeless Books, 2007.

Lang, Helen S. *The Order of Nature in Aristotle's Physics: Place and the Elements.* Cambridge and New York: Cambridge University Press. 1998.

Le Breton, David. *La Chair à vif.* Paris: Éditions A. M. Métailié, 1993.

Leder, Drew, ed. *The Body in Medical Thought and Practice.* Dortrecht and Boston: Kluwer Academic Publishers, 1992.

Lewis, Genevieve, ed. *Descartes: Correspondance avec Arnauld et Morus.* Paris: Librairie philosophique J. Vrin, 1953.

Lloyd, Genevieve. *Part of Nature: Self-Knowledge in Spinoza's Ethics.* Ithaca and London: Cornell University Press, 1994.

_____. *Routledge Philosophy Guidebook to Spinoza and the Ethics.* New York: Routledge, 1996.

_____. *Providence Lost.* Cambridge: Harvard University Press, 2008.

Lock, Margaret. *Twice Dead: Organ Transplants and the Reinvention of Death.* Los Angeles: University of California Press, 2002.

Long, A. A., and D. N. Sedley. *The Hellenistic Philosophers.* Cambridge: Cambridge University Press, 1987.

Long, A. A. *Stoic Studies.* Cambridge: Cambridge University Press, 1996.

Marchi, Dudley. *Montaigne Among the Moderns.* Providence and Oxford: Berghahn Books, 1994.

Martin, Raymond, and John Barresi. *The Rise and Fall of Soul and Self.* New York: Columbia University Press, 2006.

McTaggart, Lynne. *The Field: The Quest for the Secret Force of the Universe.* New York: HarperCollins Publishers, 2008.

Merchant, Carolyn. *The Death of Nature: Women, Ecology and the Scientific Revolution.* San Francisco: Harper & Row, 1980.

Midgley, Mary. *Evolution as Religion.* London and New York: Routledge, 1985, 2002.

———. "Souls, Minds, Bodies & Planets." *Philosophy Now*, 48 (2004), http://www.philosophynow.org/issue48/48midgley.htm (accessed January 26, 2007).

Miles, Margaret Ruth. *Augustine on the Body.* Missoula, MT: Scholars Press, 1979.

———. *Desire and Delight: A New Reading of Augustine's* Confessions. New York: Crossroad, 1992.

Montaigne, Michel de. *Essays.* Translated by M. A. Screech. London: Penguin, 1987, 1991.

Moravec, Hans. *Mind Children.* Cambridge: Harvard University Press, 1988.

Moriau, Didier. "Le corps médicalisé." In *Quel Corps?*, edited by Michel Beaulieu. Paris: Éditions de la Passion, 1986.

Nelkin, Dorothy, and Lori Andrews. "Homo Economicus: Commercialization of Body Tissue in the Age of Biotechnology." *The Hastings Center Report*, 28: 5 (1998): 30–39.

Nye, Andrea. *The Princess and the Philosopher.* Lanham, MD: Rowman & Littlefield Publishers, 1999.

O'Connor, Bonnie B. "Conceptions of the Body in Complementary and Alternative Medicine." In *Complementary and Alternative Medicine: Challenge and Change*, edited by Merrijoy Kelner and Beverly Wellman. Amsterdam: Harwood Academic Publishers, 2000.

Ogle, Martin, "Understanding Gaia Theory," http://www.gaiatheory.org/synopsis.htm (accessed November 5, 2010).

Pearsall, Paul. *The Heart's Code: Tapping the Wisdom and Power of Our Heart Energy.* New York: Broadway Books, 1998.

Pembroke, S. G. "Oikeiosis." In *Problems in Stoicism*, edited by A. A. Long. London: Athlone Press, 1971.

Plato. *The Symposium.* Translated and edited by Walter Hamilton. New York: Penguin Books, 1951.

———. *Phaedrus and Letters VII and VIII.* Translated and edited by Walter Hamilton. New York: Penguin, 1973.

———. *Phaedo.* In *Plato: Five Dialogues*, translated by G. M. A. Grube. Indianapolis: Hackett Publishing Company, 1981.

Popkin, Richard H., ed. *The Philosophy of the 16th and 17th Centuries.* New York: The Free Press, 1966.

Popkin, Richard H. *Spinoza.* Oxford: Oneworld Publications, 2004.

Remes, Pauliina. *Neoplatonism.* Berkeley and Los Angeles: University of California Press, 2008.

Richards, Jay, ed. *Are We Spiritual Machines? Ray Kurzweil vs. The Critics of Strong A.I.* Seattle: Discovery Institute, 2002.

Rist, John M. *Augustine: Ancient Thought Baptized.* Cambridge: Cambridge University Press, 1994.

———. *Man, Soul and Body: Essays in Ancient Thought from Plato to Dionysius.* Aldershot, Hampshire, UK: Ashgate, 1996.

Rist, John, ed. *The Stoics.* Berkeley: University of California Press, 1978.

Rose, Barbara. "Orlan: Is it Art?" *Art in America,* 81: 2 (February 1993): 83–125. http://www.stanford.edu/class/history34q/readings/Orlan/Orlan2.html (accessed September 21, 2010).

Rosen, Richard. *The Yoga of Breath: A Step-by-Step Guide to Pranayama.* Boston and London: Shambhala Publications, 2002.

Rosenfield, Leonora Cohen. *From Beast-Machine to Man-Machine: Animal Soul in French Letters from Descartes to La Mettrie.* New York: Octagon Books, 1968.

Sandbach, F. H. *The Stoics.* London: Chatto & Windus, 1975.

Satchidananda. *Integral Yoga: The Yoga Sutras of Patanjali.* Yogaville, VA: Integral Yoga Publications, 1985.

Sawday, Jonathan. *The Body Emblazoned: Dissection and the Human Body in Renaissance Culture.* London: Routledge, 1995.

Schacht, Richard. *Classical Modern Philosophers.* New York and London: Routledge, 1984.

Scott, T. Kermit. *Augustine: His Thought in Context.* Mahwah, NJ: Paulist Press, 1995.

Scruton, Roger. *Spinoza: A Very Short Introduction.* New York: Routledge, 1999.

Seneca. *Ad Lucillium Epistulae Morales.* Translated by R. M. Gummere. Loeb Classical Library, 1962.

Setzer, Claudia. *Resurrection of the Body in Early Judaism and Early Christianity.* Boston: Brill Academic Publishers, 2004.

Shapin, Steven. *The Scientific Revolution.* Chicago and London: University of Chicago Press, 1996.

Shusterman, Richard. *Body Consciousness: A Philosophy of Mindfulness and Somaesthetics.* New York: Cambridge University Press, 2008.

Singer, P. N. *Galen: Selected Works.* Oxford: Oxford University Press, 1997.

Singer, Peter. *Rethinking Life and Death.* New York: St. Martin's Griffin, 1994.

———. "Creating Embryos." In *Biomedical Ethics,* 5th ed., edited by Thomas Mappes and David DeGrazia. New York: McGraw-Hill, 2001.

Sivananda Radha. *Mantras: Words of Power.* Spokane, WA and Kootenay Bay, BC: Timeless Books, 1994.

———. *Hatha Yoga: The Hidden Language.* Spokane, WA and Kootenay Bay, BC: Timeless Books, 2007.

————. *Light & Vibration: Consciousness, Mysticism & the Culmination of Yoga*. Kootenay Bay, BC and Spokane, WA: Timeless Books, 2007.

Skloot, Rebecca. *The Immortal Life of Henrietta Lacks*. New York: Random House, 2010.

Slater, Lauren. "Dr. Daedalus: A Radical Plastic Surgeon Wants to Give You Wings." *Harper's* (July 2001), 57–67.

Smith, Dennis E. *From Symposium to Eucharist: The Banquet in the Early Christian World*. Minneapolis: Fortress Press, 2003.

Spinoza, Baruch. *Ethics*. Translated by Samuel Shirley. Indianapolis and Cambridge: Hackett Publishing Company, 1992.

Starobinski, Jean. *Montaigne in Motion*. Translated by Arthur Goldhammer. Chicago and London: The University of Chicago Press, 1985.

Stone, Michael. *The Inner Tradition of Yoga*. Boston and London: Shambhala Publications, 2008.

Sutton, John. *Philosophy and Memory Traces*. Cambridge: Cambridge University Press, 1999.

Sweetman, Paul. "Anchoring the (Postmodern) Self? Body Modification, Fashion and Identity." *Body & Society*, 5: 2–3 (1999): 51–76. http://bod.sagepub.com/content/5/2-3/51 (accessed 20 September 2010).

Tarnas, Richard. *The Passion of the Western Mind*. New York: Random House, 1991.

————. *Cosmos and Psyche: Intimations of a New World View*. London: Viking Penguin, 2006.

Taylor, Charles. *Sources of the Self: The Making of the Modern Identity*. Cambridge: Harvard University Press, 1989.

Timalsina, Sthaneshwar. "Meditating Mantras: Meaning and Visualization in Tantric Literature." In Jacobsen, *Theory and Practice of Yoga*, 213–34.

Tipler, Frank J. *The Physics of Immortality: Modern Cosmology, God and the Resurrection of the Dead*. New York: Anchor Books, 1995.

Toulmin, Stephen. *Cosmopolis*. Chicago: University of Chicago Press, 1990.

Vernant, Jean-Pierre. "Dim Body, Dazzling Body." In *Zone 3: Fragments for a History of the Human Body*, edited by Michel Feher, Ramona Naddaff and Nadia Taxi. New York: Zone Books, 1989.

Vivekananda. *Raja-Yoga*. New York: Ramakrishna-Vivekananda Center, 1956, 1982.

————. *Vedanta: Voice of Freedom*. St. Louis: Vedanta Society of St. Louis, 1990.

Wolff, Hans Walter. *Anthropology of the Old Testament*. Philadelphia: Fortress Press, 1974.

Woodroffe, John. *Garland of Letters: Studies in the Mantra-Sastra*. Madras: Ganesh & Co., 2004.

Worthington, Vivian. *A History of Yoga*. London: Routledge & Kegan Paul, 1982.

Wu, Harry. *Retour au laogai*. Paris: Belfond, 1997.

Yang, Kyeongra. "A Review of Yoga Programs for Four Leading Risk Factors of Chronic Diseases." *eCAM—Evidence-based Complementary and Alternative Medicine*, 4: 4 (2007): 487–91.

Yuasa, Yasuo. *The Body, Self-Cultivation, and Ki-Energy.* Albany: SUNY Press, 1993.

Youngner, Stuart J., Renée C. Fox, and Laurence J. O'Connell, eds. *Organ Transplantation: Meanings and Realities.* Madison: University of Wisconsin Press, 1996.

Zurbrugg, Nicholas. "Marinetti, Chopin, Stelarc and the Auratic Intensities of the Postmodern Techno-Body." *Body & Society*, 5: 2–3 (1999): 93–115. http://bod.sagepub.com/content/5/2-3/93 (accessed September 20, 2010).

INDEX

C

Cartesian body. *see* body-machine
(Descartes); Cartesian philosophy
Cartesian legacy of dualism and
mechanism, 2, 5–6, 9, 133–34,
197–200, 265
Cartesian philosophy
and animal souls, 67, 145
and loss of pre-modern topics, 4
body-machine and its functions
his descriptions of, 144–45
metabolism, 182
movement of the body, 147–49
perception, 149–51, 152
problems with, 152–56
the principle of life, 145–47,
181
versus Spinoza's notion of body,
181–83
Discourse on Method, 133, 135, 136,
137–38, 139
dualism
ambiguities with, 152
and modern vision of the body
machine, 5–6
cogito ergo sum, 138–40
humans *versus* animals, 145,
150–51
knowledge as activity of the
mind, 136, 140–41
versus Spinoza's monism,
170–72
legacy of
body-machine paradigm, 2,
5–6, 9, 133–34, 193–94,
197–200, 265, 290
modern concept of self, 141,
156–60, 189
modern science and medicine,
9, 197–200, 265
mechanism
and his study of the human
body, 141–42
assumptions of, 151
three basic laws of nature, 136,
143–44

method
and it's application to all areas
of science, 137
and unity of all knowledge,
135–36, 157
and unity of science, 134–35,
151, 154, 198
four main rules, 136–37
intuition and deduction, 137,
161
Principles of Philosophy, 135
Rules for the Direction of the Mind,
134
The World, 11, 142, 162, 163
Treatise on Man, 11, 142, 144, 162,
163, 199
versus Montaigne, Michel de, 121,
122, 133
Cartesian soul
human *versus* animal, 67–68, 149,
150–51, 152, 179
reduced to mind, 38, 44, 136, 151,
153, 157, 161
cell lines, 227
chain consumption argument, 90, 103
chanting mantra, 250–53
chi, 13, 15, 114, 247, 271, 285
Christian body
and original sin, 94, 99
dichotomy of good and bad, 93–94
dualism of soul and body, 79–80
nature of, before the Fall and after
the Resurrection, 95–96
paradoxical view of body, 6, 79, 84
resurrection, 84, 88–92, 99
the Eucharist, doctrine of, 83, 101
union of body and soul, 92
women, 83, 96–99, 97, 101
Christian faith
Manicheans, 85
the Eucharist, doctrine of, 83, 101
the Incarnation, 82–83, 87, 94
the Resurrection of the body, 84,
87, 89
Christian mysteries, the body in, 82–84,
92, 101, 102

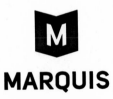